Compact Clinical Guide to

CANCER PAIN MANAGEMENT

An Evidence-Based Approach for Nurses

Pamela Stitzlein Davies, MS, ARNP, ACHPN

Yvonne D'Arcy, MS, CRNP, CNS

Yvonne D'Arcy, MS, CRNP, CNS
Series Editor

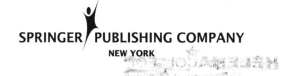

SPRINGER PUBLISHING COMPANY

NEW YORK

Springer Publishing Company, LLC
11 West 42nd Street
New York, NY 10036
www.springerpub.com

Acquisitions Editor: Margaret Zuccarini
Composition: S4Carlisle Publishing Services

ISBN: 978-0-8261-0973-6
E-book ISBN: 978-0-8261-0974-3

12   13   14/5   4   3   2   1

The author and the publisher of this Work have made every effort to use sources believed to be reliable to provide information that is accurate and compatible with the standards generally accepted at the time of publication. Because medical science is continually advancing, our knowledge base continues to expand. Therefore, as new information becomes available, changes in procedures become necessary. We recommend that the reader always consult current research and specific institutional policies before performing any clinical procedure. The author and publisher shall not be liable for any special, consequential, or exemplary damages resulting, in whole or in part, from the readers' use of, or reliance on, the information contained in this book. The publisher has no responsibility for the persistence or accuracy of URLs for external or third-party Internet websites referred to in this publication and does not guarantee that any content on such websites is, or will remain, accurate or appropriate.

Library of Congress Cataloging-in-Publication Data

Davies, Pamela Stitzlein.
  Compact clinical guide to cancer pain management : an evidence-based approach for nurses / Pamela Stitzlein Davies, Yvonne D'Arcy.
    p. ; cm.
  Includes bibliographical references.
  ISBN-13: 978-0-8261-0973-6
  ISBN-10: 0-8261-0973-X
  ISBN-13: 978-0-8261-0974-3 (E-book ISBN)
  I. D'Arcy, Yvonne. II. Title.
    [DNLM: 1. Neoplasms—nursing. 2. Pain Management. 3. Evidence-Based Nursing. 4. Palliative Care. WY 156]
  LC classification not assigned
  616.99'40231—dc23   45.00

                                                        2012014881

Special discounts on bulk quantities of our books are available to corporations, professional associations, pharmaceutical companies, health care organizations, and other qualifying groups.

If you are interested in a custom book, including chapters from more than one of our titles, we can provide that service as well.

For details, please contact:
Special Sales Department, Springer Publishing Company, LLC
11 West 42nd Street, 15th Floor, New York, NY 10036-8002
Phone: 877-687-7476 or 212-431-4370; Fax: 212-941-7842
Email: sales@springerpub.com

Printed in the United States of America by Hamilton Printing.

Contents

Foreword

One can reasonably ask the question: Is another text on cancer pain management needed in 2012? After a careful evaluation of the *Compact Clinical Guide to Cancer Pain Management: An Evidence-Based Approach for Nurses* by Davies and D'Arcy, the answer is a resounding YES! A number of reasons solidify my enthusiasm and endorsement of this new and exciting text.

First and foremost, unrelieved cancer pain remains a significant clinical problem for approximately 50% of patients during cancer treatment. In addition, approximately 25% to 50% of cancer survivors experience chronic pain related to cancer and its treatment or from other chronic medical conditions. Finally, approximately 80% of patients in the terminal phases of cancer report unrelieved pain. Of note, these percentages have not changed for over 30 years! Therefore, a moral imperative exists to provide the most up-to-date information to frontline clinicians who do pain assessments and develop pain management plans on a daily basis.

Second, a text designed specifically for nurses provides essential and practical information to the very clinicians who are most likely to have the greatest impact on improving the management of pain in oncology patients. Nurses have taken the lead in cancer pain management for the past three decades. They are intimately involved in all aspects of care for oncology patients across the trajectory of the patient's condition. Nurses are focused on the assessment and management of single and multiple symptoms. Often, they take a detailed history of the patient's pain and its impact on the patient's functional status and quality of life. They monitor the patient's level of adherence with the pain management plan, including any side effects associated with analgesic medications. They serve as the intermediary between the patient and the physician to optimize the patient's pain management plan. The evidence-based information in this text will provide nurses with strategies that they can recommend to their physician colleagues to optimize the oncology patient's pain management plan.

The third reason for my unqualified enthusiasm for this book is its emphasis on evidence-based approaches. All health care is focused on the need to implement evidence-based interventions into clinical practice. However, Davies and D'Arcy are experienced nurse practitioners who have devoted a substantial portion of their clinical careers to the care of patients in acute and chronic pain. Therefore, in addition to the evidence-based recommendations found in the book, the text is full of "clinical pearls" based on the authors' extensive clinical experience with effective and ineffective pain management interventions.

The scope of the content in this text is extremely comprehensive. Traditional content on pain assessment and on pharmacologic and nonpharmacologic interventions form the foundation for the text. Davies and D'Arcy also include content on interventional options for managing chronic pain. In addition, newer content on the effect of opioid polymorphisms, cancer pain emergencies, myofascial pain, and chronic pain in cancer survivors places this text at the forefront in terms of cutting-edge issues in cancer pain management.

The final reason for my unqualified support of this text is the emphasis on "compact." Given the hectic pace in inpatient, outpatient, and home care settings, nurses need to be equipped with texts that provide essential information that is readily available and presented in a user-friendly format. *Compact Clinical Guide to Cancer Pain Management: An Evidence-Based Approach for Nurses* fulfills this mandate.

On a personal note, I have known Pam Davies and Yvonne D'Arcy for over 20 years. Both are extremely passionate about providing optimal pain management to every patient they care for on a daily basis. In addition, both are equally passionate in their quest to educate nurses about optimal approaches to assess and manage pain in oncology. Their new book is required reading for all nurses who care for oncology patients.

Christine Miaskowski, PhD, RN, FAAN
Professor and Associate Dean for Academic Affairs
American Cancer Society Clinical Research Professor
Sharon A. Lamb Endowed Chair in Symptom
Management Research
Department of Physiological Nursing
University of California
San Francisco, California

Preface

Nursing management of cancer pain has come a long way since I started my first job in 1978 as the night nurse on Ward 7. Back then, the only nonoral route of administration for opioids was intramuscular (IM) injections. I vividly recall a young man dying of melanoma who was experiencing terrible pain. His orders were the standard of the day: Demerol 25–50 mg with Vistaril 25 mg IM every 4 to 6 hours as needed for pain. This was not only a bad drug choice, it was significantly underdosed for his needs. Additionally, in his cachectic state, all of his major muscles were rock hard from the repeated IM shots. I doubt if much of the drug was even being absorbed. His profound suffering was evident to other patients on the 52-bed open-bay ward, and throughout the night, they came to the nurse's station begging that I give him more medicine. The resident would not increase the dose despite my repeated pleas, citing concerns about addiction. So, feeling like a criminal, and worried that I might be killing him, I increased the dose to 75 mg every 3 hours, then to 100 mg every 2½ hours. Finally, he started to get a bit of relief. He died 2 days later, most of that time in severe pain.

This was a tragic and avoidable situation. The amount of agony this young man went through was indescribable, and still burns in my memory. Being a neophyte, I had not yet learned how to be an assertive advocate for the patient. Moreover, in my attempt to provide some humane relief, I put my nursing license at risk. Fortunately for me, on morning rounds the attending physician agreed to write orders to cover the increased doses.

One would hope that, three decades later, this heartbreaking story is a relic from days past. Many things *are* better now: We use the intravenous route for uncontrolled pain rather than the intramuscular route; meperidine (Demerol) is removed from most formularies, banned due to risk of buildup of the dangerous metabolite *normeperidine*; nursing and medical schools provide required education on pain; and institutional policies support improved pain management, much of it driven by the The Joint Commission standards on pain. In addition, we can be proud of the leadership and accomplishment of many nurses in the national and international field of pain management.

Since those early times working nights, I have learned not only the vital responsibility that nurses hold in pain management, but also the importance of patient advocacy for better treatment. This was highlighted for me by two additional interactions.

First, I had the wonderful opportunity to be mentored by Christine Miaskowski, PhD, RN, FAAN, in the early 1990s, while attending graduate school at the University of California, San Francisco, School of Nursing. She shared a poignant story from her early career of a patient with lung cancer. In the final months, he developed a new, severe back pain that spread in a band around his thorax, associated with new, mild lower extremity weakness and urinary retention. He sought care from his oncologist, but an evaluation was not done. Experienced oncology nurses will recognize these symptoms as an imminent spinal cord compression (SCC). This occurs when growing vertebral metastasis applies pressure on the spinal cord, resulting in paralysis if not addressed promptly. By the time the condition was recognized, the patient was permanently paralyzed, which resulted in a great deal of physical and psychic suffering. Had this been caught in time, and treated with steroids and radiation, he could have remained ambulatory for the last several months of life.

Dr. Miaskowski told this story with an evangelistic fervor, emphasizing the need for early recognition of the hallmark symptoms of SCC, and the importance of rapid treatment, while describing the essential role of nurses in the evaluation and management of cancer pain conditions. Her leadership and vision inspired me to specialize in pain management.

Finally, I witnessed the profound importance of the bedside nurse in managing pain in a personal way when my mother died of retroperitoneal leiomyosarcoma. Mom's pain was unusually difficult to control, requiring a variety of management strategies and frequent dose increases. The wisdom, resourcefulness, and dedication of the hospice nurse, Betsy Donahue, RN, CHPN, in her tireless search for pain relief, affected me immensely. What a difference *this nurse* made to my mother and our family! I will never forget her example. It inspired me to learn how to be an *active presence* in the midst of suffering and dying, to be kind and patient with demanding caregivers, and to honor and respect each person as a unique individual.

Pamela Stitzlein Davies, MS, ARNP, ACHPN

Much has been done in cancer pain management, but there is still much improvement needed. Research shows that cancer pain continues to be a significant problem worldwide. In a 2007 meta-analysis of 52 studies on cancer pain prevalence, 64% of those with advanced disease, 59% of patients on anticancer treatment, and 33% of those cured of cancer, reported pain. In addition, one third of the patients graded their pain as moderate to severe in intensity (van den Beuken-van Everdingen et al., 2007).

It is clear that we still have more to learn. The *Compact Clinical Guide to Cancer Pain Management: An Evidence-Based Approach for Nurses* is a unique volume from two experts in cancer pain management, both with decades of experience. It is intended for nurses or nurse practitioners working in oncology, surgery, medicine, rehabilitation medicine, or pain fields. Whether practicing in an outpatient oncology clinic, ambulatory infusion center, inpatient unit, ICU, primary care clinic, or palliative and hospice care, this text is intended to be a practical resource for use on a day-to-day basis at work. The compact design allows it to travel easily, and specifics of management are provided throughout to ensure appropriate understanding of treatment strategies.

It is hoped that this text will educate, as well as inspire, nurses to provide the best possible care for the patient in pain.

Pamela Stitzlein Davies, MS, ARNP, ACHPN
Yvonne D'Arcy, MS, CRNP, CNS

REFERENCE

van den Beuken-van Everdingen, M., de Rijke, J., Kessels, A., Schouten, H., van Kleef, M., & Patijn, J. (2007). Prevalence of pain in patients with cancer: A systematic review of the past 40 years. *Annals of Oncology, 18*(9), 1437–1449.

Acknowledgments

I am most grateful to the following individuals who provided support, encouragement, and critical evaluation of portions of this work:

- Hannah Linden, MD, Breast Oncology, University of Washington/Seattle Cancer Care Alliance (SCCA)
- Jennifer Jacky, MS, ARNP, SCCA Cancer Pain Clinic
- Karen Syrjala, PhD, Survivorship Program, Fred Hutchinson Cancer Research Center, Seattle
- Theresa Wittenberg, MS, PA-C, SCCA Survivorship Clinic, Fred Hutchinson Cancer Research Center, Seattle
- Heidi Trott, MS, ARNP, SCCA Breast Survivorship Clinic
- Betsy Donahue, RN, CHPN, Group Health Hospice, Seattle
- Ann Marie O'Neill, MS, ARNP, Evergreen Healthcare Inpatient Hospice Center, Kirkland, WA
- And most of all, my ever-patient husband of 26 years, Bob Davies

Pamela Stitzlein Davies, MS, ARNP, ACHPN

1

Overview of Cancer Pain

Yvonne D'Arcy

One of the most important concerns of a patient who is diagnosed with cancer is pain. In addition to questions about the diagnosis, the prognosis, and treatment options, patients will inevitably ask "Will I have pain that can be controlled?" Some patients remember friends or family with cancer who, in the past, had unrelieved pain at the end of life. That picture of unrelieved pain colors the patient's concern about pain management, even though the patient has a good prognosis for cure. Although the fear of the disease itself and the treatment options are paramount in the patient's mind, pain and the fear of pain are concomitant concerns. Some patients may not voice their concerns, not wanting to distract the health care provider from the diagnosis and treatment. Other patients do not open a discussion about pain management, fearing that they will be told that pain will be expected and that little can be done to control the pain.

What we know now is that pain relief is possible for patients with cancer. Although complete freedom from pain is not realistic, pain control that allows the patient to maintain a reasonable level of function is possible, especially with a multimodal approach. We also know that some patients have pain when they are diagnosed with cancer, while other patients develop pain from tumor progression or nerve impingement, and yet other patients develop pain from treatments such as chemotherapy or radiation. Additionally, there are many patients being seen in primary care clinics with chronic cancer pain that require attention to not only the pain but a continued focus on maintaining functionality and the highest possible level of quality of life.

PREVALENCE OF CANCER PAIN

The prevalence of pain from cancer is somewhat difficult to quantify. There are several different ways that is presented. The American Pain Society's (APS) Guidelines on Cancer Pain (2005) reports that 1.2 million Americans are diagnosed with cancer each year, while 500,000 die each year from cancer. The guidelines also indicate that pain is the problem that patients fear most when diagnosed with cancer.

The World Health Organization (WHO) reports that cancer is the leading cause of death worldwide, accounting for approximately 13% of all deaths (WHO, n.d.). Reports from the National Cancer Institute (NCI) indicate that over 1.5 million people were diagnosed with cancer in 2010 (NCI, n.d.). In another analysis, the NCI estimates that 41% of people will be diagnosed with cancer in their lifetime.

Pain can be present when the patient is first diagnosed with cancer. It is a presenting symptom in close to half of the patients diagnosed with cancer, occurring at rates from 20% to 50% (Fischer, Villines, Kim, Epstein, & Wilkie, 2010). Pain is present in approximately 20% to 75% of adult patients diagnosed with cancer (APS, 2005). Additional data indicate that 17% to 57% of patients in active treatment for cancer and 23% to 100% of patients with advanced cancer and in the terminal stages of cancer report pain (APS, 2005). Unfortunately the same types of results are found in pediatric cancer patients where cancer pain can be present at the time of diagnosis and can be found at all stages of the treatment (APS, 2005).

There are also concerns that cancer pain is being undertreated. In an early cancer pain guideline, the Agency for Healthcare Policy and Research (AHCPR) states that 90% of all patients who had cancer pain could be treated for pain with the currently available methods for pain relief (AHCPR, 1994). Pain intensities in 100 patients with cancer pain was reported to be moderate to severe for 73% of the patients, while 47% reported continuous pain, and intermittent pain was reported by 53% (Marcus, 2011). This continuing high level of pain indicates that, for some patients, getting adequate treatment for their pain remains problematic.

As people live longer, cancer is also becoming a disease of older age. In a study of 96 patients in three groups by age (40 and younger, 41 to 50, and 60 or older), constant pain was similar, while breakthrough pain episodes, and pain flares in previously controlled pain, were more common in the younger group (Green & Hart-Johnson, 2010). Although disparities in health care have been previously recognized for older adults, the impact of pain with cancer spanned all three of the study groups. The oldest group, however, had better emotional function while they had worse physical functioning (Green & Hart-Johnson, 2010). Overall, the pain related to cancer had a highly negative impact on quality of life.

The prevalence of cancer is increasing, with one estimate indicating that 17 million new cases could be expected by 2020 (Kanavos, 2006). This means that pain from cancer-related sources and treatments will be increasing dramatically as well. The impact of cancer is widespread. Depression and decreased quality of life are common. In the Indiana Cancer Pain Depression study, patients were disabled, on average, 12 to 20 days in the previous 4 weeks, while 28% to 55% reported being unable to work related to their health care issues (Kroenke et al., 2010).

The results of cancer pain itself, the undertreatment of cancer pain, and frequent breakthrough pain episodes can cause the following:

- Depression
- Needless suffering
- Anxiety
- Impaired quality of life
- Decreased functionality
- Fear of pain and the inability to control pain

In order to help patients with cancer minimize the negative impact of cancer pain and cancer pain–related conditions, aggressive treatment for cancer pain is recommended (APS, 2005). The subsequent chapters of this book will discuss treatment options, medications, and ways to improve the quality of pain relief for cancer patients of all types.

TYPES OF PAIN FROM CANCER

There are two main types of cancers: solid tumor cancers such as sarcomas, and liquid tumor cancers such as leukemia. Tumors can grow and displace organs and impinge on nerves, causing several different types of pain, while treatments for liquid cancers such as chemotherapy can cause painful neuropathies. No matter what the cause of the cancer pain is, it can be treated with some form of medication, interventions such as radiation, or surgery.

Acute pain can be the result of surgery, tissue injury, or treatment. It is a type of pain that occurs suddenly and reflects tissue injury. The patient can expect that this type of pain will not last long. It serves the purpose of letting the body know it has been injured (APS, 2008).

Chronic pain, now more correctly called persistent pain, is pain that lasts for a longer period of time, more than 3 months. This type of pain really is a result of tumor growth or treatment-related pain such as chemotherapy-related neuropathy (APS, 2008). It is a type of pain that can cause anxiety and depression as the time goes on and if relief is not adequate, the patient becomes less certain that relief can be achieved.

Neuropathic pain is pain that is the result of damage to the nervous system. Nerve damage can result in physiologic changes that activate higher levels of pain facilitation such as neuronal plasticity and wind-up, activation of NMDA receptors that heighten pain response, and allodynia and hyperalgesia. More in-depth information on neuropathic pain will be provided in Chapter 15.

Clinical Pearl	**Allodynia** is the production of a painful response to a normally nonpainful stimulus or sensation such as light touch. **Hyperalgesia** is a heightened painful response to a stimulus that is painful, such as extreme pain with an intravenous catheter insertion.

Breakthrough pain is associated with episodes of extreme pain (pain flares) in patients with well-controlled pain. This pain can be the result of increased activity or it can just occur periodically with no cause. Usually, this type of pain requires additional medication for control.

Cancer pain can occur at any time in the disease progression. To name a few examples, it can be the result of the following:

- Tumor growth
- Bony involvement
- Infections
- Surgery
- Chemotherapy
- Nerve compression
- Mucositis
- Bowel obstruction
- Ischemia
- Capsule distension
- Ascites
- Post-radiation
- Procedural pain

No matter the source or type of pain, it is important to address the pain with a multifaceted plan of care to obtain the highest level of relief possible.

PAIN TRANSMISSION

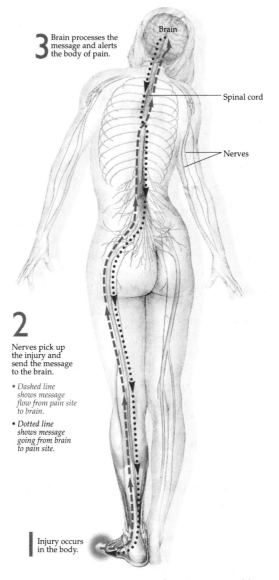

3 Brain processes the message and alerts the body of pain.

Brain

Spinal cord

Nerves

2

Nerves pick up the injury and send the message to the brain.

- *Dashed line shows message flow from pain site to brain.*

- *Dotted line shows message going from brain to pain site.*

Injury occurs in the body.

Figure 1.1 ■ Pain transmission—Exemplar. *Source:* Used by permission of Anatomical Charts, Park Ridge, IL.

The Concept of Nociception

How is pain really felt? The concept of nociception can help us determine just how pain moves through the nervous system and it can also provide us with ideas about how we can interfere with pain facilitation and inhibition. Nociception is defined as the perception of pain by sensory pain receptors called *nociceptors* located in the periphery (Sorkin, 2005). In the theory of nociception, there are four stages or levels of pain transmission (D'Arcy, 2011):

1. Transduction: A noxious stimuli converts energy into a nerve impulse, which is detected by sensory receptors called *nociceptors*.
2. Transmission: The neural pain signal moves from the periphery to the spinal cord and brain.
3. Perception: The pain impulse is transmitted to the higher areas of the brain where it is identified as pain.
4. Modulation: Facilitating and inhibitory input from the brain modulates or influences the sensory transmission at the level of the spinal cord (Berry, Covington, Dahl, Katz, & Miaskowski, 2006).

The transmission of pain is basically the passing along of a pain stimulus from the peripheral nervous system into the central nervous system, where it is translated and recognized as pain (Figure 1.1). The afferent nerve fibers are the means of moving the stimulus along the neuronal pathways.

Nociception can come from various locations: *visceral*, which is pain from body organs and is identified as crampy or gnawing pain, or *somatic*, which is pain from skin, muscles, bones, and joints identified by patients as sharp pain (Berry et al., 2006). There are several different types of receptors that can trigger a pain response:

- *Mechanoreceptors*—activated by pressure
- *Thermal receptors*—activated by heat or cold
- *Chemoreceptors*—activated by chemicals, e.g., inflammatory substances (American Society for Pain Management Nursing [ASPMN], 2010)

Peripheral Pain Transmission

Pain can first be experienced by free nerve endings or nociceptors located in the periphery of the body. When a person cuts a hand or fractures an extremity, the pain stimulus is first perceived in the nerves closest to the injury. In order for a pain stimulus to be created, the sodium ions on the nerve fiber must depolarize, which causes the pain stimulus to be produced and passed along the neural circuitry. There are two main types of nerves that transmit pain impulses or stimuli:

1. A-delta fibers are small diameter thinly myelinated nerve fibers that transmit a pain impulse rapidly. The pain transmitted on an A-delta fiber is easily localized and the patient may describe the pain as sharp or stabbing.
2. C fibers are smaller and unmyelinated, and the pain impulse is conducted at a much slower rate. Pain that is produced by C fibers is identified by patients as achy or burning in nature (ASPMN, 2010; Sorkin, 2005).

Two primary substances can help facilitate the transmission of pain from the periphery. *Substance P* is a neurotransmitter secreted by the free nerve endings of C fibers, whose function is to speed the transmission of the pain impulse. *Bradykinin* is a second type of neurotransmitter, that promotes the inflammatory response and hyperalgesia (ASPMN, 2010). Nociception can stimulate both A and C fibers for pain transmission. Other substances that participate in the facilitation of pain include the following:

- Histamine is a substance released from mast cells, and is produced in response to tissue trauma.
- Serotonin can be released from platelets, and is produced in response to tissue trauma.
- COX products include prostaglandins E_2 and thromboxane E_2, which act to sensitize and excite C fibers, causing hyperexcitability.
- Cytokines-interleukins and tumor necrosis factor can sensitize C fiber terminals and participate in the inflammatory and infection process involving mast cells.
- The calcitonin gene-related peptide (CGRP) is located at C fiber nerve endings and produces local cutaneous vasodilatation, plasma extravasation, and skin sensitzation in collaboration with substance production (ASPMN, 2010; Berry et al., 2006; Sorkin, 2005).

Once transduction takes place, the nerve impulse is passed through a synaptic junction from the peripheral nervous system to the central nervous system. This synaptic junction has a variety of functions with various substances being released. Some medications, for example, pregabalin, act by blocking calcium channels. This, in turn, can reduce the amount of neuronal firing and decrease the passage of pain stimuli. The synapse is between the peripheral neuron into the central nervous system via the dorsal root ganglion.

Central Nervous System Pain Transmission

As the pain stimulus is passed from the peripheral nervous system into the central nervous system, the signal passes through the dorsal root ganglion to a synaptic junction in the substantia gelatinosa located in the dorsal horn of the spinal cord. As the stimulus pushes the pain impulse forward and overcomes any opposing or inhibiting forces, the "gate" is opened, which allows the pain impulse to proceed up the spinal cord to the limbic system and brain.

The opening of the gate is controlled by a summing of all the forces involved in the conduction of the pain impulse. If the facilitating forces—neural excitability and pain-facilitating substances such as Substance P—predominate, the pain impulse is passed on. If pain-inhibiting forces predominate, the signal is blocked and the gate does not open. If, by chance, the pain impulse is perceived as potentially life-threatening, a reflex arc across the spinal cord will fire, causing an immediate response to protect the affected area; for example, touching a hot surface causes the body to retract and remove the hand from the hot surface. This event can take place before any central processing of the neural signal (Cervaro, 2005).

Centrally active pain-facilitating and inhibitory substances are shown in the following:

Facilitating substances include:
- Substance P
- Glutamate—responsible for communication between the peripheral and central nervous systems (Rowbotham, Kidd, & Porecca, 2006); also plays a role in activating the NMDA receptors (Mersky, Loeser, & Dubner, 2005)
- Aspartate
- Cholecystokinin
- CGRP
- Nitric oxide

Inhibitory substances include:
- Dynorphin, an endogenous opioid
- Enkephalin
- Norepinephrine
- Serotonin
- B-Endorphin, an endogenous opioid
- Gamma-aminobutyric acid (GABA) (ASPMN, 2010; Sorkin, 2005)

Also performing an inhibitory role are the opioid receptors located both presynaptically and postsynaptically that are available for binding opioid substances such as morphine and for producing analgesia. Although there are opioid receptors located at other sites in the body, we have the most information about how they function from those that are located inside the spinal cord.

As the pain impulse passes through the dorsal horn, it crosses the spinal cord to the lateral spinothalamic tracts, and ascends impulse to proceed up to the thalamus and limbic system. Here, the pain impulse activates the emotions and memories associated with pain and then proceeds to the cerebral cortex, where the pain impulse or stimulus is recognized as pain. Although this process seems complicated, the body can conduct a pain impulse in only milliseconds.

Within the central nervous system, two pain substances—norepinephrine and serotonin—are active. Current drug therapies such as tricyclic antidepressants (TCAs) and serotonin norepinepherine reuptake inhibitors (SNRIs) are aimed at this process to modulate neuronal firing at synaptic junctions. The synaptic junctions have a variety of functions: They are important not only for *producing* pain, but they are also critical sites for *reducing* pain by controlling the production of pain-facilitating substances and actions.

Once the pain stimulus reaches the cerebral cortex, the afferent pathway is completed. At that time, the efferent nerve fibers pass the neuronal response identified as pain back to the periphery. Descending nerve fibers from the locus coeruleus and periaqueductal gray matter are activated and the pain stimulus is passed back down the efferent pathway, where a response to the pain stimulus is produced, such as moving the affected area away from the pain.

It is important to remember that pain transmission not only takes place when a stimulus is created and ascends the spinal cord, but the descending neural pathways can function to inhibit or limit the pain stimulus. In the case of neuropathic pain, the descending pathways do not inhibit the pain response and the pain is more difficult to control.

In patients with cancer pain, there may several types of pain occurring at one time. As a tumor grows, it may create pressure pain on other organs or body structures and may also impinge or compress nerves. This causes both a visceral pain and a neuropathic pain. Over time, cancer pain can become chronic, creating more complicated physiologic responses to the pain stimulus. If the cancer metastasizes, or spreads to other areas of the body, it can create other types of pain and add to the complex nature of the pain presentation. Additionally, patients with cancer who are on a well-controlled opioid regimen for pain relief can have breakthrough pain episodes (pain flares) that can be incapacitating and difficult to treat. All cancer patients should have a full assessment for all the types of pain they are experiencing so adequate treatment can be implemented.

BARRIERS TO TREATING CANCER PAIN

Although it seems like a simple concept that the pain experienced by patients with cancer should be treated aggressively, there are barriers to treating the pain that come from both patients and health care providers. For health care providers, the major barrier has been identified as inadequate knowledge about pain assessment and management strategies (APS, 2005). Other health care–related barriers have been identified:

■ Poor communication
■ Preferences for a weaker analgesic
■ Lack of quality pain assessment or inconsistent use of pain assessment tools
■ Lack of knowledge about opioid dosing
■ Excessive concerns about addiction, respiratory depression, and other side effects (Marcus, 2011)
■ Fear of regulatory scrutiny
■ Time and reimbursement pressures (APS, 2005)

From the patient's side, there may be concerns that affect the quality of pain management. Since the patient has had a significant health care event with the diagnosis of cancer, the patient may be more focused on the cure for the cancer rather than treating pain. Barriers to adequate pain management that are related to the patient include:

■ Reluctance to report pain
■ Poor compliance with pain medications
■ Fear of addiction or tolerance
■ Belief that pain is just a part of having cancer and it is not treatable
■ Belief that the doctor should focus on the disease, not the pain
■ Cost of medications and lack of insurance coverage for pain medications
■ Fear of masking new symptoms
■ Concern about side effects such as constipation
■ Fear of negative feelings from family members or coworkers if opioids are being taken for pain relief
■ Lack of access to cancer pain specialists (APS, 2005; Marcus, 2011)

It is incumbent on the health care provider to open up a dialogue about pain management with patients and address any fears or concerns they may have about medications or treatments. Because the patient with cancer fears pain above all, it is important to bring the issue out and talk about what can be done to treat the pain and side effects. An open discussion about addiction and tolerance can also put the patient at ease when opioids are being used for pain relief. Some drug companies provide assistance for patients who cannot afford pain medications to get the analgesics they need for pain.

Above all, pain management should be prioritized for a patient with cancer pain. Allowing the pain to continue can lead to more chronic pain conditions that become more difficult to treat. Continued pain also causes depression, anxiety, and fears that can be alleviated with adequate pain management. The remaining chapters of this book will focus on pain assessment, medications, and other interventions that can all add to the pain management regimen for a patient with cancer and provide optimal pain relief.

Case Study

Selma Barnes is a 65-year-old patient who has had a mastectomy, completed her chemotherapy, and recently completed her radiation treatments. She had surgical pain that seemed to be significant and now she continues to complain of pain on her operative side. She describes the pain as "painful cold, aching" in her armpit and "shooting" down her arm periodically that has a severe-level pain intensity of 8 out of 10. The surgical site is very tender to touch and Selma reports that she cannot wear anything that is tight on her upper body. The pressure of the garment increases the pain. You diagnose Selma with postmastectomy pain syndrome and discuss treatment options with her. She tells you she is really concerned about continuing with her opioid medications because she is afraid of becoming addicted to them, adding that they do not seem to really help her pain anyway.

Questions to Consider

1. Does Selma have more than one type of pain? If so, how does it affect her treatment options?
2. What kinds of barriers might have affected Selma's continued pain?
3. Is Selma's fear of addiction a valid issue?
4. Why do you think Selma is telling you now that her pain medications have been ineffective?

REFERENCES

Agency for Healthcare Policy and Research (AHCPR). (1994). *Cancer pain guidelines.* Rockville, MD: Author.

American Pain Society (APS). (2005). *Cancer pain in adults and children.* Glenview, IL: Author.

American Pain Society (APS). (2008). *Principles of analgesic use in acute and cancer pain.* Glenview, IL: Author.

American Society for Pain Management Nursing (ASPMN). (2010). *Core curriculum for pain management nursing* (2nd ed.). Dubuque, IA: Kendall Hunt Publishing Company.

Berry, P. H., Covington, E., Dahl, J., Katz, J., & Miaskowski, C. (2006). *Pain: Current understanding of assessment, management, and treatments.* Reston, VA: National Pharmaceutical Council, Inc.

Cervaro, F. (2005). The gate control theory, then and now. In H. Mersky, J. Loeser, & R. Dubner (Eds.), *Paths of pain.* Seattle, WA: IASP Press.

D'Arcy, Y. (2011). *Compact clinical guide to acute pain management.* New York, NY: Springer Publishing.

Fischer, D. J., Villines, D., Kim, Y., Epstein, J., & Wilkie, D. (2010). Anxiety, depression, and pain: Differences by primary cancer. *Support Care Cancer, 18,* 801–810.

Green, C., & Hart-Johnson, T. (2010). Cancer pain: An age based analysis. *Pain Medicine, 11,* 1525–1536.

Kanavos, P. (2006). The rising burden of cancer in the developing world. *Annals of Oncology, 17,* 15–23.

Kroenke, K., Theobald, D., Wu, J., Loza, J. K., Carpenter, J. S., & Tu, W. (2010). The association of depression and pain with health related quality of life, disability, and healthcare use in cancer patients. *Journal of Pain and Symptom Management, 40,* 327–341.

Marcus, D. (2011). Epidemiology of cancer pain. *Current Pain and Headache Reports, 5,* 208–211.

Mersky, H., Loeser, J., & Dubner, R. (2005). *The paths of pain.* Seattle, WA: IASP Press.

National Cancer Institute (NCI). (n.d.). Retrieved from http://seer.cancer.gov/statfacts/html/all.html

Rowbotham, M., Kidd, B., & Porreca, F. (2006). Role of central sensitization in chronic pain: Osteoarthritis and rheumatoid arthritis compared to neuropathic pain. In H. Flor, E. Kalso, & J. Dostrovsky (Eds.), *Proceedings of the 11th World Congress on Pain.* Seattle, WA: IASP Press.

Sorkin, L. (2005). Nociceptive pain. In M. S. Wallace & P. Staats, *Pain medicine & management.* New York, NY: McGraw-Hill.

World Health Organization (WHO). (n.d.). *Cancer.* Retrieved from http://www.who.int/cancer/en/

2

Assessing Pain in Patients With Cancer

Yvonne D'Arcy

OVERVIEW

Assessing pain in patients with cancer can be difficult due to the variety of sources of pain, e.g., tumor progression, nerve impingement, or breakthrough pain. Because there are several different types of pain, nurses need to learn how to help the patient identify each type of pain for assessment. Questions related to the quality of pain and descriptors such as *burning* or *tingling* may reveal the cause as neuropathic pain, which can affect treatment options. Breakthrough pain can also have several sources such as end-of-dose failure, or sudden onset of a new pain in a patient with well-controlled pain, so a careful identification of when and how often the pain occurs is needed to differentiate from the patient's baseline pain (D'Arcy, 2011b).

From the patient's perspective, pain can also be something he or she tends to minimize or not report, fearing that pain represents a progression of the disease or a recurrence (American Pain Society [APS], 2005). Patients may also not want to distract the health care provider's focus from the curative aspect of patient–provider interactions. Although a patient may be having worsening pain that should be assessed carefully, some providers prefer that the treatment options for the cancer take precedence over the pain complaint. For each health care provider who assesses the patient, there must be an awareness of these issues so that the patient will feel comfortable talking about pain management issues with all the members of the health care group.

In addition to these assessment issues, there is also the occurrence of symptom clusters in cancer patients so that pain may be occurring with fatigue, nausea/vomiting, poor sleep, decreases in appetite, or other cancer- or treatment-related symptoms. The effect of the individual symptom is synergistic and the overall effect can be magnified. In other words, other symptoms may have a negative impact on the pain, increasing the frequency or intensity. Patients should be encouraged to report pain and any side effects to their health care team.

Pain assessment has always been challenging for nurses and other health care professionals because it relies on the patient's self-report. In a recent survey of 3,000 nurses and another survey with 400 nurse practitioners, pain assessment was cited as a major source of concern and knowledge deficit (D'Arcy, 2008, 2009). Many of the nurses who responded to the survey felt that they were not getting a pain report that was accurate. In the nurse practitioner survey, the respondents indicated they felt that their nurse practitioner education had not prepared them to treat or assess pain in patients with chronic pain (D'Arcy, 2009). There were repeated requests in the comment section of the surveys about learning to perform an accurate pain assessment and how to assess pain in patients with chronic pain and/or a history of substance abuse. Despite the years of education on pain assessment that has been provided to nurses and other health care professionals, pain assessment still remains difficult.

Pain assessment is problematic because:

- It relies on patient self-report.
- Health care providers have difficulty trusting the patient's report of pain.
- The assessment process uses an objective scale to convey a subjective experience.
- The health care provider comes to the patient interaction with bias as a result of their family and personal values and beliefs about pain (American Society for Pain Management Nursing [ASPMN], 2009; D'Arcy, 2007).

Pain assessment is the core component to developing and implementing care and providing adequate pain management for patients. Choosing a medication to treat pain is driven by the assessment process. Additionally, adjustments to the patient's plan of care are based on the patient's response to the intervention as determined by pain assessment and reassessment (Ackley, Ladwig, Swan, & Tucker, 2008; Berry, Covington, Dahl, Katz, & Miaskowski, 2006). If pain is not assessed well, it can result in undertreated or untreated pain that can have a significant effect on the patient. For patients with cancer, ongoing pain assessment is critical for identifying any new pain complaints or treatment-related painful conditions such as mucositis.

■ For acute pain, untreated or undertreated pain can limit mobility that can result in a serious complication such as pneumonia or deep vein thrombosis.

■ For patients with cancer, untreated acute pain can further diminish the patient's ability to cope with the disease both physiologically and psychologically. It can also delay discharge or impair recovery and may, in some cases, result in a difficult-to-treat chronic pain condition such as complex regional pain syndrome (CRPS; APS, 2003, 2008; D'Arcy, 2007). (See Chapter 15.)

■ For chronic pain, untreated or undertreated pain can limit functionality, increase the potential for disability, cause suffering, and decrease the patient's quality of life by causing anxiety, fear, depression, anxiety, and uncertainty (Berry et al., 2006).

■ Cancer survivors with chronic pain related to the cancer or its treatment need adequate pain treatment to maximize the patient's potential for a good quality of life.

For all pain patients, but especially patients with cancer, pain assessment is challenging because of the multifaceted nature of the pain. The patient comes to the experience with not only physiologic pain, but also depression, changes in relationships, and potential impact on lifestyle related to the inability to work and emotional needs. Because conveying those varied elements of the pain experience in a single pain intensity number is not reasonable, multidimensional pain assessment scales are needed to assess all aspects of the pain experience. For patients with chronic pain such as cancer survivors, functionality may be a better indicator of pain relief than a change in numeric intensity pain ratings (Ackley et al., 2008; D'Arcy, 2007).

Some patients do not understand the term *functionality*. The term *impact on daily activity* might be better understood. Questions that can give a good insight into the ability of the patient to perform the needed tasks of daily living include:

■ How far can you walk independently? With assistance?
■ Who does the cooking/washing/cleaning at your house?
■ How many stairs can you climb before you need to stop?
■ Do you go to the movies/church/visit family?
■ Can you go grocery shopping?
■ What can't you do now that you could do 3 months ago?
■ Are you less able to do things on the days you get chemotherapy or radiation?

If possible, it is always good to observe the patient while the patient is walking or moving from one position to another. For example, if the patient is sitting in a chair and is called into the health care provider's office, does the patient need several attempts to get into a standing position? Does the patient use the arms of the chair to push himself or herself up? Does the patient need assistive devices such as walkers to walk? Does the patient limp or favor one extremity over another? All of these examples can indicate that pain is significantly limiting the patient's ability to move freely or function. For patients with cancer, fatigue will have a significant impact on functionality. The health care team should be aware of differentiating between the impact of pain and the effect of fatigue.

For assessing functionality in patients with cancer, the Eastern Collaborative Oncology Group (EGOG) has a functional status rating scale from 0 to 5, with 0 indicating totally unimpaired and 5 indicating the patient is dead. The Karnofsky Performance Scale (KPS) is similar with a top score of 100 indicating normal functioning and 10 being moribund. These functional ratings are an important part of the overall assessment process and can help determine how much pain, fatigue, cancer, and cancer treatment are interfering with the patient's functional capacity.

> *Clinical Pearl*   When assessing a patient with chronic daily pain, always ask the patient to rate the worst daily pain level and the best daily pain level. Set a pain goal that reflects a pain level that is achievable in comparison to the best and worst pain ratings provided by the patient.

Many of the original pain assessment tools were designed for research and were one dimensional, only measuring the intensity of the pain. Because of the complexity of cancer pain, multidimensional pain assessment tools are needed to better assess pain. These more comprehensive tools include a pain intensity rating but also include questions about how effective pain medications are, the patient's mood, quality of the pain, and impact of the pain on activity (functionality). For patients who cannot use self-report such as those who are obtunded, intubated and critically ill, at end of life, or demented or cognitively impaired; behavioral scales have been developed to help assess pain. The following sections of the chapter will discuss specific pain assessment tools and techniques.

ASSESSMENT

Assessing pain is a subjective process; it is more of an art than a science. For verbal patients, self-report is the standard for assessing pain. To perform a standard pain assessment, the nurse asks the patient to rate pain intensity using a simple one-dimensional scale such as the Numeric Rating Scale (NRS). The NRS is an 11-point Likert-type scale with 10 numbers ranked from 0 ("no pain") to 10 ("worst possible pain") to indicate pain severity. The higher the number selected by the patient, the more severe the pain. This type of assessment is most useful for assessing pain intensity and medication efficacy.

The basic elements of a pain assessment for verbal patients include:

Location. Have the patient point to the area on his or her body that is painful. For multiple painful areas, have the patient locate each one individually and indicate when the pain occurs at that location. If one area is more painful than the next, make sure the most painful area is clearly identified. If there a radiation of pain, e.g., down a leg or arm, make sure the area is clearly defined so that the correct treatment options can be determined. A body diagram can be helpful when the patient is trying to locate the pain (see Figure 2.1). Using colors for pain in different parts of the body can also help determine any differences in pain intensity. Red can indicate a more severe level of pain, while blue can indicate pain that is less intense. Patients like to use different ways to communicate the exact location of their pain and intensity of pain they are experiencing.

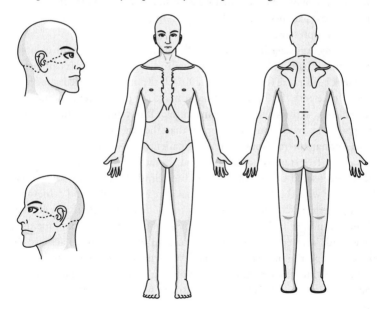

Figure 2.1 ■ Body diagram.

Duration. Ask the patient, "When did you first feel this pain?" and "How long does the pain last?" Explore any potential sources or causes of the pain. Ask if the pain intensity varies during different times of the day and how long the periods of higher intensity pain last. Ask the patient if the pain is worse when he or she is taking chemotherapy or radiation.

Intensity. Use the NRS to have the patient rate the intensity of the pain. If the patient has times during the day or night when the pain intensity is more or less severe, ask if the prescribed medication reduces the intensity of the pain. If the patient is taking pain medication, determine how effective the patient feels it is in decreasing the pain intensity. Other options for determining pain intensity if the patient cannot use the NRS are to use the terms *mild, moderate,* or *severe* to see if a range for pain intensity can be determined.

Quality/Description. Have the patient describe the quality of the pain. This may be one of the most important items in the assessment process, especially for patients who have taken vinca alkaloid chemotherapy or had a thoracotomy or mastectomy, since neuropathies can occur with these treatments. If the patient uses words like *burning, tingling,* or *painful numbness,* it may indicate a neuropathic source for the pain. It is important to allow patients to describe the pain in their own words so it is most accurately represented.

Alleviating/Aggravating Factors. All patients have some form of home treatment for pain and they most often will attempt to treat their pain before they seek health care (Roper Starch, 2001). If the patient has tried some form of pain relief, ask if it helped and did it make the pain better or worse. Ask the patient if activity made the pain worse or if rest improved the pain. Ask the patient is any one position is better than the other for relieving the pain.

Pain Management Goal. For most patients with cancer pain, achieving a pain-free state is not a valid goal. Because of tumor progression or treatment-related effects, the potential for eliminating all the pain is very low. Work with the patient to set a goal that is reasonable and achievable. Most patients with cancer pain have a pain intensity rating that will allow them to function at their highest level. Ask the patient what pain intensity they think is acceptable and then tailor pain interventions to achieve the patient's expectations. Also ask what level of medication sedation they can tolerate, because increased doses of pain medications often cause bothersome sedation. Consistent pain reassessment will track progress toward the goal that has been set.

Function Goal. Pain is dynamic and may increase with activity (Dahl & Kehlet, 2006). Ask patients how the pain interferes with their activities of daily living. Assess patients for sleep disturbances that can affect their ability to function. By setting a functionality goal, progress can be tracked at each subsequent visit.

Including the patient with cancer pain in the assessment process gives patients a feeling of validation and encourages them to work toward the pain and functional goal. Providing maximum pain relief, the highest quality of life, and functionality is the goal of any pain relief treatment for a cancer pain patient (Ackley et al., 2008; D'Arcy, 2006, 2007, 2010, 2011a; JCAHO, 2000, 2001).

These elements work well for patients who are able to self-report their pain. Using the hierarchy of pain assessment described in the following section can help delineate the assessment process for patients who are not able to report pain. Using this technique is especially helpful for patients at the end of life or who have baseline delirium or dementia.

Hierarchy of Pain Assessment

- Attempt a self-report of pain. The patient's self-report is the best way to assess for pain.
- Search for potential causes of the pain.
- Observe patient behaviors.
- Use surrogate reporting.
- Attempt an analgesic trial (Herr et al., 2006).

In addition to the hierarchy of pain assessment, using the following basic elements in practice can help standardize the assessment process for these patients.

- Use the hierarchy of pain assessment techniques.
- Establish a procedure for pain assessment.
- Use behavioral pain assessment tools, when appropriate.
- Minimize the emphasis on physiologic indicators.
- Reassess and document (Herr et al., 2006).

The most critical aspect of the pain assessment process for the nurse and other members of the health care team is to believe the patient's report of pain. Patients do the very best they can to provide you with an accurate picture of the complex pain they are experiencing. Patients with cancer are experiencing a life-changing event and will need help in describing or explaining complex pain presentations. It is extremely important for the nurse to respect the patient's report of pain as presented and then act in good faith to help relieve the pain. If the health care provider doubts or diminishes the patient's report of pain, trust will be lost and the patient will not be open to believing that the health care provider is interested in treating and managing his or her pain. This lack of trust can sabotage even the best plan of care.

Most patients with cancer pain are fearful of the pain and many are not aware of the advances in pain management. Approach the assessment process with a nonjudgmental attitude and a willingness to believe and invest time in helping patients with their pain. This personal connection with the patient who has cancer will yield tremendous benefits in creating a trusting relationship that can be useful in the long-term treatment plan for pain. The use of in-depth questions to collect all the salient information during the assessment process will help to determine the kind of interventions that will be most helpful in providing the best possible pain relief for the patient. Using a reliable and valid pain assessment tool provides objective criteria for pain assessment and a means of tracking progress toward patient goals.

Clinical Pearl	Encourage the patient with cancer to report pain honestly. Accept the patient's pain report at face value. Failure to believe the patient's report of pain will result in a faulty assessment process, which will lead to negative outcomes.

PAIN ASSESSMENT TOOLS

Many of the first pain assessment tools were developed for assessing experimentally induced pain, chronic pain, or oncology pain (Jensen, 2003). The multidimensional scales are extensions of the one-dimensional scales. The multidimensional tools were developed to assess more complex pain and included measurements of mood and psychologic elements. Today there are a wide variety of valid and reliable pain assessment tools. More recently, because The Joint Commission required that all patients have their pain assessed and adequately treated, tools for assessing pain in special populations such as the cognitively impaired, nonverbal patients, and infants have been developed to meet the needs of these patients.

One-Dimensional Pain Scales

Although unidimensional pain assessment tools are limited in scope, they are most helpful for determining if pain medication or a pain intervention is reducing the intensity of the pain. Although these tools seem very simple and the information obtained is limited, there is definitely a place for these tools in pain assessment. In order to get a more complete picture of the patient's pain, use the intensity rating as a starting point with additional questions adding more depth to the pain report. In a review of 164 journal articles on pain assessment, single-item ratings of pain intensity were reported as valid and reliable indicators of pain intensity (Ackley et al., 2008; Jensen, 2003). As an indication of efficacy, Farrar, Young, Lamoreaux, Werth, and Poole (2001) determined that a 2-point or 30% reduction in pain intensity on the NRS is a clinically significant change.

Visual Analog Scale (VAS)

Visual Analog Scale (VAS)

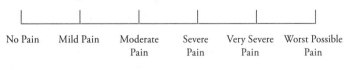

0| _____ |10

No Pain   Worst Possible Pain

Figure 2.2 ■ The Visual Analog Scale.

The Visual Analog Scale (VAS) is a 100 mm line with no pain at one end (0 mm) and worst pain possible at the other end (100 mm). See Figure 2.2. The tool was designed to be used for research where a mark could easily be measured to ascertain the intensity of the pain.

To use the VAS, the nurse asks patients to mark on the line where they feel the pain intensity is best represented. If the patient marks the line at the 50 mm position, the pain would be said to be 5/10 when compared to the NRS, or moderate-level pain.

The VAS is one of the most basic scales and has some limitations for using it clinically. Limitations to this scale include:

■ Some older adult patients have difficulty marking on the line and place the mark above or below the 100 mm line (Herr & Mobily, 1993).
■ Reassessment and comparison options are limited.

Verbal Descriptor Scale (VDS)

Verbal Descriptor Scale (VDS)

No Pain	Mild Pain	Moderate Pain	Severe Pain	Very Severe Pain	Worst Possible Pain

Figure 2.3 ■ The Verbal Descriptor Scale (VDS).

The purpose of the Verbal Descriptor Scale (VDS) is to provide a method for patient to use word descriptors to rate their pain (see Figure 2.3).

The scale is anchored on one end with "No Pain," and the opposite end indicating high-intensity pain is labeled as "Worst Pain Possible." The scale uses words such as *mild, moderate,* and *severe* to measure pain intensity. To use the scale, the nurse asks patients to select the word that best describes the pain they are experiencing. Clinically, some patients prefer to uses a word to describe their pain rather than a number. Although normally used for cognitively intact patients, Feldt, Ryden, and Miles (1998) found a 73% completion rate with the VDS in cognitively impaired patients.

   Limitations to this pain scale include:

▪ The patient must be able to understand the meaning of the words.
▪ Reassessment and comparisons are difficult.

Numeric Rating Scale (NRS)

Numeric Rating Scale (NRS)

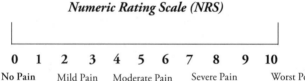

Figure 2.4 ▪ Numeric Rating Scale (NRS).

The NRS (Figure 2.4) is the most commonly used one-dimensional pain scale. It is an 11-point Likert-type scale where 0 means "no pain" and 10 means "worst possible pain." To use the scale, the nurse asks patients to rate their pain intensity from 0 to 10, where 0 is no pain and 10 is the worst possible pain. The higher the number is, the more intense the pain.

Mild pain is considered to be pain ratings in the 1 to 3 range.
Moderate pain is considered to be pain ratings in the 4 to 6 range.
Severe pain is considered to be pain ratings in the 7 to 10 range.

   Although there is discussion about whether a single-number rating of pain is accurate, the data indicate that single-item ratings can be useful. *With cancer pain, the intensity rating is only one of a number of items that are used to assess pain.* The complexity of cancer pain, which can range from acute pain during diagnosis and treatment to chronic pain in cancer survivors, requires a more detailed assessment than just a pain intensity rating. There is no good or bad, wrong or right, number for the patient to report. It is important to believe the report of pain that the patient provides. Patient self-report is still considered to be the gold standard for pain assessment (APS, 2008).

Limitations of the NRS include the following:
- It only measures one aspect of pain.

Strengths of the NRS include the following:
- It allows for reassessment and comparison of pain scores.
- It is a simple format that is easy for most patients to use.

Combined Thermometer Scale

Some patients do well when they can see a graphic pain scale. The Combined Thermometer Scale combines one-dimensional scales, the VDS and the NRS (see Figure 2.5). It was originally developed for research studies at the University of Iowa. Some patients do well with this scale and like the vertical orientation where the numbers increase from the bottom upward. The changes in color also highlight the changing pain intensity as the color merges from blue to red. (The Combined Thermometer Scale appears in color on the inside front cover.)

Pain Distress/Intensity Scale

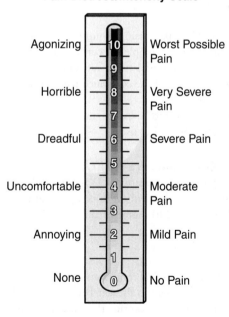

Figure 2.5 ■ Combined Thermometer Scale.

Strengths of the Combined Thermometer Scale include the following:
- It provides the ability to replicate pain ratings for reassessment.
- It is a simple, easy to use format.

Limitations include the following:
- Some patients perceive the color red to correlate to "burning/hot" pain, and blue color to "freezing/cold" pain. So, a patient with severe freezing cold pain may rate it at a lower intensity.

Multidimensional Pain Scales

Multidimensional scales are used to assess patients with chronic and cancer pain who can have a variety of pain conditions. The two scales that are most often used in the clinical setting are the McGill Pain Questionnaire (MPQ) and the Brief Pain Inventory (BPI). The difference between the one-dimensional and the multidimensional scales is the combination of indexes in the multidimensional scale to assess the following:
- Pain intensity
- Mood
- A body diagram to locate pain
- Verbal descriptors
- Medication efficacy questions

When patients rate their pain using a multidimensional pain scale, there is the opportunity to more completely convey the pain experience to the health care provider. The mood scales on some multidimensional scales can help define the impact of the continued pain on the patient's personal life and relationships.

These scales are meant to be used to measure chronic and cancer pain either for research or for clinical use.

McGill Pain Questionnaire (MPQ)

The McGill Pain Questionnaire (MPQ) is a multidimensional tool designed to measure pain in patients with complex pain conditions such as chronic pain (see Figure 2.6). Some of the areas that this pain scale has been used in include:
- Experimentally induced pain
- Postprocedural pain
- A number of medical–surgical conditions

The tool contains a VAS scale, a Present Pain Intensity (PPI) scale, and a set of verbal descriptors used to capture the sensory aspect of the pain experience. The tool has been widely used in a variety of settings and it has been

McGill Pain Questionnaire (MPQ)–Short Form

PATIENT'S NAME: _____   DATE: _____

	NONE	MILD	MODERATE	SEVERE
THROBBING	0) _____	1) _____	2) _____	3) _____
SHOOTING	0) _____	1) _____	2) _____	3) _____
STABBING	0) _____	1) _____	2) _____	3) _____
SHARP	0) _____	1) _____	2) _____	3) _____
CRAMPING	0) _____	1) _____	2) _____	3) _____
GNAWING	0) _____	1) _____	2) _____	3) _____
HOT/BURNING	0) _____	1) _____	2) _____	3) _____
ACHING	0) _____	1) _____	2) _____	3) _____
HEAVY	0) _____	1) _____	2) _____	3) _____
TENDER	0) _____	1) _____	2) _____	3) _____
SPLITTING	0) _____	1) _____	2) _____	3) _____
TIRING/EXHAUSTING	0) _____	1) _____	2) _____	3) _____
SICKENING	0) _____	1) _____	2) _____	3) _____
FEARFUL	0) _____	1) _____	2) _____	3) _____
PUNISHING/CRUEL	0) _____	1) _____	2) _____	3) _____

VAS   NO PAIN |————————————————————————————| WORST POSSIBLE PAIN

PPI

0	NO PAIN	_____
1	MILD	_____
2	DISCOMFORTING	_____
3	DISTRESSING	_____
4	HORRIBLE	_____
5	EXCRUCIATING	_____

© R. Melzack 1984

The short-form McGill Pain Questionnaire (SF-MPQ). Descriptors 1–11 represent the sensory dimension of pain experience and 12–15 represent the affective dimension. Each descriptor is ranked on an intensity scale of 0 = none, 1 = mild, 2 = moderate, 3 = severe. The Present Pain Intensity (PPI) of the standard long-form McGill Pain Questionnaire (LF-MPQ) and the Visual Analog Scale (VAS are also included to provide overall intensity scores.

Figure 2.6 ■ McGill Pain Questionnaire (MPQ). Reprinted with permission from © R. Melzack, 1984.

found to be reliable and valid. It has also been translated into a number of foreign languages (Chok, 1998; Graham et al., 1980; Melzack, 1975, 1987; McDonald & Weiskopf, 2001; McIntyre et al., 1995; Mystakidou et al., 2002; Wilkie, 1990).

Strengths of the MPQ include the following:
- It has a high level of reliability and validity.

Limitations of the MPQ include the following:
- It is difficult to score and weight the verbal descriptor section.
- It is difficult to translate the verbal descriptor section into words that indicate syndromes (Gracely, 1992; Graham et al., 1980).
  - It takes more time to complete.
  - It cannot be used if the patient has cognitive impairment.
  - The patient must be able to use paper and pen or computer to complete it.

Brief Pain Inventory (BPI)

Originally, the Brief Pain Inventory (BPI) was first used with oncology patients to assess long-term oncology pain. With further use, it has been found to be reliable and valid for assessing pain in patients with chronic pain (Daut, Cleeland, & Flannery, 1983; Raiche et al., 2006; Tan et al., 2004; Tittle et al., 2003; Williams, Smith, & Fehnel, 2006). It has also been translated into a variety of languages (Ger et al., 1999; Klepstad, 2002; Mystakidou et al., 2002; Radbruch et al., 1999). It has a simple, easy-to-use format that can be used as an interview or as a self-report completed by the patient (see Figure 2.7). The BPI includes the following:
- A pain intensity scale
- A body diagram to locate the pain
- A functional assessment
- Questions about the efficacy of pain medications

Strengths of the BPI include the following:
- It has a high level of reliability and validity.

Limitations for the BPI include the following:
- Patients must be cognitively intact to answer questions related to their individual pain condition.

Behavioral Pain Scales

In 2001, The Joint Commission applied pain standards to inpatient care that set a standard for outpatient practice as well. One of the biggest focus areas in The Joint Commission standards was pain assessment for all patients that included assessing pain in individuals who could not self-report their pain. In a study of 13,625 patients with cancer aged 65 or older, a total of 4,003 patients reported daily pain (Burnabei et al., 1998). One of the basic indicators of determining medication use with these patients was cognitive impairment or inability to report pain (Burnabei et al., 1998).

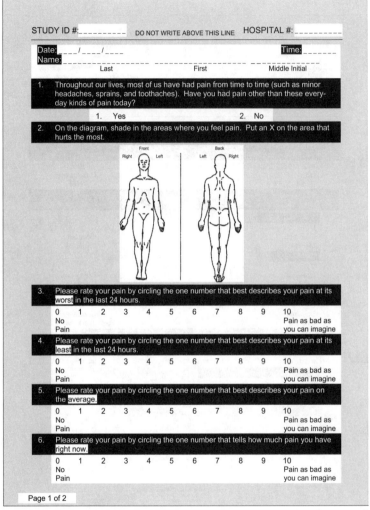

STUDY ID #:_____ DO NOT WRITE ABOVE THIS LINE HOSPITAL #:_____

Date: ____/____/____   Time: _____
Name: _____ _____ _____
      Last   First   Middle Initial

1. Throughout our lives, most of us have had pain from time to time (such as minor headaches, sprains, and toothaches). Have you had pain other than these every-day kinds of pain today?

     1.   Yes   2.   No

2. On the diagram, shade in the areas where you feel pain. Put an X on the area that hurts the most.

3. Please rate your pain by circling the one number that best describes your pain at its **worst** in the last 24 hours.

   0   1   2   3   4   5   6   7   8   9   10
   No   Pain as bad as
   Pain   you can imagine

4. Please rate your pain by circling the one number that best describes your pain at its **least** in the last 24 hours.

   0   1   2   3   4   5   6   7   8   9   10
   No   Pain as bad as
   Pain   you can imagine

5. Please rate your pain by circling the one number that best describes your pain on the **average.**

   0   1   2   3   4   5   6   7   8   9   10
   No   Pain as bad as
   Pain   you can imagine

6. Please rate your pain by circling the one number that tells how much pain you have **right now.**

   0   1   2   3   4   5   6   7   8   9   10
   No   Pain as bad as
   Pain   you can imagine

Page 1 of 2

Figure 2.7 ■ Brief Pain Inventory.   *(continued)*

(continued)

Page 2 of 2

Figure 2.7 ■ Brief Pain Inventory, page 2.

To facilitate the process, a group of pain assessment tools have been developed to use for assessing pain in the nonverbal patient.

Behavioral scales for pain assessment are some of the newest and more challenging areas of pain assessment research, and as such, the tools may not be as completely developed or refined as self-report scales that have been used for many years. Some of the tools are designed to be used for specific populations such as cognitively impaired patients or intubated, critically ill patients. This tool may be useful with critically ill oncology patients, with profound neutropenic sepsis coma in a stem cell transplant patient, or prolonged recovery after a Whipple procedure (pancreatico-duodenectomy) for pancreatic cancer where they may be unable to communicate the extent of their pain.

In order to use a behavioral scale, it is important to first identify those behaviors that indicate pain. The original research in this area was to develop a list of behaviors that were indicative of pain, the checklist of nonverbal pain indicators (CNPI). From the studies comparing pain in cognitively intact patients and similar pain experiences in patients who were cognitively impaired, a list of six behaviors was developed that were determined to indicate the presence of pain (Feldt, 2000; Feldt et al., 1998). The six behaviors were identified as follows:

- Vocalizations
- Facial grimacing
- Bracing
- Rubbing
- Restlessness
- Vocal complaints (Feldt, 2000)

Additional behaviors that were determined to be indicative of pain were listed in the American Geriatrics Society's (AGS) guideline for treating persistent pain in older persons (2002). These behaviors include the following:

- Verbalizations: moaning, calling out, asking for help, groaning
- Facial expressions: grimacing, frowning, wrinkled forehead, distorted expressions
- Body movements: rigid, tense body posture; guarding; rocking; fidgeting; pacing; massaging the painful area
- Changes in interpersonal interactions: aggression, combative behavior, resisting care, disruptive behavior, withdrawn
- Changes in activity patterns or routines: refusing food, appetite changes, increase in rest or sleep, increased wandering
- Mental status changes: crying, tears, increased confusion, irritability, or distress (AGS, 2002)

When attempting to assess pain in a nonverbal patient, the important elements are as follows:

- Attempt a self-report. (Self-report can be valid, even in advanced dementia, with use of a "yes" or "no" question.)
- Search for the potential causes of pain.
- Observe patient behaviors.

■ Use surrogate reporting by family or caregivers indicating pain and/or behavior/activity changes.

■ Attempt an analgesic trial (Herr, Bjoro, & Decker, 2006).

In order to use behaviors to identify pain, tools have developed using the behaviors and formatting the assessment in several different styles to use in different patient populations.

PAIN ASSESSMENT IN ADVANCED DEMENTIA (PAIN-AD)

	0	1	2
Breathing	Normal	Occasional labored breathing Short period of hyperventilation	Noisy labored breathing Long period of hyperventilation Cheyne-Stokes respirations
Negative Vocalization	None	Occasional moan/groan Low-level speech/negative or disapproving quality	Repeated troubled calling out Loud moaning or groaning Crying
Facial Fxpression	Smiling	Sad, frightened, frown	Facial grimacing Inexpressive
Body Language	Relaxed	Tense, distressed pacing Fidgeting	Rigid, fists clenched Knees pulled up Pulling or pushing away Striking out
Consolability	No need to console	Distracted or reassured by voice or touch	Unable to console, distract, or reassure
Total Score _____			

Figure 2.8 ■ PAIN-AD. Developed at the New England Geriatric Research Education and Clinical Center, E N Rogers Memorial Veterans Hospital, Bedford, Massachusetts. *Source:* Warden, V., Hurley, A. C., & Volicer, L. (2003). Development and psychometric evaluation of the Pain Assessment in Advanced Dementia (PAIN-AD) Scale. *Journal of the American Medical Directors Association, 4,* 9–15.

Persons with dementia are some of the most challenging patients to assess for pain, as many are nonverbal. The PAIN-AD (Figure 2.8) is a pain assessment tool created to assess pain in patients with advanced dementia and Alzheimer's disease (Lane et al., 2003; Warden, Hurley, & Volicer, 2003).

The PAIN-AD uses five behaviors common to patients with dementia who have pain, which are as follows:

▪ Breathing
▪ Negative vocalizations
▪ Facial expression
▪ Body language
▪ Consolability

To use the tool, the five behaviors are rated as follows:

▪ 0—normal, no symptoms or pain behaviors
▪ 1—occasional behaviors, slightly affected (e.g., occasional pacing, occasional moans)
▪ 2—positive behaviors (e.g., hyperventilation, body rigidity, repeated moaning or striking out)

After determining the extent of the behaviors, they are rated and a score is derived, which provides a numeric rating for the pain. Using this tool can provide a more consistent approach to assessing pain in these patients. The tool has been found to be simple and easy to use in the clinical setting, and has also resulted in increased detection of pain (Hutchinson et al., 2006).

Limitations of the PAIN-AD include the following:

▪ The caregiver assesses for pain, and caregiver assessments may not correlate well with pain.
▪ It is less comprehensive than needed for the full assessment of pain (Herr et al., 2006).

There are other tools that can be used in this patient population to assess pain, but the PAIN-AD has been used more widely.

PAYEN BEHAVIORAL PAIN SCALE (BPS)

Critically ill, intubated patients with cancer may not be able to self-report pain, especially if sedated. Many of the procedures that are performed on these patients are painful. In a large multisite study, Thunder II, pain ratings for a number of patient procedures was determined. Even as simple a task as turning a patient in bed can result in moderate-intensity pain (Puntillo et al., 2001). When these patients have baseline chronic pain or cancer pain, the new pain the patient experiences is more significant and will result in higher intensity pain.

Payen Behavioral Pain Scale		
Item	**Description**	**Score**
Facial Expression	Relaxed	1
	Partially tightened (e.g., brow lowering)	2
	Fully tightened (e.g., eyelid closing)	3
	Grimacing	4
Upper Limbs	No movement	1
	Partially bent	2
	Fully bent with finger flexion	3
	Permanently retracted	4
Compliance With Ventilation	Tolerating movement	1
	Coughing but tolerating ventilation for most of the time	2
	Fighting ventilator	3
	Unable to control ventilator	4

Figure 2.9 ■ Payen BPS. *Source:* Payen, J. F., Bru, O., Bosson, J. L., Lagrasta, A., Novel, E., Deschaux, I., … Jacquot, C. (2001). Assessing pain in critically ill sedated patients by using a behavioral pain scale. *Critical Care Medicine, 29*(12), 1–11. Used by permission of the authors.

Assessing pain in these patients requires a tool that can detect pain behaviors such as brow furrowing and can give an indication of pain intensity. The Payen Behavioral Pain Scale (BPS; Figure 2.9) is designed specifically for unresponsive, critically ill intubated patients and includes a section that is designed to assess compliance with ventilation. The three assessment categories for this scale include the following:

■ Facial expression
■ Upper limb movement
■ Compliance with ventilation

To score each category, a 4-point scale is used that ranges from 1 (relaxed, no movement, tolerating movement) to 4 (grimacing, permanently retracted, unable to control ventilation).

In the original validation study, 30 critically ill, intubated patients were divided into three groups based on sedation levels: mild, moderate, or heavy. Findings from the study indicate that in each of the groups there was a sufficient correlation with the NRS when a pain stimulus such as a turn in bed was performed (Payen, 2001; Purdum & D'Arcy, 2006). The effect of the sedation was apparent but there was still a fair correlation with the NRS, even in the group of heavily sedated patients. The tool is reliable and valid for assessing pain in this patient population. A replication study by Aissaoui (2005) had similar results.

There are other critical care pain assessment tools, such as the Gelinas CPOT, that use behavioral observation to estimate pain intensity (Gelinas, Fillion, Puntillo, Viens, & Fortier, 2006). Although these tools are not perfected, they do provide a means of assessing pain in patients who were once thought to be unassessable (Hutchinson et al., 2006).

MEASURES OF FUNCTIONALITY

Because success with chronic pain treatment plans relies so heavily on functionality, it is important to get a baseline measure of functionality and continue to track progress throughout the treatment period. There are two measures that are used most often for both research and clinical practice: the Owestry Disability Index and the SF-36, or its shorter version, the SF-12.

The Owestry Disability Index

This tool is a reliable and valid measure of functionality. It was designed for use as a functional outcome measure for patients with low back pain. The tool consists of 10 sections with 6 questions in each that relate to pain intensity, ability to perform personal care, sleeping, sitting, and social life, to name a few. Each section has a series of questions that indicate how long the person can sustain the activity, e.g., sitting, medication use for pain relief, or level of activity such as traveling.

Patients complete the assessment tool and select the answer that most closely represents their pain or limitation within the last week or two. If two answers seem to fit the best response, the patient is instructed to select the answer with the highest point value. Disability is calculated by taking the point total, dividing by 50, and multiplying by 100. This provides the percent disability. After scoring the tool, disability is rated according to the following scale:

- 0% to 20%—minimal disability, no treatment indicated except for advice on lifting, sitting, and exercise
- 21% to 40%—moderate disability, difficulty with sitting, lifting, standing (may be disabled from work); management is conservative treatment
- 41% to 60%—severe disability; pain is main problem, activities of daily living affected
- 61% to 80%—crippled; pain affects all areas of the patient's life; positive intervention required
- 81% to 100%—either bed bound or exaggerating symptoms (Owestry Disability Index, n.d.)

SF-36 or SF-12 Questionnaires

The original form of the SF questionnaire was the 36-item survey that assessed eight domains of health such as physical functioning, bodily function, role limitation, and social functioning. It is a generic measure that determines the burden of disease on an individual patient.

A shorter version of the SF-36, the SF-12, uses 12 items taken from the original 36-question format. The shorter form has the questions from the eight domains and can reproduce the physical and mental health summary measures with at least 90% accuracy (IQOLA, n.d.). Using either of these tools allows the health care practitioner to screen individual patients, and assess the health and relative burden of disease while differentiating the benefits of various treatment options (IQOLA website).

ASSESSING PAIN IN SPECIALTY POPULATIONS

There are some patient populations in which pain assessment is more difficult: children, older adults, and patients with a history of substance abuse. These patients have special needs and understanding when it comes to assessing pain and there are some tools and concepts that are helpful for these groups of patients.

Assessing Pain in Older Adults

Older patients have usually experienced pain before. They have any number of chronic pain conditions (such as osteoarthritis or angina) and comorbidities (such as chronic renal failure or atrial fibrillation on warfarin) that can make selecting pain medication difficult. Adding cancer pain to the baseline pain conditions can mean a dramatic decrease in the patient's overall functional ability. Older patients may be reluctant to report pain, not wanting to be seen as complainers or due to concerns about adding costly medications for pain to their already crowded medication regimen (Bruckenthal & D'Arcy, 2007).

To get a good pain assessment in older patients, make sure that any assistive devices such as glasses and hearing aids are in place. Convey to the patient that you have an interest in his or her pain, would like to help relieve the pain, and have the time to talk. Educate the patient about pain assessment. Help the patient to understand that a good pain assessment is the best way to determine what medications and interventions could be helpful for pain relief. Include the family when it is appropriate.

Assessing Pain in Patients With a Substance Abuse History

Illicit substance abuse and prescription drug abuse and misuse has been steadily increasing at an alarming rate. Patients who have a history of substance abuse are difficult to assess for pain because they often will report continued levels of high-intensity pain despite efforts to control the pain. Since opioid use for pain control is so prevalent in patients with cancer, the issue of prior illicit drug use or prescription drug misuse can impact the way the patient reports the pain, how well the pain medications work, and pain reassessment ratings.

It can be very frustrating for a nurse to give large doses of pain medication to these patients and have them continue to report high-intensity pain. Some of this response is related to theorized alterations in the patient's physiology caused by continued use of opioid medications or illicit substances, making the patient's body more sensitive to pain. This heightened sensitivity to pain is called *hyperalgesia* and it can occur as soon as 1 month after opioid use/abuse begins (Chu, Clark, & Angst, 2006). It would then be expected that these patients would report higher pain levels and require more pain medication to control their pain.

To perform a pain assessment in a patient who is actively using illicit substances or has a history of substance abuse, it is important to remember the following:

- A nonjudgmental approach is best. In order to get accurate information, patients should feel that they can trust you with the information and they will not be judged.
- Determine when the patient last used an illicit substance.
- Determine what the substance is and how much the patient uses every day.
- Assess for any co-substance abuse, such as combinations of alcohol, heroin, marijuana, cocaine, and so on.
- Reassure the patient that you need this information to help determine what types of medication or interventions will help to control the pain.
- Reassess the patient's pain at regular intervals to determine if the pain medication has been effective in reducing pain.
- Remember that these patients may have had bad experiences with other health care providers; try to gain their trust so that patients feel comfortable talking to you about their pain. (More information on treating patients with cancer pain in the setting of substance use is provided in Chapters 12 and 13.)

BARRIERS TO PAIN ASSESSMENT

There are some barriers that make accurate pain assessment challenging for nurses, as shown in the following list:

- Bias
- Cultural influences
- Family values
- Belief systems (Harrison, 1991)

Research indicates that nurses still have difficulty accepting the patient's report of pain as valid and credible (Berry et al., 2006; D'Arcy, 2008, 2009; Donovan, Dillon, & Mcguire, 1987; Drayer, Henderson, & Reidenberg, 1999; Grossman, Sheidler, Sweeden, Mucenski, & Piantadosi, 1991; Paice, Mahon, & Faut-Callahan, 1991). In order to minimize the effects of these factors on pain assessment, it is important for the nurse to recognize these factors and consciously work to derive as accurate a pain assessment as possible.

Today's nurses are being held accountable for the quality of their pain management, including assessment. It is incumbent on each nurse who performs a pain assessment to attempt to get as accurate a pain assessment as possible. When pain assessment is poorly done, it can affect the patient's plan of care and adversely impact outcomes.

Focusing on pain relief as the primary end to the assessment process and treatment selection will help control fears and bias that can negatively affect patient care. Accepting and believing the patient's report of pain are essential to performing a good pain assessment. Using a recognized, reliable, and valid pain assessment tool, believing the patient, and accepting the patient's report of pain in a nonjudgmental fashion will provide the patient with the best chance for adequate pain relief.

Case Study

Peter Smith is an infusion center patient who is receiving chemotherapy for lung cancer. He says the chemotherapy makes him nauseated and tired but his main complaint is pain that radiates across his chest. He says it destroys his sleep and is there all the time. When he rates the pain, it is an 8/10 at the worst and 5/10 at the best. It is getting more difficult for Peter to manage his pain. The medications they give for the pain do not help and recently his health care provider started him on a long-acting opioid along with his short-acting opioid medication. When Peter describes his pain, he tells you "The pain across my chest feels like there is a blow torch moving back and forth across the area where I had my thoracotomy. I can manage the effects of the chemotherapy but this pain is making me weary and depressed since no pain medication seems to be able to relieve it." How will you assess Peter's pain and what are some important elements of his description?

Questions to Consider

1. What is the best tool to use to assess the pain Peter is having?
2. You assess Peter's pain as severe, constant, and located at the surgical site on his chest with neuropathic descriptors. Since the pain seems to be neuropathic, is it surprising that the opioid medications are not providing that pain relief you expected?
3. What are the biggest elements in the assessment process for Peter? Pain intensity, loss of sleep, depression, or fatigue?
4. What are some of the outcomes of the poorly relieved pain that Peter is experiencing?
5. Use the BPI to assess the pain Peter is having and determine what the major effect of the pain is on his life.

REFERENCES

Ackley, B., Ladwig, G., Swan, B. A., & Tucker, S. J. (2008) *Evidence-based nursing care guidelines.* St. Louis MO: Mosby Elsevier.

American Geriatrics Society (AGS). (2002). The management of persistent pain in older persons—The American Geriatrics Society Panel on Persistent Pain in Older Persons. *Journal of the American Geriatrics Society, 50*(6), 205–224.

American Pain Society (APS). (2005). *Cancer pain in adults and children.* Glenview, IL: Author.

American Pain Society (APS). (2008). *Principles of analgesic use in the treatment of acute and cancer pain* (6th ed). Glenview, IL: Author.

American Society for Pain Management Nursing. (2010). *Core curriculum for pain management nursing.* Dubuque, IA: Kendall Hunt Publications.

Aissaoui, Y., et al. (2005). Validation of a behavioral pain scale in critically ill, sedated and mechanically ventilated patients. *Anesthesia & Analgesia, 101*(5), 1470–1476.

Berry, P. H., Covington, E., Dahl, J., Katz, J., & Miaskowski, C. (2006). *Pain: Current understanding of assessment, management, and treatments.* Reston, VA: National Pharmaceutical Council, Inc. and The Joint Commission on Accreditation of Healthcare Organizations.

Bruckenthal, P., & D'Arcy, Y. (2007). Assessment and management of pain in older adults: A review of the basics. *Topics in Advanced practice Nursing* ejournal 2007 (1). Retrieved September 17, 2009, from http://www.medscape.com/viewarticle/556382

Burnabei, R., Gambassi, G., LaPane, K., Landl, F., Gatsonis, C., Dunlop, R., . . . Mor, V. (1998). Management of pain in elderly patients with cancer. *Journal of the American Medical Association, 279,* 1877–1882.

Chok, B. (1998). An overview of the Visual Analogue Scale and the McGill Pain Questionnaire. *Physiotherapy Singapore, 1*(3), 88–93.

Chu, L., Clark, D., & Angst, M. (2006). Opioid tolerance and hyperalgesia in chronic pain patients after one month of oral morphine therapy: A preliminary prospective study. *The Journal of Pain, 7*(1), 43–48.

Dahl, J. B., & Kehlet, H. (2006), Postoperative pain and its management. In S. B. McMahon & M. Kolzenburg (Eds.), *Wall & Melzack's textbook of pain* (5th ed.). Philadelphia, PA: Churchill Livingstone.

D'Arcy, Y. M. (2006). Pain assessment and management. In *Medical legal aspects of medical records.* Tucson, AZ: Lawyers and Judges Publishing Company, Inc.

D'Arcy, Y. (2007). *Pain management: Evidence-based tools and techniques for nursing professionals.* Marblehead, MA: HcPro.

D'Arcy, Y. (2008). Be in the know about pain management. Results of the pain management survey. *Nursing 2008, 38*(6), 42–49.

D'Arcy, Y. (2009). Be in the know about pain management. Results of the pain management survey. *The Nurse Practitioner, 34,* 43–47.

D'Arcy, Y. (2010). Pain assessment. In *American Society for Pain Management Nursing core curriculum* (Ch. 13). Dubuque, IA: Kendall Hunt Publishing.

D'Arcy, Y. (2011a). *Compact clinical guide to chronic pain management.* New York, NY: Springer Publishing Company.

D'Arcy, Y. (2011b, December). Breakthrough pain in cancer. *Pain Medicine News.*

Daut, R. L., Cleeland, C. S., & Flannery, R. (1983). Development of the Wisconsin Brief Pain Questionnaire to assess pain in cancer or other diseases. *Pain, 17,* 197–210.

Dochterman, J. M., & Bulechek, G. M. (Eds.). (2004). *Nursing Interventions Classification (NIC)* (4th ed.). St. Louis, MO: Mosby.

Donovan, M., Dillon, P., & Mcguire, L. (1987). Incidence and characteristics of pain in a sample of medical-surgical inpatients. *Pain, 30*(1), 69–78.

Drayer, R., Henderson, J., & Reidenberg, M. (1999). Barriers to better pain control for hospitalized patients. *Journal of Pain and Symptom Management, 17*(6), 434–440.

Farrar, J. T., Young, J. P., Lamoreaux, L., Werth, J. L., & Poole, R. M. (2001). Clinical importance of changes in chronic pain intensity measured on an 11 point numerical pain rating scale. *Pain, 94,* 149–158.

Feldt, K. S., Ryden, M. B., & Miles, S. (1998). Treatment of pain in cognitively impaired compared with cognitively intact older patients with hip fractures. *Journal of the American Geriatrics Society, 46,* 1079–1085.

Feldt, K. S. (2000). The checklist of non-verbal pain indicators (CNPI). *Pain Management Nursing, 1*(1), 13–21.

Gelinas, C., Fillion, L., Puntillo, K., Viens, C., & Fortier, M. (2006). Validation of the Critical Care Pain Observation Tool in adult patients. *American Journal of Critical Care, 15*(4), 420–427.

Ger, L., Ho, S., Sun, W., Wang, M., & Cleeland, C. (1999). Validation of the Brief Pain Inventory in a Taiwanese population. *Journal of Pain and Symptom Management, 18*(5), 316–322.

Gracely, R. H., & Dubner, R. (1987). Reliability and validity of verbal descriptor scales of painfulness. *Pain, 29,* 175–185.

Graham, C., Bond, S., Gerkovich, M., & Cook, M. (1980). Use of the McGill Pain Questionnaire in the assessment of cancer pain: Replicability and consistency. *Pain, 8,* 377–387.

Grossman, S., Sheidler, V., Sweeden, K., Mucenski, J., & Piantadosi, S. (1991). Correlation of patient and caregiver ratings of cancer pain. *Journal of Pain and Symptom Management, 6*(2), 53–57.

Jensen, M. P. (2003). The validity and reliability of pain measures in adults with cancer. *Journal of Pain, 4*(1), 2–21.

Harrison, A. (1991). Assessing patient's pain: Identifying reasons for error. *Journal of Advanced Nursing, 16,* 1018–1025.

Herr, K. A., & Mobily, P. (1993). Comparison of selected pain assessment tools for use with the elderly. *Applied Nursing Research, 6*(1), 39–46.

Herr, K., Bjoro, K., & Decker, S. (2006). Tools for assessment of pain in nonverbal older adults with dementia: A state-of-the-science review. *Journal of Pain and Symptom Management, 31*(2), 170–192.

Herr, K., Coyne, P., Key, T., Manworren, R., McCaffery, M., Merkel, S., . . . Wild, L. (2006). Pain assessment in the nonverbal patient: Position statement with clinical practice recommendations. *Pain Management Nursing, 7*(2), 44–52.

Hutchinson, R., Tucker, W., Kim, S., & Gilder, R. (2006). Evaluation of a behavioral assessment tool for the individual unable to self report pain. *American Journal of Hospice and Palliative Medicine, 23*(4), 328–331.

IQOLA. (n.d.). Retrieved from http://www.iqola.org/instruments

Joint Commission on Accreditation of Healthcare Organizations (JCAHO). (2000). *Pain assessment and management: An organizational approach.* Oakbrook Terrace, IL: JCAHO.

Klepstad, P., Loge, J., Borchgrevink, P., Mendoza, T., Cleeland, C., & Kaasa, S. (2002). The Norwegian Brief Pain Inventory Questionnaire: Translation and validation in cancer pain patients. *Journal of Pain and Symptom Management, 24*(5), 517–525.

MacIntyre, D., Hopkins, P., & Harris, S. (1995). Evaluation of pain and functional activity in palletofemoral pain syndrome: Reliability and validity of two pain assessment tools. *Physiotherapy of Canada, 47*(3), 164–170.

McDonald, D. D., & Weiskopf. C. S. A. (2001). Adult patients' postoperative pain descriptions and responses to the Short Form McGill Pain Questionnaire. *Clinical Nursing Research, 10*(4), 442–452.

Melzack, R. (1975). The McGill Pain Questionnaire: Major properties and scoring methods. *Pain, 1,* 277–299.

Melzack, R. (1987). The Short Form McGill Pain Questionnaire. *Pain, 30,* 191–197.

Mystakidou, K., Mendoza, T., Tsilika, E., Befon, S., Parpa, G., Bellos, G., Valhos, L., & Cleeland, C. (2001). Greek Brief Pain Inventory: Validation and utility in cancer pain. *Oncology, 60*(1), 35–42.

Mystakidou, K., Parpa, E., Tsilka, E., Kalaidopoulou, O., Georgaki, S., Galanos, A., & Vlahos, L. (2002). Greek McGill Pain Questionnaire: Validation and utility in cancer patients. *Journal of Pain and Symptom Management, 24*(4), 370–387.

Owestry Disability Index. (n.d.). Retrieved from http://www.chirogeek.com/001_Owestry_20htm

Paice, J., Mahon, S., & Faut-Callahan, M. (1991). Factors associated with adequate pain control in hospitalized postsurgical patients diagnosed with cancer. *Cancer Nursing, 14*(6), 298–305.

Payen, J. F., Bru, O., Bosson, J. L., Lagrasta, A., Novel, E., Descheaux, I., . . . Jacquot, C. (2001). Assessing pain in critically ill sedated patients by using a behavioral pain scale. *Critical Care Medicine, 29*(12), 1–11.

Puntillo, K., White, C., Morris, A., Purdue, S., Stanik-Hutt, J., Thompson, C., & Wild, L. (2001). Patients perceptions and responses to procedural pain: Results of the Thunder II project. *American Journal of Critical Care, 10*(4), 238–251.

Purdum, A., & D'Arcy, Y. (2006). *A comparison of two behavioral pain scales with intubated intensive care patient.* San Antonio, TX: American Pain Society.

Radbruch, L., Liock, G., Kienke, P., Lindena, G., Sabatowski, R., Grond, S., Lehmann, A., & Cleeland, C. (1999). Validation of the German version of the Brief Pain Inventory. *Journal of Pain and Symptom Management, 18*(3), 180–187.

Raiche, K., Osborne, T., Jensen, M. P., & Cardenas, D. (2006). The reliability and validity of pain interference measures in persons with spinal cord injury. *Journal of Pain, 7*(3), 179–186.

Tan, G., Jensen, M. P., Thornby, J., & Shanti, B. (2004). Validation of the Brief Pain Inventory for chronic non-malignant pain. *Journal of Pain and Symptom Management, 5*(2), 133–137.

Tittle, M., McMillan, S., & Hagan, S. (2003). Validating the Brief Pain Inventory for use with surgical patients with cancer. *Oncology Nursing Forum, 30*(2), 325–330.

Roper Starch Worldwide, Inc. (2001). *Chronic pain in America: Roadblocks to relief.* Retrieved from www.painfoundation.org/page.asp?file.

Warden V., Hurley A. C., & Volicer, L. (2003). Development and psychometric evaluation of the Pain Assessment in Advanced Dementia (PAIN-AD) Scale. *Journal of the American Medical Directors Association, 4*, 9–15.

Wilkie, D., Savedra, M., Holzmer, W., Tesler, M., & Paul, S. (1990). Use of the McGill Questionnaire to measure pain: A meta-analysis. *Nursing Research, 39*(1), 36–41.

Williams, V., Smith, M., & Fehnel, S. (2006). The validity and utility of the BPI interference measures for evaluating the impact of osteoarthritis pain. *Journal of Pain and Symptom Management, 31*(1), 48–57.

ADDITIONAL RESOURCES

Gordon, D., Pellino, T., Miaskowski, C., McNeill, J. A., Paice, J., Laferriere, D., & Bookbinder, M. (2002). A 10-year review of quality improvement monitoring in pain management: Recommendations for standardized outcome measures. *Pain Management Nursing, 3*(4), 116–130.

Herr, K., & Garand, L. (2001). Assessment and measurement of pain in older adults. *Clinics in Geriatric Medicine, 17*(4), 1–22.

Merkel, S., Voepel-Lewis, T., Shayevitz, J., & Malviya, S. (1997). The FLACC: A behavioral scale for scoring postoperative pain in young children. *Pediatric Nursing, 23*, 293–297.

Weiner, D. K., Herr, K., & Rudy, T. (2002). *Persistent pain in older adults: An interdisciplinary guide for treatment.* New York, NY: Springer Publishing Company.

3

Using Nonopioid Medications for Cancer Pain Management

Yvonne D'Arcy

OVERVIEW OF MEDICATION MANAGEMENT

Drug treatment is the mainstay of cancer pain management (World Health Organization [WHO], 1996). Because the sources of cancer pain are varied, a variety of medications and combinations of medications may be needed to provide the best possible pain relief. Although opioids alone can control up to 85% of the pain in cancer patients, the addition of multimodal approaches, such as adding nonopioid medications and other modalities such as neural blockade, can provide pain control for up to 95% of patients with cancer pain (Thapa, Rastogi, & Ahuja, 2011).

Treating the acute pain of cancer during diagnosis and active treatment is of paramount importance, but many cancer survivors are left with chronic pain conditions such as neuropathies. As the survivors live longer, they also develop non–cancer-related chronic pain conditions such as arthritis and low back pain. These patients may not require opioids but may benefit from adjuvant medications that reduce pain to tolerable levels and allow for maximum functionality.

For some conditions such as acute low back pain, the current recommendation by pain societies is acetaminophen and nonsteroidal anti-inflammatory drugs (NSAIDs) and continued activity, rather than opioids and bedrest (Chou et al., 2007). About 15% of the patients who have acute low back progress to chronic low back pain and that is when medication management is recommended and a plan of care that includes medications along with other therapies such as physical therapy and counseling is developed. Opioids currently are reserved in most cases of chronic low back pain for severe pain that is impairing functionality (Chou et al., 2009). For cancer patients who had ready access to opioids during their treatment phase for cancer, this change in thinking may be difficult to process.

To treat cancer pain with medications requires a pain assessment, history and physical examination, and medication review that includes over-the-counter medications, herbal supplements, and vitamins (WHO, 1996). Patients who have been treated for cancer pain have personal experience using pain medications. When patients share information about medications that are effective for relieving their pain, consider this to be information that is similar to what a diabetic provides about their daily insulin doses to a new health care provider. Just because a patient is familiar with medication names and doses does not make him or her a "drug seeker."

There are genetic factors that influence the effectiveness of pain medications in a specific individual, so when a patient says, "the only medication that works for me is morphine," it may really be a reflection of how his or her genetic makeup has reacted to medications tried in the past. The patient should never be penalized or labeled for providing information on how specific medications have worked in the past.

This section of the book will provide information about using pain medications of various types—NSAIDs, opioids, and other coanalgesics such as antidepressants. The information will be taken from current guidelines developed by the American Pain Society (APS), the American Geriatrics Society (AGS), the WHO, the American Academy of Pain Medicine (AAPM), and other national organizations. The topics of addiction, dependency, and tolerance will be discussed in the other chapters of this book. Information on integrative therapies that can be combined with medication management will be provided in Chapter 7.

GENERAL GUIDELINES

All patients have the right to have their pain treated and most health care providers make honest efforts at getting the patient's pain to a tolerable level (Brennan, Carr, & Cousins, 2007). Most chronic pain patients with acute or surgical pain realize that "pain free" is not a reasonable goal to set and that a risk–benefit analysis is used to determine what type of medication management will provide the best outcome for the patient. However, the prevalence of pain in cancer patients requires consideration of a variety medications and techniques to provide adequate pain relief. Combining nonopioid medications, opioid analgesics, and coanalgesics in conjunction with interventional treatments may make dealing with cancer pain a more intensive endeavor.

Most prescribers have very little concern when opioids are needed for short-term pain management, but when opioid therapy is required long term, their concern increases and fears of addicting the patient or fear of increased regulatory oversight can affect the prescriber's willingness to continue providing opioid medications to the patient with chronic noncancer pain (D'Arcy, 2009). For acute pain, this issue is not as significant, but there are still some health care providers (HCPs) who feel that they are contributing to addiction when opioids are used in the acute care setting. This can lead the prescriber to consider the nonopioid medications as first-line treatment when an opioid may be indicated. Or prescribers may try an opioid that they perceive has a lower potential for abuse or addiction such as acetaminophen with codeine, even though the patient may be reporting severe pain. Selecting a medication that will be effective for the patient's pain complaint can be a trial-and-error process until the right medication and dose are found.

Some patients who have acute pain during active treatment will progress to chronic pain as cancer survivors. Even in the setting of active cancer treatment, it is wise to screen all patients who are being considered for chronic opioid therapy (COT) for risks that include opioid misuse, development of aberrant medication taking behaviors, and addiction (Chou et al., 2009). The development of a comprehensive treatment plan that includes the use of various medications is extremely important to the success of pain management (Institute for Clinical Symptoms Improvement [ICSI], 2008). If long-term opioids are being considered, an opioid agreement may be created that outlines when the medications will be refilled, the risks and benefits of the medications, the use of random urine screens, and the consequences of violating the agreement (Trescot et al., 2008). A sample opioid agreement can beobtained at the website of the American Academy of Pain Medicine.

At the other end of the spectrum, the undertreatment of cancer pain can produce a plethora of unwanted side effects, especially with older patients. Some of the significant consequences of undertreated pain include the following:
- Depression
- Impaired cognition
- Sleep disturbances
- Poorer clinical outcome
- Decreased functional ability
- Decreased quality of life
- Anxiety
- Decreased socialization
- Increased health care utilization and costs (AGS, 2002; Brenann et al., 2007; D'Arcy, 2007; Karani & Meier, 2004)

In a recent survey of patients with chronic noncancer pain conducted by Stanford University, 40% of the respondents reported that pain interfered with enjoyment of life and pleasurable activities, plus chronic pain adversely affected their mood (Stanos, Fishbain, & Fishman, 2009). Although 63% of the survey respondents indicated that they had gone to their health care provider, only 31% of the patients reported that they had either complete or a great deal of pain relief with less than 50% reporting a lot of control over their pain. What this tells us about pain that progresses to chronic pain and its management is that the problem is very big and the ability of the health care provider to control the pain is limited.

Among pain specialists, there is currently a movement toward considering chronic pain as a disease in and of itself (Brennan et al., 2007). There is also evidence to support the idea that untreated or undertreated acute pain can lead to more difficult-to-treat chronic pain syndromes. The effect of chronic pain on the patient is so profound that it constitutes a major threat to health and wellness. Unrelieved chronic pain can affect many different physiologic systems. This includes the following:

- Reduced mobility
- Loss of strength
- Disturbed sleep
- Decreased immune function
- Increased susceptibility to disease
- Dependence on medications for pain relief
- Depression and anxiety (Brennan et al., 2007)

Because of the magnitude of the problem of pain and the impact on the individual patient's well-being, health care providers need to become proficient in prescribing and dosing medications for pain of all types. It is distressing for the patients with cancer who finish active treatment and then find that they are in daily chronic pain related to the disease itself or the treatment. The WHO developed an analgesic ladder that can provide guidance to prescribers about their choices of pain medications. Although the ladder was originally developed for cancer pain, it has been adapted for use in many areas of pain management to include acute pain (see Figure 3.1).

WHO Level I Medications—Mild to Moderate Pain

Medications on the first step of the ladder, mild to moderate pain, include acetaminophen, NSAIDs (both selective and nonselective), and adjuvant medications, or coanalgesics. These medications can add to pain relief

World Health Organization
Step Approach to Cancer Pain

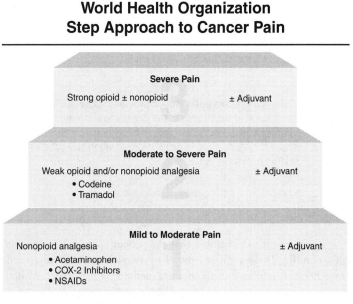

Severe Pain

Strong opioid ± nonopioid   ± Adjuvant

Moderate to Severe Pain

Weak opioid and/or nonopioid analgesia   ± Adjuvant
- Codeine
- Tramadol

Mild to Moderate Pain

Nonopioid analgesia   ± Adjuvant
- Acetaminophen
- COX-2 Inhibitors
- NSAIDs

Figure 3.1 ▦ Analgesic ladder.

although they are not primarily classified as pain medications. These medications include antidepressants, anticonvulsants, muscle relaxants, and topical medications.

WHO Level II Medications—Moderate to Severe Pain

On the middle step of the ladder are medications for moderate to severe pain, such as combination medications with an opioid such as hydrocodone or oxycodone and acetaminophen. In addition, tramadol and tapentadol (a mixed mu agonist and serotonin-norepinephrine reuptake inhibitor [SNRI]) are included in this level for moderate pain. Adjuvant medications may include the drugs listed on Level I.

WHO Level III Medications—Severe Pain

Patients who are reporting severe pain require strong opioid medications for pain relief. Included in this group are: morphine, fentanyl, hydromorphone, and methadone. As with the other steps, adjuvant medication should be continued to this point to help reduce opioid needs and provide additional pain relief (adapted from D'Arcy, 2007).

Clinical Pearl	Although the analgesic ladder provides some guidance with the choice of medications, the overall assessment, source of cancer pain, history and physical with comorbidities, and organ functions need to be considered when selecting a medication for pain.

It is important to remember that the patient's report of pain is more than a number. There are many pieces of the patient puzzle that need to fit together just right to find an effective method for pain relief. Although the severity ratings of the analgesic ladder provide a guide to choosing the correct medication, the practitioner should individualize the medication selection. The efficacy of the medication is an individualized response based on the patient's report of decreased pain or increased functionality (D'Arcy, 2007).

NONOPIOID ANALGESICS FOR PAIN (ACETAMINOPHEN AND NSAIDs)

Although acetaminophen and NSAIDs are considered to be weaker medications for pain, they can provide a good baseline of relief that can help decrease the amount of opioid required to treat pain. Both acetaminophen and NSAID medications are seriously overlooked and underutilized as co-analgesics when higher intensity pain is reported. Multimodal analgesia, which is recommended for complex pain needs and for postoperative pain relief, may consist of any combination of medications that may include the use of acetaminophen and NSAIDs. However, there are some important considerations when adding these medications into a pain regimen. These medications are not benign and have a risk potential that should be considered prior to use in all patients. Patients with cancer may have coagulopathies that make the use of NSAIDs contraindicated. These medications also have maximum dose levels referred to as a *ceiling dose*.

Acetaminophen (APAP, Paracetamol)

Acetaminophen is used the world over to treat pain. Known as paracetamol in Europe, it is associated with the Tylenol brand in the United States and is widely added to many over-the-counter pain relievers such as Excedrin, Midol, and the various Tylenol products. It is available as tablets, gel caps, elixirs, and as pediatric formulations. The newest FDA-approved form is intravenous acetaminophen provided as a infusion called Oramev. This is helpful for patients who cannot take oral medications such as cancer patients with chemotherapy-related nausea/vomiting. Most home medicine chests have some type of acetaminophen compound that the family uses for relief of minor aches and pains. Because it is so popular and easy to obtain, some 24.6 billion doses were sold in 2008 (Pan, 2009).

Acetaminophen is classified as a para-acetaminophen derivative (*Nursing 2010 Drug Handbook*, 2009) and it has a similar pain relief profile to aspirin without the potential to damage the gastric mucosa (APS, 2008). Pain relief is superior to placebo, but slightly less than NSAIDs (APS, 2008). The action of the medication is thought to be inhibition of prostaglandins and other pain-producing substances (*Nursing 2010 Drug Handbook*, 2009). It is entirely metabolized in the liver and can cause blood pressure elevations (Buvenendran & Lipman, 2010).

Advantages of acetaminophen over NSAIDs include the following:

- Fewer gastrointestinal (GI) adverse effects
- Fewer GI complications
- Decreased risk of renal impairment

In general, acetaminophen is safe and effective when used according to the directions and labeling on over-the-counter preparations and any prescription-strength medication information. There are serious concerns today about acetaminophen overdose, both intentional and unintentional. The Food and Drug Administration (FDA) has been holding hearings and is considering reducing the recommendations for the daily total dose from 4,000 mg per day to a lower limit. They are also considering making the 500 mg strength tablets available only with prescription and limiting the number of doses in each package (Alazraki, 2009).

The concerns underlying these fears are related to some very serious statistics about the increase in liver disease related to acetaminophen use. There is a clear connection to acetaminophen overuse to liver disease and failure. Total acetaminophen doses should not exceed 4,000 mg per day, including any combination medication being taken by the patient that may include acetaminophen (Trescot et al., 2008). Even at this dose, there is an associated risk of hepatotoxicity (APS, 2008).

From 1998 to 2003, acetaminophen was the leading cause of acute liver failure in the United States (*Daily Finance*, 2009). Between 1990 and 1998, there were 56,000 emergency department visits, 26,000 hospitalizations, and 458 deaths reportedly connected to acetaminophen overdoses (Alazraki, 2009). Many of these overdoses were unintentional and caused by a knowledge deficit about the "hidden" acetaminophen found in combination medications. Some of the most common prescription strength combinations with acetaminophen include the following:

- Tylenol #3
- Vicodin
- Percocet
- Ultracet

Other, over-the-counter medications that can contain hidden acetaminophen include the following:

- Alka-Seltzer Plus
- Cough syrups such as NyQuil/DayQuil cold and flu relief
- Over-the-counter pain relievers such as Pamprin and Midol maximum-strength menstrual formula

Care should be taken with older patients, patients with impaired liver function, and any patient who uses alcohol regularly (AGS, 2009; APS, 2008). In these cases, acetaminophen doses should not exceed 2,000 mg/day or should not be used at all (AGS, 2009). The risk of liver failure is very real. It is imperative for all patients who are taking acetaminophen to read and understand the medication administration guidelines and recommendations. Exceeding daily recommended doses of acetaminophen can have deadly consequences.

One little-known effect is the effect of acetaminophen on the anticoagulant warfarin. Careful monitoring of anticoagulation should take place when a patient is taking both acetaminophen and warfarin since acetaminophen is an underrecognized cause of excessive anticoagulation when both medications are being used concomitantly (APS, 2008).

Aspirin (ASA)

Aspirin is one of the oldest pain relievers known to man. It is classified as a salicylate (*Nursing 2010 Drug Handbook*, 2009). Before the beginning of modern medicine, salicylate-rich willow bark was used as one of the earliest forms of pain relief. Most Americans use aspirin for minor aches and pains, and because of its action on platelet activity, it has been promoted for early in-the-field treatment for patients who are experiencing a heart attack. It was traditionally used for pain relief of osteoarthritis, rheumatoid arthritis, and for other inflammatory conditions but has been replaced by NSAIDs (APS, 2008; *Nursing 2010 Drug Handbook*, 2009).

Aspirin is available in many different doses but the most common dose is 500 to 1,000 mg every 4 or 6 hours, with a maximum dose of 4,000 mg per day (APS, 2009). It is available as buffered, sustained-release, and chewable formulations.

Despite its easy availability and widespread use, there are some serious adverse events connected with regular aspirin use. These include the following:

- GI distress
- GI ulceration and bleeding
- Prolonged bleeding times
- Reye's syndrome
- Aspirin hypersensitivity
- Nephrotoxicity

These adverse reactions to aspirin are quite serious and in some cases can be life-threatening. GI ulceration and bleeding can cause death. Aspirin is not recommended for children under the age of 12 due to the potential for Reye's syndrome, which can develop when a child has a viral illness and aspirin is given for pain relief (APS, 2008). Aspirin hypersensitivity reactions can be minor or very severe. A minor reaction presents as a respiratory reaction with rhinitis, asthma, or nasal polyps. A smaller group of patients can get more serious reactions that include the following:

- Urticaria
- Wheals
- Angioneurotic edema
- Hypotension
- Shock and syncope (APS, 2008)

Although aspirin seems like a very simple analgesic, care should be taken with use. Aspirin is not typically used for analgesia in the cancer setting.

Nonsteroidal Anti-Inflammatory Drugs (NSAIDs)

NSAIDs of all types are commonly used for pain that is mild to moderate in intensity. They can be used for pain that is from an inflammatory source, as the primary analgesic for mild pain, or as coanalgesics. They are available in many different combinations in both prescription strength and over-the-counter preparations. One of the newest ways to use NSAIDs is the topical formulations that can be used at the site of the pain. Oral NSAIDs do have a maximum dose that limits escalation beyond the dose ceiling.

NSAIDs have two different types of actions, selective and nonselective:
1. *Nonselective NSAIDs* affect all types of prostaglandins found in the stomach, kidneys, heart, and other organs of the body.
2. *Selective NSAIDs* (COX-2) protect the prostaglandins that coat the stomach lining but do affect the other types of prostaglandins found elsewhere in the body.

The most common use of NSAIDs is to treat pain that is caused by inflammation such as arthritis or common musculoskeletal injuries (APS, 2008; D'Arcy, 2007). In the cancer setting, they are useful for treating pain from bone metastasis.

NSAIDs have long been a standard for pain relief in older patients. Relatively inexpensive they are easily accessible at most supermarkets or drug stores. They are available as over-the-counter formulations and in prescription strength, as well.

As mentioned, there are two basic classes of NSAIDs, nonselective and selective. The nonselective NSAIDs such as ibuprofen (Motrin, Advil), naproxen (Naprosyn), and ketoprofen (Orudis) affect production of the prostaglandins that coat and protect the lining of the stomach and those that are found in other organs of the body such as the kidneys and heart. Another class of NSAIDs is COX-2 selective medications. The only COX-2 medication available at this time is celecoxib (Celebrex), which spares the stomach prostaglandins and does not affect platelet aggregation, so blood clotting is not affected. Mechanisms for both types of NSAIDs can be found at www/fda/gov.

Newer research from the FDA indicates that all NSAIDs, not only the COX-2 selective medications such as Celebrex, have the potential for increased cardiovascular risk, renovascular risk, stroke, and myocardial infarction (MI; Bennet et al., 2005; D'Arcy, 2007). GI bleeding with NSAIDs continues to be a risk; for those patients who are taking aspirin as a cardiac prophylaxis, the risk increases several-fold with concomitant NSAID and aspirin use (D'Arcy, 2007).

Gastrointestinal Risks With NSAIDs

One of the major risks with nonselective NSAIDs is gastric ulceration. Gastric ulcers develop within a week in about 30% of patients started on nonselective NSAIDs (Wallace & Staats, 2005). Most patients with these ulcers are asymptomatic and only seek medical care when the bleeding becomes obvious with tarry stools or hematemesis.

In an effort to lessen the risk of GI bleeding, some practitioners use a proton pump inhibitor (PPI) such as omeprazole (Prilosec), which only provides protection for the upper GI system. Patient adherence to taking a PPI for protection is a concern. A recent study found the nonadherence rate for use of PPIs with NSAIDs was 60.8% (Sturkenboom et al., 2003).

Since many older patients are also using an aspirin a day for cardio-protective effect, adding the incidence of ulcer formation with aspirin to the NSAID risk only increases the potential for GI bleeding. Higher doses and older age are associated with a higher incidence of GI side effects (Perez-Gutthan, Garcia Rodriguez, & Raiford, 1997). Additionally, chronic alcohol use with NSAIDs increases the risk for GI bleeding and ulceration. Whether GI issues are a consideration depends largely on the individual patient's history and medical situation.

Cardiovascular Risks With NSAIDs

There are certain patient groups who are a higher risk for cardiovascular events and for whom NSAIDs are not recommended, including those patients who have had recent heart bypass surgery, patients with heart disease, and patients who have had transient ischemic attacks (TIAs) or strokes. In a sample of chronic NSAID users (882) and intermittent users (7,286) in hypertensive patients with coronary artery disease, NSAID use was associated with an increased risk of adverse events such as cardiovascular mortality (Bavry et al., 2011). For patients with multiple cardiac risk factors in a study of 23,728 patients, no association was found between NSAID use and MI, cardiovascular death, or stroke but there was an increased risk profile for patients with stable atherothrombosis (Barthelemy et al., 2011). For these at-risk patients, an alternate form of analgesic is recommended.

When trying to determine which NSAID to offer a patient, consider that there are indications that naproxen interferes with the inhibitory effect of aspirin (Capone et al., 2005) and the same effect may be seen with concomitant use of ibuprofen, acetaminophen, and diclofenac (Catella-Lawson et al., 2001). Overall, for patients taking aspirin for cardiac prophylaxis, there is an increased risk for GI events, and using NSAIDs may decrease the effectiveness of the aspirin.

In general, the recommendations for using NSAIDs for pain relief indicate that the medication should be used at the lowest dose for the shortest period of time (Bennet et al., 2005). That being the case, older patients should be aware that continuing to take NSAIDs long term for arthritis or other chronic conditions could cause serious, life-threatening effects. NSAIDs are generally contraindicated when a patient is taking anticoagulants or steroids.

New Developments With NSAIDs

Newer forms of NSAIDs have come to market recently. These types of NSAIDs are called *targeted topical medications* and are applied directly at the site of pain. Some of the medications are applied as liquids, while others have been made into patches. The newest formulation is a liquid made of diclofenac sodium, a topical solution called Pennsaid. The liquid can be applied directly to the knees for osteoarthritis patients. Diclofenac also comes as a 1% gel formulation that is rapidly absorbed and is recommended for use on joints with osteoarthritis. The patient will need to apply the solution or gel to the affected joint four times per day.

A patch containing diclofenac epolamine 1% (Flector) has been used successfully for minor orthopedic injuries such as strains and sprains. The patch should be applied directly to the site of the injury. Despite the topical application, each medication has recommendations to use the smallest dose possible for the shortest period of time and gastrointestinal effects, though rare, cannot be excluded.

In a Cochrane Review with 47 studies comparing all types of targeted topical NSAID preparations, topical diclofenac, ibuprofen, ketoprofen, and piroxicam all had efficacy but indomethacin and benzydamine had no better results than placebo (Massey, Derry, Moore, & McQuay, 2010). The number needed to treat to achieve 50% pain relief was 4.5 for 6 to 14 days. The conclusions of the Cochrane authors related to the use of topical NSAIDs was that they could provide a good level of pain relief without systemic adverse effects associated with oral NSAID use in the treatment of acute musculoskeletal conditions (Massey et al., 2010).

Case Study

Sabrina T. is a 65-year-old breast cancer survivor who has osteoarthritis in her knees and who has recently been complaining about new back pain. Her back pain started 2 weeks ago after she worked in her garden pulling weeds, although she notices it still is present at night and she cannot get comfortable in her bed. She has been suffering from lost sleep and feels fatigued. She has lost some weight lately but attributes it to her lack of appetite. She tried to treat the pain at home with acetaminophen and some Advil but she is still having difficulty moving around her house. The pain is constant and achy and she rates it at 6/10. She comes into your office asking for help with her pain. How will you help Sabrina with her pain?

Questions to Consider

1. Is the back pain inflammatory or musculoskeletal? Could it be a recurrence of cancer?
2. Sabrina's knee pain is inflammatory. What medications could you recommend for her if she has a history of GERD and hypertension?
3. Would you consider any of the new targeted medications such as a Flector patch for the back pain?
4. Would acetaminophen or aspirin be good choices for the back pain Sabrina is experiencing?
5. How will you educate Sabrina about taking over-the-counter medications considering her GERD and hypertension?

REFERENCES

Alazraki, M. (2009). *The risk of over the counter meds: How many Tylenols have you taken today?* Retrieved from http://www.dailyfininace.com/2009/06/30

American Geriatrics Society (AGS). (2002, 2009). *Persistent pain in the older patient.* New York, NY: Author.

American Pain Society (APS). (2008). *Principles of analgesic use in the treatment of acute pain and cancer pain.* Glenview, IL: Author.

Barthelemy, O., Limbourg, T., Collet, J., Beygui, F., Silvain, J., Bellemain-Appaix, A., . . . Montalescot, G. (2011). Impact of non-steroidal anti-inflammatory drugs (NSAIDs) on cardiovascular outcomes in patients with stable atherothrombosis or multiple risk factors. *International Journal of Cardiology.* June 28 [ePub ahead of print].

Bavry, A., Khlaiq, A., Gong, Y., Handberg, E., Cooper-DeHoff, R., & Pepine, C. (2011). Harmful effects of NSAIDs among patients with hypertension and coronary artery disease. *The American Journal of Medicine, 124*, 614–620.

Bennet, J. S., Daugherty, A., Herrington, D., Greenland P., Roberts, H., & Taubert K. (2005). The use of non-steroidal anti-inflammatory drugs (NSAIDs): A science advisory from the American Heart Association. *Circulation, 111*(13), 1713–1716.

Brennan, F., Carr, D., & Cousins, M. (2007). Pain management: A fundamental human right. *Anesthesia & Analgesia, 105*(10), 205–221.

Buvanendran, A., & Lipman, A. (2010). Nonsteroidal anti-inflammatory drugs and acetaminophen. In *Bonica's management of pain* (4th ed.). Philadelphia, PA: Lippincott, Williams and Wilkins.

Capone, M., Sciulli, M., Tacconelli, S., Grana, M., Ricotti, M., Randa, G., . . . Patrignani, P. (2005). Pharmacodynamic interactions of naproxen with low-dose aspirin in healthy subjects. *Journal of the College of Cardiology, 45*(8), 1295–1301.

Catella-Lawson, F., Reilly, M., Kapoor, S., Cucchiara, A., Demarco, S., Tournier, B., . . . FitzGerald, G. (2001). Cyclooxygenase inhibitors and the antiplatelet effects of aspirin. *New England Journal of Medicine, 345*(25), 1809–1817.

Chou, R., Qaseem, A., Snow, V., Casey, D., Cross, J. T., Jr., Shekelle, P., Owens, D. K.; Clinical Efficacy Assessment Subcommittee of the American College of Physicians; American College of Physicians; American Pain Society Low Back Pain Guidelines Panel. (2007). Diagnosis and treatment of low back pain: A joint clinical practice guideline from the American College of Physicians and the American Pain Society. *Annals of Internal Medicine, 147*(7), 478–491.

Chou, R., Fanciullo, G., Fine, P., Adler, J., Ballantyne, J., Davies, P., . . . Miaskowski, C. (2009). Opioid treatment guidelines: Clinical guidelines for the use of chronic opioid therapy in chronic noncancer pain. *The Journal of Pain, 10*(2), 113–130.

Daily Finance. (2009). *Acetaminophen & liver failure.* Retrieved January 31, 2012, from www.Dailyfinance.com

D'Arcy, Y. (2007). *Pain management: Evidence based tools and techniques for nursing professionals.* Marblehead, MA: Hc Pro.

D'Arcy, Y. (2009). Be in the know about pain management. *The Nurse Practitioner, 34*(4), 43–47.

Institute for Clinical Systems Improvement (ICSI). (2008). *Assessment and management of chronic pain.* Bloomington, MN: Author. Retrieved from www.guideline.gov

Karani, R., & Meier, D. (2004). Systematic pharmacologic postoperative pain management in the geriatric orthopedic patient. *Clinical Orthopedics and Related Research, 425,* 26–34.

Massey, T., Derry, S., Moore, R. A., & McQuay, H. (2010). Topical NSAIDs for acute pain in adults. *Cochrane Database of Systematic Reviews, 6.* doi:10.1002/14651858.CD007 402.pub.2

Nursing 2010 Drug Handbook. (2009). Philadelphia, PA: Wolters Kluwer/Lippincott Williams and Wilkins.

Pan, G. J. (2009). *Acetaminophen: Background and overview.* Retrieved January 12, 2012, from www.fda.gov

Perez-Gutthan, S., Garcia Rodriguez, L., & Raiford, D. (1997). Individual nonsteroidal and anti-inflammatory drugs and other risk factors for upper gastrointestinal bleeding and perforation. *Epidemiology, 8,* 18–24.

Stanos, S., Fishbain, D., & Fishman, S. (2009). Pain management with opioid analgesics: Balancing risk and benefit. *Physical Medicine & Rehabilitation, 88*(3, Suppl. 2), S69–S99.

Sturkenboom, M., Burke, T., Tangelder, M., Dieleman, J., Walton, S., & Goldstein, J. (2003). Adherence to proton pump inhibitors or H2-receptor antagonists during the use of non-steroidal anti-inflammatory drugs. *Alimentary Pharmacology and Therapeutics, 18*(11–12), 1137–1147.

Thapa, D., Rastogi, V., Ahuja, V. (2011). Cancer pain management—current status. *Journal of Anesthesiology and Clinical Pharmacology, 27*(2), 162–168.

Trescot, A., Helm, S., Hansen, H., Benyamin, R., Glaser, S., Adlaka, R., . . . Manchikanti, L. (2008). Opioids in the management of chronic non-cancer pain: An update of the American Society of Interventional Pain Physicians (ASIPP) guidelines. *Pain Physician, 11*(Suppl. 2), S5–S62.

Wallace, M., & Staats, P. (2005). *Pain medicine & management.* New York, NY: McGraw-Hill.

World Health Organization (WHO). (1996). *Cancer pain relief* (2nd ed.). Geneva, Switzerland: Author.

4

Opioid Medications for Cancer Pain

Yvonne D'Arcy

OVERVIEW

Opioids have long been considered the mainstay for treating cancer pain (American Pain Society [APS], 2005). In the early days, opioids were given as intramuscular injections but today there is a wide variety of routes for delivering the medications including oral, nasal, sublingual, intravenous, subcutaneous, intrathecal, and rectal. Additionally, there are many more formulations of opioids to use for analgesia than morphine, which was considered the best medication to use for analgesia. This chapter will provide information on a wide variety of opioids that can be used to treat pain in patients with cancer.

The term *opiate* denotes a class of medications that are derived from the latex sap of *Papaver somniferum*, the opium poppy. The term *opioid* refers to synthetic or semisynthetic analogs to these natural substances. Opium has a two-sided history: one as a potent analgesic and the other as a recreational drug. For example, it was smoked for its euphoric effect in the opium dens of China. Early herbalists recognized the pain-relieving potential of opium and used it to treat many different types of pain in their patients.

Morphine was first isolated in 1895 in Germany, where the medication was thought to be useful as a cure for opium addiction (Fine & Portenoy, 2007). The development of the hypodermic syringe in the mid-19th century gave medical practitioners another route for delivering opioid medications, which they injected directly into the site of the pain.

By the 20th century, opioid use was not only seen as beneficial for treating pain, it had become problematic as opioid abuse increased. The United States passed the first two acts for controlling the use of these substances, The Pure Food and Drug Act (1906) and the Harrison Narcotics Act (1914). These were the first two attempts at controlling the use and prescribing of opioid substances. As late as 1970, the federal Controlled Substances Act provided standards for monitoring, manufacturing, prescribing, and dispensing of opioids and created the five-level division of controlled substances that we use today. Today, the FDA has issued a mandate that all long-acting opioids need to have a Risk Evaluation and Mitigation Strategy (REMS) for prescribers who write prescriptions for long-acting opioids.

Opioids are the best medications we have to control cancer pain. They come in a variety of formulations and they have a good profile for adverse side effects when compared to other medication types.

Natural derivatives of the opium include morphine, codeine, and heroin. Synthetic analogs such as fentanyl (Sublimaze) and meperidine (Demerol) were developed much later as attempts to perfect compounds for better pain relief. Following are characteristics that these compounds all have in common:

■ They activate by binding sites in the body called *mu receptors* to produce analgesia. Mu receptors are found in many places in the body, including the brain and spinal column neurons.
■ Their main action is analgesia.
■ Side effects such as sedation, constipation, and nausea are common with all members of the drug class.
■ They all have the potential for addiction.

The Various Forms of Opioids

Some of the opioids are used in their natural form such as morphine and heroin. Other natural opium alkaloids include codeine, noscapine, and thebaine (www.opiates.com). These alkaloids can be further reduced into more common analgesic compounds. The alkaloid thebaine is used to produce semisynthetic opioid morphine analogues such as oxycodone (Percocet, Percodan), hydromorphone (Dilaudid), and hydrocodone (Vicodin/Lortab). Other classes of morphine analogues include the 4-diphenylpiperidines such as meperidine (Demerol), and diphenylpropylamines such as methadone (Dolophine) (www.opiates.com). Each of these compounds was developed to either increase analgesic effect or reduce the potential for addiction.

Although all of the opioid substances can be classified as analgesics, they vary in potency. To be classified as a morphine, the drug must have a piperidine ring in the chemical configuration or a greater part of the ring must be chemically present (www.opiates.com).

As mentioned, the main binding sites for opioids are receptor sites called mu receptors (Holden, Jeong, & Forrest, 2005). These receptors are found in the following locations:
- Brain cortex
- Thalamus
- Periaqueductal gray matter
- Spinal cord—substantia gelatinosa (Fine & Portenoy, 2007)

Secondary binding sites include the *kappa* and *delta* sites. *Kappa* sites are found in the brain (hypothalamus), periaqueductal gray matter, claustrum, and spinal cord (substantia gelatinosa) (Fine & Portenoy, 2007). The *delta* receptors are located in the pontine nucleus, amygdala, olfactory bulbs, and the deep cortex of the brain (Fine & Portenoy, 2007). Recently, an opioid receptor-like site was discovered and called *opioid receptor-like 1 (ORL1)*. The activity at this site is thought to be related to central modulation of pain but does not appear to have an effect on respiratory depression (Fine & Portenoy, 2007).

When an opioid is introduced into a patient's body, it looks for the binding site that conforms to a specific protein pattern that will allow the opioid to bind to the receptor site and create an agonist action, analgesia. At one time, the binding action for opioids was believed to be a simple lock-and-key effect—e.g., inject the medication, find the receptor binding site, and bind, thus creating analgesia. Today, we know that the process is much more specific and more sophisticated than a simple lock-and-key effect.

Once the opioid molecule approaches the cell, it looks for a way to bind. On the exterior of each cell are ligands, or cellular channel mechanisms connecting the exterior of the cell with the interior that convey the opioid molecule into the cell. The ligands are affiliated with the exterior receptor sites and can contain a variety of G-proteins. These G-proteins couple with the opioid molecule and mediate the action of the receptor (Fine & Portenoy, 2007). "One opioid receptor can regulate several G proteins, and multiple receptors can activate a single G protein" (Fine & Portenoy, 2007, p. 31). As efforts progress to better identify the process, greater than 40 variations in binding site composition have been identified (Pasternak, 2005). These differences explain some of the variation in patient response to opioid medications.

The body also has natural pain-facilitating and pain-inhibiting substances. These include the following:
- Facilitating: Substance P, bradykinin, and glutamate
- Inhibiting: Serotonin (central), opioids (natural or synthetic), norepinephrine, GABA (D'Arcy, 2007)

When these substances are activated or blocked, pain can be relieved or increased. These more complex mechanisms are difficult to clarify and trying to link them to a specific mechanism of analgesia and opioid effect can be misguided.

Formulations of Opioid Medications

Opioid medications are very versatile in that they can be given as a standalone medication such as oxycodone, or combined with another type of nonopioid medication such as an NSAID; for example, oxycodone combined with ibuprofen (Combunox), or oxycodone combined with acetaminophen (Percocet). Opioids can be formulated as elixirs (such as morphine [Roxanol]), or a suppository form such as hydromorphone (Dilaudid) suppositories. Since the elixir form can be very bitter, adding a flavoring available at most pharmacies can help the patient tolerate the taste of the medication.

The duration of the oral short-acting preparations are usually listed as 4 to 6 hours but each patient has an individual response and ability to metabolize medications. For example, the duration of action of short-acting morphine may be 3 to 7 hours (Quill et al., 2010).

Most of the combination medications are considered as short acting and the combination of another dose-limited medication such as acetaminophen limits the amount of medication that can be taken in a 24-hour period. Those that are combined with acetaminophen are limited to the recommended dose for daily acetaminophen use to 4,000 mg/d maximum (APS, 2008; D'Arcy, 2007).

Many opioids are created in a long-acting (LA), sustained-release (SR), and extended-release (ER) formulation that can be dosed every 12 to 24 hours. Examples include oxycodone SR (Oxycontin), oxymorphone ER (Opana ER), and morphine (Kadian, Avinza). These extended-release medications are particularly helpful for patients when cancer pain is present throughout the day. They are not designed to be used in patients who are opioid naïve, but for those who have been taking the short-acting medications regularly to control their pain.

Some long-acting opioid medications such as the fentanyl (Duragesic) patch have specific short-acting medication requirements before they can be started. For example, before initiating the fentanyl 25 mcg/hr patch, the patient must have been using a total daily dose of at least 60 mg morphine, or 30 mg oxycodone, or 8 mg hydromorphone by mouth per day for 2 weeks prior to patch application (www.duragesic.com). Every patient who uses an extended-release opioid medication for cancer pain should have a short-acting medication available to take for worsening pain. Referred to as *breakthrough pain*, this is an increased intensity of pain that occurs spontaneously, with increased activity, or from end-of-dose failure of the long-acting agent (APS, 2008).

Opioid naïve refers to patients who are not chronically taking opioid medications on a daily basis.

Opioid tolerant refers to patients who take opioid medication regularly for 1 week or longer, in these doses or higher (FDA, 2011; NCCN, 2011; Stokowski, 2010; see Chapter 14 for further information):

- 60 mg/d of oral morphine
- 25 mg/hr of transdermal fentanyl
- 30 mg/d of oral oxycodone
- 8 mg/d of oral hydromorphone
- 25 mg/d of oral oxymorphone
- An equianalgesic dose of any other opioid

No matter what type or form of opioid medication is being considered for use, the health care prescriber should be aware of the risks and benefits of each medication and weigh the options carefully. A full history and physical should be performed. A detailed risk assessment for possible opioid misuse should be done, even in the setting of cancer pain management. Information on opioid prescribing safety will be provided in a later chapter of this book.

Short-Acting Medications

Short-acting pain medications last for several hours at the recommended doses. For most patients with cancer, a short-acting medication is appropriate when pain is less severe and does not last throughout the day or night. Some patients with cancer do not have high levels of pain and short-acting opioids may be all that is needed to control the pain. Patients with more severe pain intensities and consistent daily pain require a more complex medication regimen to control their pain effectively.

Most short-acting medications are oral, as either pills or elixirs. Some patients with cancer may have difficulty swallowing pills but can tolerate an elixir, either swallowed or sublingual. Intramuscular (IM) administration of opioids is no longer recommended because the IM route causes irregular absorption and tissue sclerosis. Therefore, most national guidelines have removed the IM route from their recommendations (APS, 2008; D'Arcy, 2007).

Cancer pain may be continuous, and often requires ongoing opioid administration to control pain. For these patients, a careful assessment of pain patterns and intensities throughout the day will help determine when and how the opioid medication will be prescribed. For some, movement can be very painful, while others cannot tolerate standing or lying in a bed. Pain medication should be chosen to have the full dose effect at these particularly painful times. If the pain is only episodic or present at certain times of day, a short-acting medication may provide all the pain relief that is needed. However, patients with continuous cancer pain will benefit from adding an extended-release medication.

Most short-acting opioid medications are designed for moderate to severe pain intensities. Onset of action is usually 10 to 60 minutes with a short duration of action, 2 to 6 hours (Katz, McCarberg, & Reisner, 2007).

Overall advantages to short-acting medications include a synergistic effect if combined with acetaminophen or ibuprofen to improve pain relief and provide a better outcome. However, if the patient has liver impairment from his or her disease, the use of acetaminophen products is discouraged.

Medications

Morphine *(MSIR [immediate-release morphine], Roxanol [elixir])*

Morphine is the gold standard for pain relief. It is the standard for equianalgesic conversions and has a long history of use in many different forms for pain control. It is available in many different forms—pills, elixir, intravenous, and suppository. It is indicated for severe pain. The biggest drawback to morphine is the side effect profile: Constipation, nausea/vomiting, delirium, and hallucinations are some of the most commonly reported adverse effects. For patients with cancer pain, morphine is widely used but other medications such as Dilaudid can be substituted for morphine if side effects are problematic.

Oxycodone-Containing Medications *(Oxycodone, Percocet, Roxicet, Percodan, Oxifast)*

Medications with oxycodone are designed for treating moderate pain. They are commonly used for patients with higher pain intensities and for patients with chronic pain. Percocet is a combination medication with 5 mg of oxycodone and 325 mg of acetaminophen. (Percodan is oxycodone combined with aspirin. Aspirin is generally avoided in patients in active cancer treatment.) If the patient requires a higher dose of medication for pain control, combining an oxycodone 5 mg tablet with a combined form such as Roxicet (5 mg oxycodone/325 mg acetaminophen) will provide additional pain relief but still maintain the acetaminophen dose at 325 mg. To help patients tolerate the medication without nausea, giving the medication with milk or after meals is recommended (*Nursing 2010 Drug Handbook*, 2009).

Oxymorphone-Containing Medications (Opana)

Opana is a medication designed to treat moderate to severe pain. The short-acting medication has a longer half-life (4-6 hours) than other medications of the same class, resulting in a decreased need for breakthrough medications (Adams & Abdieh, 2004; Adams, Pienazek, Gammatoni, & Abdieh, 2005). The medication should be taken 1 hour before or 2 hours after a meal (*Nursing 2010 Drug Handbook*, 2009).

Hydromorphone (Dilaudid)

Dilaudid is an extremely potent analgesic and it is designed for use with severe pain. In the oral form, it comes in 2 mg, 4 mg, and 8 mg tablets. It also comes in a suppository form. In the IV form, 0.2 mg of Dilaudid is equal to 1 mg of IV morphine. Because of the strength of this medication, it is possible to give small amounts, get good pain relief, and potentially have fewer side effects. It is not available in combination form with acetaminophen; therefore, doses can be titrated as needed to achieve adequate pain relief.

Fentanyl (Sublimaze [intravenous]; Duragesic [transdermal]; Onsolis [transmucosal]; Actiq & Fentora [buccal]; Lasanda [nasal])

There is no oral formulation for fentanyl. The route of administration is either buccal (Actiq, Fentora), transmucosal (Onsolis), nasal (Lasanda), or intravenous. This is not true. Nurses give IV push and we use PCA all the time. When used buccally for breakthrough pain in opioid-tolerant patients, the transmucosal medications can be rubbed across the buccal membrane and absorbed directly into the circulation. The fast absorption makes this medication a risk for oversedation so that the indication is only for breakthrough pain in opioid-tolerant cancer patients who take opioid medications on a daily basis.

If the entire dose of an Actiq oralet is not used, it should be dissolved under hot running water, or temporarily placed in a childproof container until properly disposed. Lasanda should be stored in the locked container provided with the medication. The transmucosal, buccal and nasal medications are not meant to be used for acute or postoperative pain (*Nursing 2010 Drug Handbook*, 2009) or in opioid-naïve patients, since serious oversedation can occur (Fine & Portenoy, 2007).

Hydrocodone-Containing Medications *(Vicodin, Lortab, Norco, Lortab elixir)*

Hydrocodone-containing medications are designed to be used for moderate pain. They usually contain 5 to 10 mg of hydrocodone with 325 mg or 500 mg of acetaminophen. Many patients tolerate the medication very well for intermittent pain or for breakthrough pain. It has an elixir form that is very effective and can be used with patients who have difficulty swallowing pills or who have enteral feeding tubes.

Other Drugs
Tramadol *(Ultram, Ultracet);* Tapentadol *(Nucynta)*

Not typically used in cancer pain settings, tramadol and tapentadol are a unique class of drug with weak (tramadol) or moderate (tapentadol) mu agonist (opioid-like) properties and tricyclic antidepressant-type structure (D'Arcy, 2007). It is designed for use with moderate pain. Doses should be reduced for patients with increased creatinine levels, cirrhosis, and in older patients. It may increase the risk for seizures and serotonin syndrome (*Nursing 2010 Drug Handbook*, 2009). Patients should be instructed to taper off the medication gradually when discontinuing the medication. It should not be stopped suddenly (*Nursing 2010 Drug Handbook*, 2009). Because of the chemical structure with similarities to tricyclic antidepressants, tramadol and tapentadol use is not recommended in patients receiving active chemotherapy.

Extended-Release Medications—Pain Relief for Consistent Pain and Around-the-Clock Pain Relief

For patients with cancer pain, extended-release medication can give a consistent blood level of medication that can provide a steady comfort level. This may increase functionality and improve quality of life, enhance sleep, and let the patient participate in meaningful daily activities. Extended-release medications have a slower onset of action of 30 to 90 minutes with a relatively long duration of action of up to 72 hours (Katz et al., 2007).

When a patient has pain that lasts throughout the day, is taking short-acting medications regularly, and has reached the maximum dose limitations of the nonopioid medication, the prescriber should consider switching the patient to an extended-release or long-acting medication. Some of the short-acting medications have an extended-release (ER) formulation such as Opana ER, Ultram ER, OxyContin, Kadian, Avinza, and MS Contin. Most are pure mu agonist medications such as morphine with an ER action that allows the medication to dissolve slowly in the gastrointestinal tract. Some ER medications are encapsulated into beads that allow gastric secretions to enter the bead and force the medication out. Other ER formulations have a coating around an ER plasticized compound that keeps the medication from dissolving too quickly. When ER medication is being started, the patient should be instructed on the important aspects of the medications, which include the following:

- ER medications of all types should never be broken, chewed, or degraded in any way to enhance the absorption of the medications. To do so runs the risk of all the medication being given at one time and there is a high risk for potentially fatal oversedation.
- ER medications should not be taken with alcohol. To do so modifies the ER mechanism and allows for a faster absorption of medications, which can cause potentially fatal oversedation.
- ER medications are not meant to be injected.
- ER medication should not be crushed and inserted into enteral feeding tubes.
- Enteral administration of the long-acting morphine (Kadian ER) is an option when a 16 Fr or larger gastrostomy tube is present. Kadian ER capsules are filled with pellets. The capsules are opened and mixed into 10 mL of water. Per the Kadian package insert, this is poured into the gastrostomy tube through a funnel, followed by a 10 mL flush of water. Both Kadian ER and Avinza ER pellets may also be sprinkled onto applesauce if the patient can swallow some food. These brand-name formulations are more expensive.
- ER medications are meant to be used on a scheduled basis, not an "as-needed" basis (APS, 2008).
- If the patient experiences end-of-dose failure several hours before the next dose of medication is due, the interval should be shortened (e.g., every 8 hours instead of every 12 hours) or the dose should be increased (APS, 2008).

When converting a patient from short-acting medications, the rule of thumb is as follows:

- If the medication is the same (oxycodone short acting and oxycodone SR), the equivalent doses of the medication can be prescribed. For example, if the patient is taking 5 mg oxycodone tablet, 4 tablets per day, the patient can be safely started on 10 mg oxycodone SR (OxyContin) twice a day.
- If the medication is a different drug—for example, oxycodone short acting to morphine CR (MS Contin)—the daily dose should be calculated using

the equianalgesic conversion table (see Tables 4.1 and 4.2) and reduced, usually by 30%. To ensure that adequate pain relief is maintained, additional doses of breakthrough medication should be prescribed, about 5% to 15% of the total daily dose to be taken every 2 hours as needed (APS, 2008).

Table 4.1 ◼ *Basic Intravenous Conversions*

Morphine	1 mg IV
Hydromorphone	0.2 mg IV
Fentanyl	10 mcg IV

Table 4.2 ◼ *Basic Oral and Transdermal Conversions*

Morphine	30 mg oral
Oxycodone	20 mg oral
Hydromorphone	7.5 mg
Hydrocodone	30 mg
Fentanyl patch TD	12 mcg/hr transdermal

Because these ER medications are potent, the use of tamper-resistant formulas is highly recommended. Some medication now will dissolve into a gumlike substance when there is an attempt to crush the medication for abuse. This does not allow the opioid component to be used. Other formulas contain a mu antagonist medication such as naltrexone that will activate and neutralize the opioid effect of the medication when tampering is attempted.

Methadone (Dolophine, Methadose)

Methadone is considered to be a long-acting medication because it has an extended half-life of 15 to 60 hours (APS, 2008). However, pain relief for the oral form is less extended at 6 to 8 hours (*Nursing 2010 Drug Handbook*, 2009). Therein is the danger. If the half-life is long and the pain relief is shorter, dosing must be done carefully to avoid oversedating the patient, which may become apparent only a day or two after the doses are given. Dose escalation should be done no more often than every 5 to 7 days (APS, 2008).

Methadone can be prescribed legally by physicians, nurse practitioners, and physician assistants in primary care and oncology for pain relief. It is also used for opioid substitution therapy (e.g., methadone maintenance) to control addiction in heroin and other opioid addicts. A special license is required to prescribe methadone for addiction management. The addiction program has no connection to prescribing methadone for pain management. However, since there is such a risk with this medication, the current recommendation of the American Pain Society is that only pain management practitioners or those skilled and knowledgeable about the use of methadone prescribe the drug (Chou et al., 2009; D'Arcy, 2009a).

An additional risk factor for methadone is the potential for QTc interval prolongation. This puts the patient at risk of the potential deadly ventricular arrhythmia of *torsades de pointes* (APS, 2008). Health care providers are advised to obtain a baseline ECG for patients who are receiving methadone with periodic monitoring of ECG. At a QTc prolongation of greater than 450, consideration should be given to reducing the dose of methadone or switching to another drug (APS, 2008). Combinations of drugs that cause risk of QTc prolongation require more careful monitoring.

Fentanyl Transdermal Patch *(Duragesic)*

Fentanyl patches can provide a high level of pain relief and are used for a variety of chronic pain conditions. It is the only transdermal (TD) opioid application that is available for use. The fentanyl TD (Duragesic) patch is a delivery system that contains a specified dose of fentanyl in a gel formulation. It is designed for use with opioid-tolerant patients and should never be used for acute pain or with opioid-naïve patients.

The fentanyl TD patch should be applied to clean, intact, nonhairy skin. It delivers the specified amount of medication for 72 hours, such as 25 mcg/hr (D'Arcy, 2007). The systemic medication effect begins after the medication depot develops in the subcutaneous fat, which can take from 12 to 18 hours after application (D'Arcy, 2007, 2009b). It can also take up to 48 hours for steady-state blood levels to develop, so when the fentanyl TD patch is being started, the patient may need additional short-acting pain medication to control breakthrough pain (D'Arcy, 2009a).

There are some safety concerns with fentanyl TD patch use. More than 100 patients have died related to fentanyl patch use and misuse. When a TD patch is prescribed for pain relief, education of the patients should include the following:

- **Do not cut the patch.** To do so will result in a dose-dumping effect where all the medication is released at one time, resulting in an overdose.
- **Do not apply heat over the patch.** Use of heating pads will result in accelerated medication delivery that could result in an overdose.
- **Dispose of the patch properly.** Seal in a baggy with kitty litter or used coffee grounds. Bag the garbage and put it in an outside garbage receptacle with a sealed lid immediately. There is about 16% of the dose remaining in the patch

after use and an animal or small child could remove the patch and chew or place it on themselves, resulting in overdose (D'Arcy, 2009a). Since there is medication left in the patch, safe disposal is necessary to avoid diversion.

■ **Fentanyl patches should only be started on an opioid-tolerant patient.** In order to start a 25 mcg/hr fentanyl patch, the patient should be taking one of the following oral dosages: 30 mg of oxycodone per day for 2 weeks, 8 mg of hydromorphone per day for 2 weeks, or 60 mg of oral morphine per day for 2 weeks (www.duragesic.com).

Rapid-Acting Fentanyl Products for Breakthrough Cancer Pain *(Onsolis, Lasanda, Oralets)*

■ Fentanyl (Actiq) Oralets are a form of rapid-onset fentanyl. These are rubbed against the buccal membrane, which releases the prescribed dose of medication. The Oralets come in 200, 400, and 800 mcg. The Oralet may be used up to four times per day. Patients must be taught to "paint" the buccal surface with the Oralet, and keep it in constant motion. They should not "suck" on the Oralet as a candy sucker. It takes about 15 to 20 minutes to use the medication. Unused medicine should be dissolved under very hot water. Partially used Oralets must destroyed and not be left lying around, as a child or pet could die from ingestion of leftover medicine.

■ Fentanyl (Onsolis) buccal film is a small strip that is applied to the buccal membrane and slowly releases the prescribed dose of medication. The starting dose of Onsolis is 200 mcg, which is equivalent to 200 mcg Actiq.

■ Fentanyl (Lasanda) nasal spray uses a pectin base that has an extremely rapid onset of action, 15 minutes, and is well tolerated by patients. The starting dose of Lasanda is 100 mcg.

■ Fentanyl (Fentora) buccal tablet is a dissolvable tablet of fentanyl that rapidly dissolves when placed against the buccal membrane. The starting dose of Fentora is 100 mcg, which is equivalent to 200 mcg Actiq.

Medications That Are No Longer Recommended

There are two pain medications that are no longer recommended for use related to toxic metabolites, poor pain relief, or high profile for side effects.

Codeine-Containing Medications: *Codeine, Tylenol #3 (Codeine 30 mg Combined With Acetaminophen 325 mg)*

Codeine use is discouraged, especially in cancer pain settings. It is effective only for mild pain, and causes significant nausea and constipation. In addition, many authors believe that, unlike other opioids, codeine has an analgesic ceiling (meaning that higher doses of the drug do not provide more analgesia). In addition, the number needed to treat is high, at 11. This means you would see the first effective analgesic effect in the 12th patient who was given the medication for pain relief. About 10% of the people lack the enzyme needed to convert codeine to the active metabolite of morphine (APS, 2008).

Meperidine

Meperidine (Demerol) has also fallen out of favor. It is no longer considered a first-line pain medication (APS, 2008; D'Arcy, 2007). Meperidine has a toxic metabolite, normeperidine, that accumulates with repetitive dosing (APS, 2008). This metabolite can cause tremors and seizures. Other drawbacks include the need to use high doses to achieve an analgesic effect that is accompanied by sedation and nausea (D'Arcy, 2007). If meperidine is to be used, there are certain recommendations that include the following:

■ Meperidine should never be used with children and infants.
■ It should never be used in patients with renal impairment, such as in patients with sickle cell anemia or multiple myeloma or older patients.
■ A potentially fatal hyperpyrexic syndrome with delirium can occur if meperidine is used in patients who are taking monoamine oxidase inhibitors.
■ If used, it should never be for more than 1 to 2 days at doses not to exceed 600 mg/24 hours (APS, 2008).

Mixed Agonist/Antagonist Medications

There is a group of medications that have both an agonist and antagonist action at the various binding sites throughout the body. These medications are termed *mixed agonist/antagonist* medications. These medications include the following:

■ Buprenorphine (Buprenex injection or Butrans TD patch)
■ Nalbuphine (Nubain)
■ Pentazocine (Talwin)

These medications act at the kappa receptor sites, so the potential for respiratory depression is believed to be less. Since these medications have both agonist and antagonist actions, they have the potential for reversing the opioid effect of pure opioid agonists such as morphine. If a patient is taking morphine, giving a mixed agonist/antagonist medication will reverse the effect of the morphine and pain relief is lessened. This group of medications also has a high profile for adverse side effects such as confusion and hallucinations and has dose ceilings that limit dose escalations (APS, 2008).

Buprenorphine is used in chronic pain management, but has less of a role in cancer pain management. Use of pentazocine is no longer recommended.

Selecting an Opioid

Selecting an opioid for an individual patient can involve a trial-and-error process. Each individual has a genetic preference for one or more types of opioids. It is just a matter of determining which opioid works best for the patient.

Many patients with cancer pain have tried opioids before for surgery or acute pain from injuries. They may know which one works best and which ones do not work at all. If the patient can provide you with information on the efficacy of pain medications, it should not be considered as drug seeking or potential addiction. If the patient has used a medication successfully, starting with one that was effective will in many cases provide the best outcome.

Conversely, if the patient tells you he or she has tried a medication but it did not work, get more information about when, for what indication, and what doses were tried. In many cases, patients with pain have been underdosed with medications and they then feel they are "not working" or are ineffective. If the correct dose of medication had been provided, the medication could have provided good pain relief. It is always wise to revisit the use of a medication that has been underdosed, using appropriate doses for treating pain unless there are side effects that would contraindicate the use of the drug.

Risk Evaluation and Mitigation Strategies (REMS)

Although REMS is a new concept for opioids, it has been used for years for medications such as thalidomide for multiple myeloma treatment, so that prescribers have the knowledge to prescribe medications that have been identified with special risk factors. For opioids, long-acting formulations and newer medications such as some of the rapid-acting fentanyl drugs had been identified as having higher risks and so the FDA has asked the manufacturers to develop REMS programs for their medications.

Most REMS programs consist of an educational component that the prescriber must complete correctly to be allowed to prescribe the medication. This has a two-sided effect. The positive side is the extra education that these providers get about the medication they are prescribing. The other side is the need to have a REMS certificate makes it less likely that long-acting opioids will be prescribed, and more likely that short-acting opioids will be given instead.

In the best-case scenario, the prescriber can consider that the extra education is helpful in ensuring that these potent medications are prescribed correctly. In the worst-case scenario, REMS may limit the prescribing practice of health care providers. But overall the use of REMS should make prescribing practice safer for both the health care provider and the patient.

Opioids in the Older Patient

Older patients have a large number of conditions such as osteoarthritis and other painful comorbidities. Choosing a medication to treat pain in these patients is more of a challenge. The myth that older patients do not tolerate pain medications is just that—a myth. Older patients can use opioid medication to manage cancer pain with good effect with careful dosing and titration.

The American Geriatrics Society (AGS) updated their pain management guidelines for persistent noncancer pain in older patients in 2009. These guidelines indicate that opioids are an option for the older patient when moderate to severe pain is present.

For older patients, pain is experienced in the same way, but aging can change the way the nervous system perceives the pain and transmission may be altered (Huffman & Kunik, 2000; McLennon, 2005.) Aging can also change the way the older patient's body processes pain medications and can increase the potential for adverse effects. Some of the reasons an older patients may experience adverse effects from opioids include the following:

- Muscle-to-fat ratios change as a patient ages, causing the body fat composition to be altered.
- Poor nutrition can decrease protein stores, which in turn can decrease the binding ability of some medications.
- Because of the changes in the protein-binding mechanisms, drugs may need to compete for binding sites, making one or more of patient's medications ineffective.
- Aging affects the physiologic functions of metabolism, absorption, and medication clearance, including a slowed gastrointestinal motility, decreased cardiac output, and decreased glomerular filtration rate.

▪ Baseline changes in sensory and cognitive perception such as sedation or confusion can increase the risk for some patients to experience side effects such as sedation and confusion related to opioid use.

▪ Drug excretion and elimination are reduced by 10% for each decade after 40 because of decreased renal function (Bruckenthal & D'Arcy, 2007; D'Arcy, 2009b; Horgas et al., 2003).

The old adage of "start low and go slow" still applies to starting opioid therapy in older adults. Older patients are not all the same, and bodies age in different ways. Using conservative doses and monitoring the patient carefully for side effects can help ensure that opioids are being used to provide the highest possible pain relief but are also being used safely.

Tips for Starting Analgesic Medication in the Older Patient

Since the older patient has pain control needs, yet requires more monitoring of dosing and adverse effects, starting new medications can be somewhat complicated. Recommendations for pain medications for the older adult include the following:

▪ Reduce the maximum daily acetaminophen dose from 4,000 mg per day to 1,000 to 2,000 mg per day.

▪ Decrease the acetaminophen dose even further or do not use at all if the patient has a history of alcohol use/abuse, or liver or renal impairment (AGS, 2002, 2009).

▪ Reduce beginning opioid doses by 25% to 50% to decrease the potential for oversedation.

▪ Scheduling medication may provide better pain relief and reduce the likelihood of needing increased doses for uncontrolled pain.

▪ Monitor older adults closely when they are started on opioid therapy since organ impairment may decrease the elimination of the medication.

▪ For older patients, avoid the use of the following medications because of unwanted side effects and/or toxic metabolites: meperidine, pentazocine, indomethacin, and amitriptyline (McLennon, 2005).

▪ (D'Arcy, 2009b)

Treating Opioid Side Effects

All opioids have the potential for side effects. There is no opioid pain medication that does not have the potential for constipation, sedation, or pruritis. See the chapter on medication side effects for treatment options if side effects such as constipation occur with opioid use.

Mark is a 48-year-old truck driver with chronic low back pain. He was diagnosed with prostate cancer 1 year ago, and underwent a prostatectomy and external beam radiation. His main complaint is chronic low back pain that radiates to his hips and down his leg. He feels like the pain is present all the time and is achy, with a pain intensity of 8/10. The pain has been thoroughly worked up, and there is no evidence of residual or recurrent cancer. Mark reports that Percocet worked well to relieve his postoperative pain. Now he has tried using the same medication for this chronic low back and hip pain, but it does not seem to work as well. He is currently taking six oxycodone 5 mg/acetaminophen 325 mg tablets per day, and a muscle relaxant, Robaxin. He cannot drive his truck any longer because he cannot pass the required urine drug screens at work. In addition, he does not feel safe due to medication side effects of sedation. This change in his lifestyle has left him depressed and he feels this may be a pain that cannot be managed. He cannot sleep well and hopes that you can help manage his pain better. What types of medications would you choose for Mark?

Questions to Consider

1. Should you begin an extended-release pain medication such as oxycodone ER or morphine ER? Which do you think would be the best one to trial?
2. Should you add a neuropathic pain medication? Would you recommend starting with an anticonvulsant (such as gabapentin), or an antidepressant (such as duloxetine or amitriptyline)?
3. Should you continue the oxycodone/acetaminophen for breakthrough pain? Would you consider using a rapid-acting fentanyl product for breakthrough pain?
4. Should you continue the muscle relaxant for muscle spasms? Do you think it makes any difference for the pain related to muscle spasms?

REFERENCES

Adams, M., & Abdieh, H. (2004). Pharmokinetics and dose proportionality of oxymorphone extended release and its metabolites: Results of a randomized crossover study. *Pharmacotherapy, 24*(4), 468–476.

Adams, M., Pienazek, H., Gammatoni, A., & Abdieh, H. (2005). Oxymorphone extended release does not affect CVP2C9 or CYP3A4 metabolite pathways. *Journal of Clinical Pharmacology, 45*, 337–345.

American Geriatrics Society (AGS). (2002). Persistent pain in the older patient. *Journal of the American Geriatrics Society, 50*, S205–S224.

American Geriatrics Society (AGS). (2009). The pharmacological management of persistent pain in older persons. *Journal of the American Geriatrics Society, 57*, 1331–1346.

American Pain Society (APS). (2005). *Cancer pain in adults and children*. Glenview, IL: Author.

American Pain Society (APS). (2008). *Principles of analgesic use in the treatment of acute pain and cancer pain*. Glenview, IL: Author.

Bruckenthal, P., & D'Arcy, Y. (2007). Pain in the older adult. *Topics in Advanced Practice ejournal*. Retrieved April 1, 2008, from http://www.medscape.com

Chou, R., Fanciullo, G., Fine, P., Adler, J., Ballantyne, J., Davies, P., . . . Miaskowski, C. (2009). Opioid treatment guidelines: Clinical guidelines for the use of chronic opioid therapy in chronic noncancer pain. *The Journal of Pain, 10*(2), 113–130.

D'Arcy, Y. (2007). *Pain management: Evidence based tools and techniques for nursing professionals*. Marblehead, MA: HcPro.

D'Arcy, Y. (2009a). Avoid the dangers of opioid therapy. *American Nurse Today, 4*(5), 16–22.

D'Arcy, Y. (2009b). *Pain in the older adult*. Indianapolis, IN: Sigma Theta Tau.

Fine, P. G. Opioid induced hyperalgesia and opioid rotation. *Journal of Pain & Palliative Care Pharmacology, 18*(3), 75–79.

Food and Drug Administration (FDA). (2011, October 2). *FDA for health professionals*. Retrieved from www.Janssen.com

Holden, J., Jeong, Y., & Forrest, J. (2005). The endogenous opioid system and clinical pain management. *AACN Clinical Issues, 16*(3), 291–301.

Horgas, A. (2003). Pain management in elderly adults. *Journal of Infusion Nursing, 26*(3), 161–165.

Huffman, J., & Kunik, M. (2000). Assessment and understanding of pain in pain with dementia. *The Gerontologist, 40*(5), 574–581.

Katz, N., McCarberg, B., & Reisner, L. (2007). *Managing chronic pain with opioids in primary care*. Newton, MA: Inflexxion.

McLennon, S. M. (2005). Persistent pain management. National Guideline Clearinghouse. Retrieved April 1, 2008, from http://www.guideline.gov

National Comprehensive Cancer Network (NCCN). (2011). *National Comprehensive Cancer Network Guidelines: Adult cancer pain*. Retrieved from http://www.nccn.org/professionals/physician_gls/f_guidelines.asp

Nursing 2010 Drug Handbook. (2009). Philadelphia, PA: Lippincott Williams & Wilkins.

Pasternak, G. W. (2005). Molecular biology of opioid analgesia. *Journal of Pain and Symptom Management, 29*(5S), S2–9.

Quill, T. E., Holloway, R. G., Shah, M. S., Caprio, T. V., Olden, A. M., & Storey, J. C. (2010). *Primer of palliative care* (5th ed.). Glenview, IL: American Academy of Hospice and Palliative Medicine.

Stokowski, L. (2010). *Opioid-naive and opioid-tolerant patients.* Retrieved from http://www .medscape.com/viewarticle/733067_2

Websites:

The Plant of Joy: A Brief History of Opium. Retrieved from http://www.opiates.net/

Opium: Opium History up to 1858 AD by Alfred McCoy. Retrieved from http://opioids .com/opium/history/index

ADDITIONAL RESOURCES

Fine, P., & Portenoy, R. (2007). *A clinical guide to opioid analgesia.* New York, NY: Vendome Group, LLC.

Institute for Clinical Systems Improvement (ICSI). (2008). *Assessment and management of chronic pain.* Bloomington, MN: Author. Retrieved from www.guideline.gov

Snyder, S., & Pasternak, G. (2003). Historical review: Opioid receptors. *Trends in Pharmacological Sciences, 24*(4), 198–205.

Stanos, S., Fishbain, D., & Fishman, S. (2009). Pain management with opioid analgesics: Balancing risk and benefit. *Physical Medicine & Rehabilitation, 88*(3, Suppl. 2), S69–S99.

5

Coanalgesics for Additive Pain Relief in Cancer Patients

Yvonne D'Arcy

OVERVIEW

Coanalgesics comprise a varied group of medications that can provide additive pain relief when they are added to nonsteroidal antiinflammatory drugs (NSAIDs) or opioids (American Pain Society [APS], 2008). They can have independent analgesic activity for some painful complaints and can counteract select adverse effects of analgesics (APS, 2008). This group of medications was developed originally to treat a wide variety of conditions such as seizures, depression, or muscle spasms. However, patients reported pain relief with these medications and health care providers realized their additional application.

Opioids are the mainstay of pain relief for cancer patients, but addition of a coanalgesic may help decrease pain, have an opioid-sparing effect, or help to treat depression. The three main indications for using adjuvant medications to treat cancer pain include the following:

- To enhance pain relief
- To treat concomitant psychologic disturbances such as insomnia, anxiety, depression, and psychosis
- To provide an opioid-sparing effect (APS, 2008; Fitzgibbon, 2010)

As with any medication, weighing the risks and benefits of adding medications to an analgesic regimen should be carefully considered and outcomes evaluated.

There are no adjuvant medications with Food and Drug Administration (FDA) approval specifically for cancer pain management. Although some classes of these medications are not used specifically for pain, there are some that can be used effectively to help treat pain on an *off-label* basis. If pain has been determined to have a neuropathic source, medications such as antidepressants, antiseizure medications, or topical medications such as lidocaine 5% (Lidoderm) patches can be tried to see if there is any improvement of the pain. An example of neuropathic pain is a patient who has a large amount of tissue damage or swelling from tumor growth, where nerves are being compressed causing additional pain.

Medications that are considered to be coanalgesics for pain management include the following:

- Antidepressants
- Anticonvulsants
- Muscle relaxants
- Topical agents
- Cannabinoids
- Corticosteroids
- Ketamine
- Antihistamines
- NMDA receptor blockers
- Alpha$_2$ adrenergic agonists
- Benzodiazepines
- Antispasmodic agents
- Stimulants (Aiello-Laws et al., 2009; APS, 2008)

Adjuvant analgesics have been used for adjunct pain relief and found to be effective. For some medications, improvement in pain was so notable that the manufacturers received FDA indication for pain management. For example, duloxetine has an indication for diabetic peripheral neuropathy, chronic musculoskeletal pain, and fibromyalgia; pregabalin for diabetic peripheral neuropathy and fibromyalgia; and gabapentin for postherpetic neuralgia. Many patients with neuropathic pain benefit greatly from the addition of these agents to help decrease pain. Since persons with chronic cancer pain are often depressed, the use of serotonin-norepinephrine reuptake inhibitors (SNRIs) or tricyclic antidepressants (TCAs) has improved the quality of pain relief and enhanced sleep.

When the World Health Organization (WHO) analgesic ladder was developed with medication choices for pain management (see Chapter 2), the focus was on escalating steps in the approach for cancer pain, with higher steps using stronger opioid medications. However, the ladder also includes adjuvant medications, also known as coanalgesics, on each step of the ladder. The broad classes of these medications are listed, but no specific medications are given; therefore the choice of coanalgesic is patient dependent (Dalton & Youngblood, 2000).

Trying to group these medications into a single class, coanalgesics, is difficult. They all have such different mechanisms of action and application. These medications can enhance the effect of opioids or other medication being used for pain relief, or they can stand alone as single-agent pain relievers (APS, 2008).

No matter which medication is selected or combined, each patient's comorbidities need to be assessed and evaluated before adding a new medication to the pain management medication regimen. The following sections of the chapter will discuss different classes of coanalgesic that can be used for additional pain relief. Evidence-based ratings for coanalgesics are located in Table 5.1.

Table 5.1 ■ *Recommendations for Practice*

Effective	*Nociceptive Pain*		
Acetaminophen	*Likely to be effective*	Benefits balanced	*Effectiveness not*
NSAIDs	*for nociceptive*	with harm	*established*
Corticosteroids	*pain*	Spinal opioids	Ketamine
Local anesthetics	Bisphosphonates	Caffeine	Antihistamines
Opioids	Radionuclides		Dextroamphetamine
			Topical agents
			Skeletal muscle
			relaxants

Effective	*Neuropathic Pain*	
Anticonvulsants	*Effectiveness unlikely*	*Not recommended*
Antidepressants	*for neuropathic pain*	*for practice*
Serotonin-	Antiarrhythmics	Mixed agonists and
norepinephrine	Calcitonin	antagonists
reuptake	Dextromethorphan	Meperidine
inhibitors	Capsaicin	Propoxyphene
Tricyclic		Codeine
antidepressants		Placebos
Tramadol		Phenothiazine
		Carbamazepine
		Intramuscular (IM)
		route
		Carisoprodol (Soma)

Source: Adapted from Aiello-Laws et al. (2009) as adapted from the Oncology Nursing Society, *Putting Evidence into Practice* (ONS PEP) quick resource.

ANTIDEPRESSANT MEDICATIONS

Antidepressants are most commonly used as adjunct medications for neuropathic-type pain such as postherpetic neuralgia, painful diabetic neuropathies, and neuropathic syndromes associated with cancer treatments such as chemotherapy, and surgical syndromes such as postmastectomy syndrome (Lynch & Watson, 2006). They are also good adjuncts in patients with cancer and neuropathic pain when opioids have provided suboptimal pain relief (APS, 2008).

Classes of Antidepressant Medications

- Serotonin-norepinephrine reuptake inhibitors (SNRIs): duloxetine (Cymbalta), venlafaxine (Effexor)
- Tricyclic antidepressants (TCAs): amitriptyline, desipramine, nortriptyline
- Selective serotonin reuptake inhibitors (SSRIs): citalopram, paroxetine

Antidepressant medications have several different mechanisms of action. The TCAs such as amitriptyline, desipramine, or nortriptyline inhibit presynaptic uptake of norepinephrine and serotonin, as do the SNRIs such as duloxetine. Other less-studied actions for TCAs include a mild opioid action at the mu binding sites, sodium and calcium channel blockade, NMDA site antagonism, and adenosine activity (Lynch & Watson, 2006). The SSRI medications such as citalopram (Celexa) inhibit serotonin at presynaptic junction sites (Ghafoor & St. Marie, 2009).

Serotonin-Norepinephrine Reuptake Inhibitors (SNRIs)		
SNRIs	Starting Dose	Effective Dose
venlafaxine (Effexor)	37.5 mg daily	150–225 mg daily
duloxetine (Cymbalta)	20 mg daily	60 mg daily

Source: APS, 2008.

The SNRI medications have fewer anticholinergic side effects compared to the TCA medications. They are effective for a variety of neuropathic pain conditions such as diabetic neuropathy, postherpetic neuralgia, and atypical facial pain (Lynch & Watson, 2006). Venlafaxine has shown an effect on hyperalgesia and allodynia, both preventing the occurrence and decreasing the pain (APS, 2008; Wallace & Staats, 2005). Effective doses of venlafaxine for pain relief range from 150 mg to 225 mg, with a starting dose of 37.5 mg.

Duloxetine has received FDA approval for treating painful diabetic peripheral neuropathy (DPN) and chronic pain. For duloxetine, the starting dose of 20 mg/day may decrease the incidence of side effects, with pain relief experienced at 60 mg/day. Careful titration of the medications and slow dose increases will help decrease some of the side effects such as somnolence, nausea, and sweating. There have been no identified increased cardiovascular risks associated with the use of duloxetine (APS, 2008).

There are some drawbacks with both venlafaxine and duloxetine. There is an increased risk for suicidal ideation and behavior in children and adolescents with major depressive disorders and these drugs are not approved for pediatric patients. Care should also be taken with patients who have liver disease or use alcohol consistently (Cymbalta package insert, www.cymbalta.com). To avoid the development of serotonin syndrome, a rare but serious side effect, patients on SNRIs should not also take SSRI medications, unless supervised by a psychiatrist.

The noradrenergic effect of SNRIs may increase blood pressure. Patients should have regular blood pressure screenings to assess for this. Cardiac changes are also possible with AV block and increases in blood pressure (Lynch & Watson, 2006). Five percent of venlafaxine-treated patients developed changes on ECG (APS, 2008). As a result, patients who are taking venlafaxine who also have diabetes mellitus, hypertension, hypercholesterolemia, or are currently smoking should have ECG monitoring while on the antidepressant medication (APS, 2008) and should be assessed regularly for any signs of cardiac changes. Careful dose tapering should take place when these medications are being discontinued to avoid discontinuation syndrome, insomnia, lethargy, diarrhea, nausea, dizziness, or paresthesia (APS, 2008).

Tricyclic Antidepressants (TCAs)		
Common TCAs	*Starting Dose*	*Effective Dose*
amitriptyline (Elavil)	10–25 mg hs	50–150 mg hs
desipramine (Norpramin)	10–25 mg qd	50–150 mg qd
nortriptyline (Pamelor)	10–25 mg hs	50–150 mg hs

Source: APS, 2008.

The TCAs have the best profile for use in treating neuropathic pain conditions, and were at one time first-line treatment for neuropathic pain such as postherpetic neuralgia or postmastectomy pain syndromes. The starting doses are low, 10 to 25 mg titrated up to 150 mg/day (APS, 2008; Wallace & Statts, 2005). Antidepressants should be titrated no more often than every 1 to 2 weeks (Chen et al., 2004). The doses required for pain management are lower than the antidepressant doses of 150 to 300 mg/day. Of note, the pain relief action of these medications is independent of any effect there may be on mood (Lynch & Watson, 2006).

A meta-analysis of the TCA medications indicates that TCAs are effective for use in treating neuropathic pain (APS, 2008). Amitriptyline is the best known and most studied of the TCAs. It is also a primary recommendation for the treatment of fibromyalgia pain (D'Arcy & McCarberg, 2005). However, TCA use in active cancer treatment is limited due to drug interactions with chemotherapy, potential hematologic side effects, and adverse reactions. Analgesic response is usually seen within 5 to 7 days (APS, 2008). Adverse effects for TCAs include the following:

- Sedation
- Dry mouth
- Constipation
- Urinary retention
- Orthostatic hypotension
- Anticholinergic side effects
- Caution in patients with heart disease, symptomatic prostatic hypertrophy, neurogenic bladder, dementia, narrow-angle glaucoma
- Increased suicide behavior in young adults (Institute for Clinical Systems Improvement [ICSI], 2007)

These side effects make TCAs undesirable for use in the elderly, especially when they are used in combination with opioid analgesics.

TCAs can prolong the QTc and increase the risk for cardiac arrhythmias in patients who are on concomitant methadone or those with underlying conduction abnormalities. Use caution with desipramine in children; anecdotal reports of sudden death have been reported (APS, 2008). Although these drugs are inexpensive and readily available, they do have some very significant adverse effects. However, each patient being considered for TCAs should have a thorough assessment for any risk factors such as cardiac conduction abnormalities. When starting TCA therapy, the current recommendation is to screen all patients over 40 years of age via ECG to evaluate for conduction abnormalities or QTc prolongation (APS, 2008).

TCA medications are not recommended for use in elderly patients due to the high incidence of undesirable side effects and the potential for increased fall risk related to early morning orthostatic hypotension (American Geriatrics Society [AGS], 2002, AGS, 2009; Lynch & Watson, 2006).

The greatest benefits of using TCAs for pain relief are improved sleep, (Wilson et al., 1997) relief of neuropathic pain, and improved mood (D'Arcy, 2007).

When caring for a patient who is taking TCAs as adjuvant pain medication, patients should be carefully instructed regarding the risk of orthostatic hypotension, especially in the morning. Nurses have an important role in cautioning patients to sit on the side of the bed before trying to stand. Some patients complain of sleepiness with these medications and if this is problematic, the patient should be instructed to take the medication earlier in the evening rather than at bedtime hoping to decrease the early morning sedation that can be experienced. For older men, urinary retention can be problematic and urinary status should be carefully checked. For the dry mouth associated with TCA use, hard candies or gum can ease the dry feeling.

Patients should always be told the rationale for prescribing an antidepressant medication for pain so they are comfortable taking the medication. The onset of analgesic effect may take 2 to 4 weeks, and patients should be encouraged to extend a trial of these medications to this period of time to see if analgesia occurs.

Selective Serotonin Reuptake Inhibitors (SSRIs)		
Common SSRIs	*Starting Dose*	*Effective Dose*
paroxetine (Paxil)	10–20 mg daily	20–40 mg daily
citalopram (Celexa)	10–20 mg daily	20–40 mg daily

Source: APS, 2008.

There is no evidence that SSRIs have any effect on neuropathic pain (Max et al., 1992; Rowbotham, Reisner, Davies, & Fields, 2005), but they are useful as antidepressants (APS, 2006). When compared to placebo, these medications did not have any significant advantage for pain relief. Given the lack of efficacy for pain relief, and the side effect profile of sexual dysfunction, anxiety, sleep disorder, and headache, SSRI use should be limited to management of depression, anxiety, or insomnia (APS, 2008). In the oncology setting, citalopram is the drug of choice for depression management, as it has the fewest interactions with chemotherapy. In addition, SSRIs may limit the effectiveness of tamoxifen and aromatase inhibitors.

ANTICONVULSANT MEDICATIONS

Anticonvulsants are commonly used to treat neuropathic pain of many different types such as postherpetic neuralgia (PHN), painful diabetic peripheral neuropathy (DPN), and trigeminal neuralgia (APS, 2006). The original premise for use was that if these medications could control the erratic neuronal firing in seizures, it could be applied for controlling neuronal discharge from pain stimuli. Research has shown that this is essentially true and one of the primary mechanisms of these medications is to reduce neuronal excitability and spontaneous firing of cortical neurons (APS, 2008). These drugs are thought to decrease the neuronal firing after nerve damage, are used for neuropathic pain, and are used to decrease neuronal sensitization that leads to chronic neuropathic pain (APS, 2008).

Anticonvulsant Medications		
Common Anticonvulsants	*Starting Dose*	*Effective Dose*
gabapentin (Neurontin)	100–300 mg hs	300–1,200 mg TID
pregabalin (Lyrica)	25–75 mg BID	150–300 mg BID
carbamazepine (Tegretol)	100–200 mg daily	300–600 mg BID
topiramate (Topamax)	25 mg daily	100 mg BID

Anticonvulsant agents are commonly used as coanalgesics for managing neuropathic pain. Gabapentin is FDA approved for use in postherpetic neuralgia and painful diabetic peripheral neuropathy. It is also useful for management of postmastectomy and postthoracotomy pain, phantom limb pain, and pain from neuropathic cancer pain and acute and chronic spinal cord injury (APS, 2008; ICSI, 2007).

Both gabapentin and pregabalin act by blocking neuronal calcium channels, the alpha$_2$-delta subunit specifically, thereby reducing the release of glutamate, norepinephrine, and substance P (APS, 2008). Because the drugs are renally excreted, dose reductions are advised for patients with renal impairment. The one drawback to gabapentin is the length of time needed to reach effective dose strength. Since medication response is patient dependent, it takes weeks to reach a dose of gabapentin that will provide pain relief. Pregabalin as an alternate option can provide a faster response for pain relief since therapeutic doses can be given earlier in the treatment.

For acute pain, gabapentin and pregabalin have demonstrated an opioid-sparing effect of up to 60% when the medications are given preoperatively at doses of 1,200 mg and 300 mg, respectively. The drawback is the increased sedation that has also been reported.

There is a new long-acting formulation of gabapentin (Gralise) available. It has an indication for postherpetic neuralgia and is designed as a once-daily dose. It is not interchangeable with other gabapentin products because of the differing pharmacokinetic profiles that affect the frequency of administration. The medication is provided in 300 and 600 mg strengths. The dose should be titrated up to a dose of 1,800 mg taken once daily with the evening meal. As with all extended-release products, Gralise tablets should be swallowed whole and never crushed or chewed. Gralise should not be stopped abruptly, and should be tapered over a minimum of 1 week or longer (per Gralise prescribing information).

The older anticonvulsants such as carbamazepine (Tegretol) have not been studied for pain relief and thus have only weak evidence for their use as coanalgesic medications for pain. There is a need for further research data. One early meta-analysis (McQuay, Carroll, Jadad, Wiffen, & Moore, 1995) of four anticonvulsants including phenytoin, carbamazepine, clonazepam, and valproate determined that these anticonvulsants were effective for relieving the pain of trigeminal neuralgia, diabetic neuropathy, and migraine prophylaxis. Given the high profile for serious adverse side effects of the older anticonvulsants, as well as potential drug interactions with chemotherapy, newer anticonvulsants are recommended for treating neuropathic pain in the cancer setting (APS, 2008).

One of the major drawbacks to anticonvulsant medications is their high side effect profile for adverse side effects. These include the following:

- Somnolence
- Dizziness
- Fatigue
- Edema
- Nausea
- Weight gain
- Increased risk of suicidal behavior or ideation

The older anticonvulsants may cause the following:

- Stevens-Johnson syndrome (rare)
- Aplastic anemia and agranulocytosis (ICSI, 2007)

The serious nature of the adverse side effects of this class of medications makes it imperative that a full baseline history is taken from the patient when starting these medications. Careful monitoring is required and the patients should be instructed to report the occurrence and severity of any adverse effect if it occurs.

TOPICAL ANALGESICS

Lidocaine 5% Patch (Lidoderm)

The lidocaine patch (5%) is a soft flannel-backed patch that is applied over the painful area. The FDA indication is for use with postherpetic neuralgia. Off label, it has been studied in painful diabetic neuropathy, complex regional pain syndrome, postmastectomy pain, and HIV-related neuropathy (APS, 2008). In addition, some clinicians have found success in using it to treat myofascial trigger points or tender points.

The directions for use of the patch is to use for 12 hours, then remove for at least 12 hours. However, patients have worn the patch for 24 hours with no ill effects (APS, 2008; D'Arcy, 2007). The maximum dose of Lidoderm is up to three patches at one time. The patches should be replaced daily and placed only on intact skin. Measurable serum levels of lidocaine with patch use are minimal (APS, 2008). Patients tolerate topical treatments well. The one side effect from the Lidoderm patch that has been reported is rare instances of skin irritation at the site of patch application.

Capsaicin Cream (Zostrix)

A topical cream that can reduce the secretion of substance P at peripheral nerve endings is derived from hot peppers and is called *capsaicin*. It is sold over the counter as Zostrix 0.025% and Zostrix-HP 0.075% cream. The neuropathic conditions for which this cream has been most helpful include postmastectomy pain, other peripheral neuropathic conditions, and neck and arthritis pain (APS, 2008).

When the cream is applied, it causes a burning sensation in the application area. Patients should be warned to expect this sensation and gloves should be used to apply the cream. It should not be applied near the eyes or on mucous membranes, and care should be taken to wash hands thoroughly before touching any other part of the body such as the eyes. The patient must be dedicated and willing to persevere with applying the cream three to four times per day for 2 weeks to see if there is any analgesic benefit.

A new 8% capsaicin patch called Qutenza is used for postherpetic neuralgia. It needs to be applied by a health care provider who has been trained in the technique. Local anesthetic is applied over the site of the pain, then the patch is applied for an hour and removed. This form of capsaicin can provide up to 12 weeks of pain relief. It has not been studied in cancer-related neuropathic pain conditions.

MUSCLE RELAXANTS

Although referred to as "skeletal muscle relaxants," these drugs do not "relax" muscles, with the exception of baclofen. They are highly sedating, and increase the risk of falls. Therefore, they should be cautiously added to a pain regimen, especially in frail and older adults. As functionality declines, patients with cancer may have limited mobility and face long periods of time confined to bed. For pain that is defined as cramping or spasms, a muscle relaxant can be tried. The skeletal muscle relaxants consist of several different groups of medications: benzodiazepines, sedatives, antihistamines, other centrally acting medications (APS, 2008).

Skeletal Muscle Relaxants

Name	Starting Dose (oral)	Effective Dose
cyclobenzaprine (Flexeril)	5 mg TID	10 mg TID
orphenadrine (Norflex)	100 mg BID	100 mg BID
tizanidine (Zanaflex)	2 mg hs	8 mg TID
metaxalone (Skelaxin)	400 mg TID–QID	800 mg TID–QID
methocarbamol (Robaxin)	500 mg QID	500–750 mg QID
Other:		
Antispasmodic: baclofen	5 mg TID	10–20 mg TID
Benzodiazepine: diazepam	1 mg BID	2–10 mg BID–QID

Source: APS, 2008.

Although there is no indication that these medications relax skeletal muscles, they are commonly used for spasms and muscle tightness (APS, 2008). After 1 to 2 weeks, the action of the medication shifts to a central activity rather than skeletal muscle activity (APS, 2008). The most common side effect of this group of medications is sedation. If they are being used concomitantly with opioid analgesics, the sedative effect is cumulative. There is the potential for abuse in patients who are predisposed to this problem, so intermittent or short-term use is advised. In particular, carisoprodol (Soma) is highly abused, and its use is not recommended. This drug has been removed from the market in many European countries. Many states have reclassified it as a Schedule IV or V drug due to the risk of abuse.

PSYCHOTROPIC DRUGS

For some cancer patients with intractable nausea and vomiting or agitation, a medication to control these effects is needed. In patients with cancer pain, the starting dose may need to be reduced (Fitzgibbon, 2010). Concomitant use of two psychotropic medications or a combination of an opioid with a psychotropic medication can cause sedation in acutely ill and malnourished cancer patients (Fitzgibbon, 2010). For delirium and agitation, the choice of medications is limited, with haloperidol being the first choice and lorazepam the second related to the sedating effect of the medication.

OTHER COANALGESICS

There are a variety of other medications that can be used as coanalgesics ranging from cannabinoids, dronabinol, which are recommended for neuropathic pain from multiple sclerosis, to NMDA receptor blockers, ketamine, dextromethorphan, and amantadine, which are used for centrally mediated neuropathic pain and hyperalgesia. These agents are not recommended for first- or second-line use, but rather for patients who have failed all other attempts for pain relief. There is little research to support their use, with the literature primarily focusing on case reports and anecdotal reports.

These medications also have significant adverse side effects. Dronabinol use can cause cognitive impairment, psychosis, and sedation (APS, 2008).

The NMDA receptor blockers have significant adverse side effects as well; ketamine may cause hallucinations and memory problems, and has abuse potential; amantadine and dextromethorphan are associated with less severe side effects such as dizziness, insomnia, and nausea (*Nursing 2010 Drug Handbook*, 2009).

When considering using a coanalgesic, the health care provider needs to fully assess the patient and consider all the comorbidities and potential drug–drug interactions. The use of these medications is highly individual and doses may vary according to the patient's ability to tolerate the medications. Starting at lower doses and escalating slowly can help reduce the seriousness of the side effects. Since analgesic effect can take time to become apparent, patients should be encouraged to use these medications for at least 2 weeks before deciding they are not effective for pain relief.

Case Study

Sally B. is a 65-year-old patient with metastatic ovarian cancer. She has been on opioids for pain relief for a few months. As the disease progressed and metastasized to her liver and bones, she has had increased abdominal swelling and has some changes in respiration requiring supplemental oxygen. She has become delirious and moans periodically. A thoracentesis provided a short period of relief, but the pain is increasing. The health care providers are concerned about increasing the opioids because her respiratory status seems tenuous. Other than increasing the opioid that is indicated, what other types of coanalgesics might be helpful?

Questions to Consider

1. What type of opioid will you use—more orals, IV, PCA, or epidural?
2. Would you consider adding a medication for her delirium?
3. What other types of coanalgesics would you consider to treat the pain of the abdominal distension and metastatic disease?

REFERENCES

Aiello-Laws, L., Reynolds, J., Delzer, N., Peterson, M., Ameringer, S., & Bakitas, M. (2009). *Putting evidence into practice: What are the pharmacologic interventions for nociceptive and neuropathic cancer pain in adults?* Retrieved from http://www.guideline.gov

American Geriatrics Society (AGS). (2002). The management of persistent pain in older persons. *Journal of the American Geriatrics Society, 50*, S205–S224.

American Geriatrics Society (AGS). (2009). The pharmacological management of persistent pain in older persons. *Journal of the American Geriatrics Society, 57*, 1331–1346.

American Pain Society (APS). (2006). *Pain control in the primary care setting.* Glenview, IL: Author.

American Pain Society (APS). (2008). *Principles of analgesic use in the treatment of acute and cancer pain.* Glenview, IL: Author.

Chen, H., Lamer, T., Rho, R., Marshall, K., Sitzman, T., Ghazi, S., & Brewer, R. (2004). Contemporary management of neuropathic pain for the primary care physician. *Mayo Clinic Proceedings, 79*(12), 1533–1545.

Dalton, J. A., & Youngblood, R. (2000). Clinical application of the World Health Organization analgesic ladder. *Journal of IV Nursing, 23*(2), 118–124.

D'Arcy, Y. (2007). *Pain management: Evidence-based tools and techniques for nursing professionals.* Marblehead, MA: HcPro.

D'Arcy, Y., & McCarberg, B. (2005). New fibromyalgia pain management recommendations. *The Journal for Nurse Practitioners, 1*(4), 218–225.

Fitzgibbon, D. (2010). Cancer pain: Principles of management and pharmacotherapy. In *Bonica's management of pain* (pp. 582–590). Philadelphia, PA: Lippincott Williams & Wilkins.

Ghafoor, V., & St. Marie, B. (2009). Overview of pharmacology. In *Core curriculum for pain management nursing.* Indianapolis, IN: Kendall Publications.

Institute for Clinical Systems Improvement (ICSI). (2008). *Assessment and management of chronic pain.* Retrieved from http://www.guideline.gov

Lynch, M., & Watson, C. (2006). The pharmacotherapy of chronic pain: A review. *Pain Research & Management; The Journal of the Canadian Pain Society, 11*(1), 11–38.

Max, M. B., Lynch, S. A., Muir, J., Shoaf, S. E., Smoller, B., Dubner, R. (1992). Effects of desipramine, amitriptyline, and fluoxetine on pain in diabetic neuropathy. *NEJM, 326,* 1250–1256.

McQuay, H., Carroll, D., Jadad, A. R., Wiffen, P., Moore, A. (1995). Anticonvulsant drugs for management of pain: A systematic review. *British Medical Journal, 311,* 1047.

Nursing 2010 Drug Handbook. (2009). Philadelphia, PA: Wolters Kluwer/Lippincott.

Rowbotham, M. C., Reisner, L. A., Davies, P. S., & Fields, H. L. (2005). Treatment response in antidepressant-naïve postherpetic neuralgia patients: Double-blind, randomized trial. *Journal of Pain, 6*(11), 741–746.

Wallace, M., & Staats, P. (2005). *Pain medicine & management.* New York, NY: McGraw-Hill.

Wilson, P., Caplan, R., Connis, R., Gilbert, H., Grigsby, E., Haddox, D., . . . Simon, D. (1997). Practice guidelines for chronic pain management: A report by the American Society of Anesthesiologists Task Force on Pain Management, Chronic Pain Section. *Anesthesiology, 86*(4), 995–1004.

6

Management of Side Effects From Pain Medications

Pamela Stitzlein Davies

OVERVIEW

Prevention and management of side effects from pain medications, especially those caused by opioids, are key to successful cancer pain management. It is common for the nurse to hear a patient complain, "I won't take those pain medicines because they block me up so bad!" Sadly, this situation may occur simply because the patient did not receive appropriate instructions. Advising the patient about strategies for constipation prevention and management, as well as other side effects such as nausea and sedation, will significantly improve the patient's quality of life. The nurse is in an ideal position to provide that instruction, thereby improving the chances that patients will continue on their prescribed pain medications.

Opioids are the most effective medications for moderate to severe cancer pain (Miaskowski et al., 2008; World Health Organization [WHO], 1986). However, other classes of analgesics are commonly utilized, including steroids, nonsteroidal anti-inflammatory drugs (NSAIDs), acetaminophen, adjuvant agents such as anticonvulsants and antidepressants, bisphosphonates, and topical agents such as lidocaine or capsaicin. Many of these medications, such as antidepressants and anticonvulsants, have adverse reaction profiles similar to opioids.

COMMON SIDE EFFECTS FROM PAIN MEDICATIONS

Given the large number of potential side effects from pain medications, this section reviews some of the more commonly occurring side effects that create a heavier symptom burden for the patient.

Constipation

Dame Cicely Saunders, founder of the modern hospice movement, was known to have repeatedly stated, "Nothing matters more than the bowels!" (Quill et al., 2010).

Constipation is the most bothersome side effect of opioid therapy for many patients (Bell et al., 2009; Cook et al., 2008; Rosti, Gatti, Costantini, Sabato, & Zucco, 2010; Sykes, 2005; Thomas, 2008). Other drugs causing slow passage of stool include serotonin norepinephrine reuptake inhibitors (SNRI) drugs, such as duloxetine; and tricyclic antidepressant (TCA) drugs, such as amitriptyline or desipramine (Mays, 2006). Some chemotherapy agents, such as vincristine, as well as some antiemetics ($5-HT_3$ serotonin receptor antagonist agents such as ondansetron), also cause constipation.

Age impacts the incidence of constipation. Many older adults struggle with infrequent passage of stool at baseline (Mugie, Benninga, & DiLorenzo, 2011). The National Cancer Institute (NCI) Surveillance Epidemiology and End Results (SEER) reported that 77% of all cancers are diagnosed in persons 55 years and older (NCI, 2012). Therefore, the nurse can anticipate that constipation will impact the majority of oncology patients (Economou, 2010; Klaschik, Nauck, & Ostgathe, 2003). In addition, the presence of bulky tumor in the abdomen or pelvis (e.g., from melanoma or renal tumors), carcinomatosis (peritoneal seeding of the tumor leading to bowel dysfunction, such as in ovarian or colorectal cancer), or ascites, will increase the incidence constipation in advanced cancer (Chi, Phaeton, Miner, Kardos, & Diaz, 2009).

Concurrent diseases will increase the potential for development of constipation. Examples include diabetes, hypothyroidism, irritable bowel syndrome, depression, and neurologic conditions such as multiple sclerosis or autonomic neuropathy (Sykes, 2005). Conditions seen in malignancy also contribute to slowed gut motility, including dehydration, anorexia, hypercalcemia, hypokalemia, and spinal cord compression (Economou, 2010; Sykes, 2006). Vigilance is important to prevent this common but extremely uncomfortable problem.

In the setting of advanced cancer, upward titration of opioid pain medications may result in obstipation (severe constipation). It can become so severe that it necessitates an emergency department evaluation and hospital admission.

Bowel obstruction may occur, occasionally requiring surgical intervention for treatment or prevention of bowel perforation (Chi et al., 2009). This only adds to the physical, emotional, and financial burdens suffered from the cancer diagnosis. In addition, creation of a colostomy for management of bowel perforation can have a profoundly negative impact on quality of life (Beaver et al., 2010).

An assessment of bowel function is required prior to instituting a bowel regimen, but many patients are embarrassed to discuss this with their health team. The nurse can help relieve the embarrassment with a proactive and straightforward approach to questioning, or use of a symptom rating scale that includes constipation. Use of a visual scale, such as the Bristol Stool Scale (Lewis & Heaton, 1997) may aid in discussion of stool characteristics and patterns.

Clinical Pearl	The key to constipation management is *prevention*. The key to constipation prevention is *education*.

Nurses are uniquely positioned to assist the cancer patient with bowel management because of the discipline's focus on patient education. Classes of laxatives are discussed in Table 6.1.

Table 6.1 ■ *Classification of Laxatives*

Laxative Class	Effect and Mechanism of Action	Examples of Drugs Belonging to Class
Surfactant/detergents	Soften stool by reducing surface tension, allowing absorption of water and fats into stool	Docusate
Bowel stimulants	Work directly on colon to induce peristalsis; may cause cramping	Senna, bisacodyl (Dulcolax)
Osmotic laxatives	Nonabsorbable sugars exert an osmotic effect primarily in the small intestine; also lowers ammonia levels, which can improve confusion from hepatic encephalopathy	Polyethylene glycol (MiraLax) Lactulose Magnesium hydroxide (Milk of Magnesia), magnesium citrate Glycerine suppositories

(continues)

Table 6.1 (continued)

Laxative Class	Effect and Mechanism of Action	Examples of Drugs Belonging to Class
Bulk laxatives	Provide bulk to increase stool mass, which stimulates peristalsis; requires significant fluid intake; generally not recommended in advanced cancer or significant nausea and vomiting	Dietary fiber (bran) Psyllium (Metamucil) Methylcellulose (Citrucel)
Lubricant laxatives	Lubricates the stool surface, which softens stool; generally not recommended due to risk of malabsorption, aspiration pneumonitis (in frail elderly), and risk of development of lipoid granuloma in intestinal wall when combined with docusate; short-term use can be helpful in advanced cancer setting	Mineral oil
Opioid antagonists		Methylnaltrexone (Relistor) Alvimopan (Entereg) (indicated for postop ileus following partial large or small bowel resection with primary anastomosis) Oral naloxone, oral naltrexone: not recommended due to reversal of systemic analgesia

Source: Adapted from Economou, 2010; Pasero & McCaffery, 2011.

All patients at risk for medication-induced constipation should be started on a basic bowel regimen. A handy bowel program mnemonic that patients can easily remember (and usually get a chuckle from) is *"Mush," "Push," and "Gush"* (see Clinical Pearl).

> *Clinical*
> *Pearl*
>
> BASIC BOWEL REGIMEN: MUSH, PUSH, GUSH
>
> The following bowel regimen mnemonic is easy for patients to remember.
>
> "*Mush*": Docusate, a stool softener, acts as a detergent to break up and "soften" the stool. Take 1 to 2 capsules once or twice a day.
>
> "*Push*" is the colonic stimulant effect provided by senna or bisacodyl, which acts like a "whip" on the bowel to get it moving. Take 1 to 2 tablets at bedtime.
>
> "*Gush*" refers to an osmotic laxative, such as polyethylene glycol (MiraLax), which works by drawing fluid into the colon. Mix a 17 g scoop in juice and drink daily.

The 2009 Cochrane Review reports that there is insufficient evidence to support the use of any particular bowel regimen over another for management of constipation in palliative care patients (Miles, Fellowes, Goodman, & Wilkinson, 2009). A variety of laxative regimens exists, and typically starts with stool softener and stimulant (Economou, 2010; Quill et al., 2010). An osmotic laxative (such as polyethylene glycol) may be added next (Fleming & Wade, 2010). Extra fluids should be encouraged, and a daily serving of prunes or prune juice is very helpful. For more severe constipation, bisacodyl suppository, enema, or manual disimpaction may be required (Clemens & Klaschik, 2008; Sykes, 2005). See Table 6.2.

Methylnaltrexone (Relistor) is a new agent on the market for refractory opioid-induced constipation in a palliative care setting. This agent selectively binds the peripheral mu-opioid receptor in the gut. As it does not cross the blood–brain barrier, systemic opioid analgesia is maintained, even after 3 months of regular use (Lipman, Karver, Austin, Stambler, & Israel, 2011). In two initial studies, 62% and 48% of patients who received methylnaltrexone had a bowel movement within 4 hours of the first injection. Of those patients who responded within 4 hours, 50% experienced laxation within 30 minutes of injection (Salix Pharmaceuticals, n.d.). Currently, methylnaltrexone is only available as a subcutaneous injection, but studies are currently in progress on an oral preparation. Although methylnaltrexone has good results for many patients, it is an expensive treatment option, and should be considered when standard laxative therapies are not effective. However, in overall cost consideration, the drug is significantly more cost effective than inpatient medical or surgical treatment of obstipation. Methylnaltrexone should not be given if the patient is not on opioids, or if a bowel obstruction is suspected.

Table 6.2 ◼ *Prevention and Management of Opioid-Induced Constipation*

1. **Goal:** The goal of a bowel regimen is a soft, formed stool that is easy to pass daily or every other day without straining.
   a. Encourage regular fluid intake, as tolerated, to improve bowel function.
   b. Encourage daily walking, if able, as this stimulates peristalsis.
   c. Patients with advanced cancer should pass a small bowel movement every several days, even with limited food and fluid intake, due to normal secretory output of the bowels.
2. **Step 1**: All patients taking regular doses of opioid or other constipating medicine should be started on one of the following bowel regimens, taken on a regularly scheduled basis (not prn).
   a. A combined stool softener and mild peristaltic stimulant, such as Senekot-S (docusate 50 mg + senna 8.6 mg) 1 to 2 tablets daily at bedtime; may increase to 2 to 3 tablets BID.
   b. Polyethylene glycol (MiraLax) 1 scoop or 1 packet (17 g) mixed in juice daily.
   c. Prunes (6) or prune juice (6 oz) once or twice daily may suffice for some.
   d. Note: Fiber supplements (such as psyllium [Metamucil] or methylcellulose [Citrucel] should be avoided in the setting of advanced cancer, abdominal or pelvic cancers, or in patients with significant nausea/vomiting. Patients unable to ingest the required higher fluid intake to flush the fiber through the gut may be at increased risk of obstruction from high fiber intake.
3. **Step 2:** For worsening constipation (no bowel movement in any 48-hour period, or hard stools that are difficult or painful to pass), combine all three of the following on a regular basis:
   a. "Mush": Stool softener (docusate): If stool is hard and/or small pellets, increase docusate to a 250 mg capsule, 1 to 2 capsules BID.
   b. "Push": Stimulant: Choose one of the following:
      i. Bisacodyl (Dulcolax) 5 mg tablet, 2 to 3 tablets BID
      ii. Senna 8.6 mg 2-3 tablets BID
   c. "Gush": Osmotic laxative: Choose one of the following:
      i. Polyethylene glycol (MiraLax) 1 scoop or packet (17 g) mixed in juice daily or BID
      ii. Lactulose (10 g/15 mL) 15 to 30 mL daily to QID
4. **Step 3:** If no bowel movement in 72 hours:
   a. Perform a rectal examination to rule out impaction/stool in the rectal vault.
5. **Step 4:** If not impacted/no stool in the rectal vault, add one or two of the following agents to Step 2 above:
   a. Bisacodyl (Dulcolax) suppository 10 mg rectally, may repeat in 24 hours if no results
   b. Magnesium citrate 8 oz bottle, may repeat in 24 hours if no results
   c. Milk of Magnesia 25 mL + cascara 50 mg (5 mL) suspension
   d. Fleet enema
6. **Step 5:** If rectal exam in Step 3 reveals stool in the rectal vault with impaction, patient will require manual disimpaction:

(continued)

Table 6.2 *(continued)*

   a. Premedicate with analgesic and anxiolytic.

   b. If the stool is hard, administer a glycerin suppository or oil retention enema to soften the stool prior to disimpaction.

   c. Manually disimpact.

   d. Follow up with tap water or castile soap enemas, repeated until effluent is clear.

   e. Increase the bowel regimen (Step 2) and monitor the patient's evacuations closely until stable.

7. **Step 6:** For refractory constipation/obstipation:

   a. Consult with a health care provider.

   b. Consider abdominal X-ray to assess for ileus or bowel obstruction.

   c. Consider worsening abdominal or pelvic disease, development of carcinomatosis or ascites.

   d. Consider surgical consultation for impending bowel obstruction.

   e. For patients on opioid therapy, consider methylnaltrexone (Relistor) subcutaneous injection every 24 to 48 hours. Dose is weight based:

     i. Patient weight of 84 to 135 lb (38 to 61 kg): 8 mg (0.4 mL) subcutaneous

     ii. Patient weight of 136 to 251 lb (62 to 114 kg): 12 mg (0.6 mL) subcutaneous

     iii. For patient weight less than 84 lb (less than 38 kg) or more than 251 lb (114 kg), see package insert for dosing information

     iv. Methylnaltrexone is contraindicated in bowel obstruction.

Source: Economou, 2010; Sykes, 2005; Quill et al., 2010; Pasero & McCaffery, 2011; Clark, Urban, & Currow, 2010; Lipman, Karver, Austin, Stambler, & Israel, 2011; NCCN, 2011; Saliz Pharmaceuticals, n.d.

A new opioid antagonist to treat postoperative constipation is alvimopan (Entereg). This is a peripheral mu antagonist, and is approved to accelerate the time to upper and lower gastrointestinal recovery following partial large or small bowel resection surgery with primary anastomosis (Entereg-Home, n.d.). Patients are given a 12 mg capsule orally 30 minutes to 5 hours prior to surgery, and twice daily up to a maximum of 7 days. Its FDA approved use is restricted to inpatient perioperative settings.

Persons with constipation who receive diarrhea-inducing chemotherapy may experience a frustrating "roller coaster effect" from the many drugs that impact their bowel function through the treatment cycle. For an example of this, see the Case Study at the end of the chapter.

When a patient calls with an unexpected complaint of "diarrhea," the astute nurse will recognize the need to assess for a phenomenon called "overflow diarrhea" (Sykes, 2004). This occurs when the patient is so severely constipated that nothing gets through except a small amount of thin watery liquid. There may occasionally be incontinence of stool.

It is important to recognize that the source of this so-called "diarrhea" is actuallyobstipation, and an aggressive bowel program is indicated. A bowel history and medication review will help to separate true diarrhea from "overflow diarrhea." In the latter, the patient will report progressive worsening of constipation in the setting of medications, such as opioids, that slow gut transit. Importantly, the patient must be clearly instructed to avoid antidiarrheal agents, as that will only make the condition worse (Economou, 2010).

Nausea and Vomiting From Opioid and Other Pain Medications

Nausea is a common early side effect of opioids, but will typically improve after a few days of therapy initiation or dose increase (De La Cruz & Bruera, 2010). However, 15% to 30% of cancer patients on chronic opioid therapy continue to experience chronic nausea (Cherny et al., 2001). Persons at higher risk to develop opioid-induced nausea and vomiting include patients with a prior history, those who are constipated, or those who are receiving highly emetogenic chemotherapy (Miaskowski et al., 2008).

The clinician must keep in mind that nausea and vomiting is often multifactorial. Clinical experience reveals that patients frequently blame nausea and vomiting on the opioid therapy, when it is actually caused by other sources, such as the following (Berger & Berger, 2007; De La Cruz & Bruera, 2010; King & Dana, 2010):

- Other medications:
  - Chemotherapy
  - Antibiotics
  - Antifungals
- Physiologic processes:
  - Constipation
  - Gastroparesis
  - Dehydration
  - Ascites
  - Sepsis
  - Carcinomatosis, progression of disease involving tumor seeding in the abdominal cavity
  - Cerebral edema
  - Brain metastasis
  - Leptomeningeal carcinomatosis (spread of disease to the meninges and spinal fluid)

- Metabolic abnormalities
  - Hypercalcemia
  - Hypokalemia
  - Uremia
  - Liver failure
- Psychologic processes
  - Anxiety
  - Fear
  - Grief

Taking a careful history and being sensitive to the patient's concerns will help sort out other causes of nausea and vomiting besides the pain medication.

Strategies for management of opioid-induced nausea include the following (Berger & Berger, 2007; Harris & Kotob, 2006; King & Dana, 2010; Miaskowski et al., 2008):

- Medication:
  - Take an antiemetic 30 to 60 minutes prior to the scheduled opioid dose (e.g., prochlorperazine 5 to 10 mg PO QID, ondansetron 4 to 8 mg PO TID)
  - Metoclopramide 5 to 10 mg QID 30 to 60 minutes prior to eating to promote gastric emptying
  - Scopolamine transdermal patch 1.5 mg TID every 3 days
- Rotation to another opioid may help, as an individual may tolerate one opioid better than another
- Prevention and management of constipation
- Nonpharmacologic:
  - Take opioid with small amounts of food
  - Eat frequent, small meals
  - Complementary therapies such as deep breathing, relaxation
- Psychologic therapy
  - Management of anxiety, fear, grief
- "Tincture of time"
  - Most opioid-induced nausea and vomiting resolves spontaneously within 1 to 2 weeks

Somnolence and Fatigue From Opioid and Other Pain Medications

Somnolence (sleepiness) and fatigue (tiredness) are bothersome side effects of opioids (Hanks, Cherny, & Fallon, 2005). Other pain medications may also cause problems, these include tricyclic antidepressants (TCAs; e.g., amitriptyline, nortriptyline), serotonin–norepinephrine reuptake inhibitors (SNRIs; e.g., duloxetine, venlafaxine), dual-mechanism agents (e.g., tramadol, tapentadol), anticonvulsants (e.g., gabapentin, pregabalin), and muscle relaxants (e.g., cyclobenzaprine, methocarbamol) (de Leon-Casasola, 2006). The most troublesome effects usually improve after 1 to 2 weeks, especially if the drugs are initiated at low doses and titrated slowly. However, sedation and fatigue may continue for many weeks and may never completely resolve for some patients (Hanks et al., 2005). Patients must be advised to stop driving if are excessively sleepy. Management options for sedation and fatigue include:

- If taken only once daily, give the sedating drug in the evening or bedtime.
- For drugs taken several times daily, use asynchronous dosing if possible, with a higher dose in the evening or bedtime:
  - For example, gabapentin 100 mg in a.m., 300 mg at dinner, 900 mg at bedtime
- Slowly titrate the drug over weeks or months instead of days to weeks.
- Try a different drug in the same class:
  - For example, desipramine is less sedating than amitriptyline.
  - Pregabalin may be less sedating for some individuals than gabapentin.
- Add a psychostimulant to counteract the sedation effects. The last dose should be by 6 p.m. to prevent insomnia:
  - Caffeine (coffee, tea, soda, energy drinks)
  - Methylphenidate (Ritalin) 2.5 to 5 mg PO each morning and midday, up to 60 mg daily (Quill et al., 2010, p. 80)
  - Modafinil (Provigil) 100 mg daily PO, titrate to effect (Miaskowski et al., 2008)
  - Atomoxetine (Strattera) currently FDA approved for attention deficit disorder

Cognitive Changes From Opioid and Other Pain Medications

Similar to the adverse effects noted earlier, cognitive changes from opioid and other pain medicines are quite bothersome, and may have a profound impact on quality of life. It may prevent the cancer pain patient from being able to safely drive or function at work or home. One patient described the cognitive effects of topiramate (Topamax) for management of neuropathic pain as giving her "cotton brain," adding "my thoughts and words just get tangled up and won't come out."

It is important to recognize that cognitive impairment is common in the setting of advanced cancer, whether or not someone is receiving opioids or other sedating medication (Bruera et al., 1992). In a study by Kurita et al. (2011), one-third of patients on opioid therapy who were being treated for cancer had cognitive dysfunction. Those at highest risk were patients with lung cancer, those on morphine oral daily equivalent of more than 400 mg/day, older adults, and those with poor performance scores.

Other sources of cognitive changes include (De La Cruz & Bruera, 2010; Lawlor, 2002):

- Brain metastasis:
  - Most likely to occur in lung, breast, prostate, and melanoma cancer
- Electrolyte abnormalities and metabolic disorders:
  - Hypercalcemia, hyponatremia
- Liver failure
- Renal failure
- Sepsis
- Dehydration
- "Chemo brain"
- Sleep deprivation
- Combination with other medicines (e.g., benzodiazepines)
- Substance use (alcohol, cannabis)

Options for management of cognitive changes from opioids and other pain medications are noted in the next section. It must be emphasized that cognitive problems are usually multifactorial, and the clinician should carefully consider the contribution of many factors before changing medications (Fitzgibbon & Loeser, 2010; Harris & Kotob, 2006):

- Trial rotation to another opioid, anticonvulsant, or antidepressant.
  - Drug rotation may allow for overall decreased doses, which may improve mentation. This should be done in a sequential fashion, testing one drug at a time, not multiple drug changes at once.
- Asymmetrical dosing of opioids and other pain medications may improve cognition, with lower doses in the morning, and higher doses in the afternoon, evening, and bedtime:
  - Many patients are willing to put up with more pain in the early part of the day in order to have improved mental functioning.
- Psychostimulants (such as methylphenidate [Ritalin]; see the earlier section on fatigue and sedation)
- Dose reduction of opioid or other pain medication:
  - This should be paired with concomitant aggressive use of nonpharmacological methods of pain management (such as relaxation and breathing exercises). However, the patient must be very committed to alternate therapies to make this strategy work well.
- Change of route of opioid:
  - Intravenous to oral
  - Oral to epidural or intrathecal

▓ Interventional pain management options (Fitzgibbon & Loeser, 2010):
  ▓ Celiac plexus block for pancreatic cancer
  ▓ Superior hypogastric plexus block for pelvic organ pain (cervical, bladder, prostate, rectum)

Driving Safety

Driving safety must be addressed in all patients who are receiving sedating pain medications, especially those who complain of cognitive dulling (Ersek, Cherrier, Overman, & Irving, 2004). Indeed, some studies have suggested that *all* patients with advanced cancer, as well as all in active cancer treatment, are at risk of significant impairment in driving ability, whether taking sedating medications or not (De La Cruz & Bruera, 2010; Sjogren, Olsen, Thomsen, & Dalberg, 2000). Although some studies have shown that patients on *stable* doses of opioids for chronic *noncancer* pain may be able to drive safely (Byas-Smith, Chapman, Reed, & Cotsonis, 2005), others have shown that the reaction time may be in the range of an older adult after a stroke (Galski, Williams, & Ehle, 2000). Cancer patients have additional challenges beyond the sedating effects of opioids, such as "chemo brain," profound fatigue (which worsens cognition), and sedating premedications (such as diphenhydramine or lorazepam), all of which create risk of unsafe driving (Brandman, 2005).

Ideally, counseling regarding safe driving habits should be provided to all cancer patients while in treatment and those with advanced disease (Borgeat, 2010). However, special education should be given to patients who have the following characteristics:

▓ Those who recently had a dose increase of opioid or other sedating pain medication
▓ Those who receive diphenhydramine, lorazepam, or other sedating medications as treatment premedications
▓ Those who complain of fatigue
▓ Those who appear to have trouble staying awake during the clinic visit ("nodding off")

Specific patient education for diving safety includes the following (AAA Foundation for Traffic Safety, 2012):

▓ Do not drive if sleepy. Do not drive after receiving sedating medications such as diphenhydramine or lorazepam for chemotherapy, blood products, or procedure premedication.
▓ Do not talk on the cell phone while driving, even with a headset. Avoid talking to passenger if traffic is heavy.

- Plan driving between 10 a.m. to 2 p.m. Avoid driving during rush hour. Avoid driving after dark.
- Stick with familiar driving routes. Avoid left turns. Allow more space between the car infront of you.
- Be honest with yourself. Consider the safety of those around you on the road. If other drivers are frequently honking their horn at you, honestly assess your driving ability. Ask a family member or a neighbor to ride along and give an honest appraisal of your driving ability.
- Don't be embarrassed to ask for help if you don't feel safe driving. There may be volunteer drivers available to bring you to your oncology appointments.

Dry Mouth From Opioid and Other Pain Medications

Xerostomia (dry mouth) is a common side effect of many medications used for cancer pain management, especially opioids, as well as TCA and SNRI antidepressants. Persons who undergo surgery or radiation involving the salivary glands are likewise affected. Although some professionals may discount it as a mere trifle, dry mouth can have significant impact on a cancer patient's ability to maintain protein and calorie intake. Xerostomia impacts the ability to speak normally, results in difficulty with chewing and swallowing, causes changes in taste acuity, and leads to significant oral discomfort and ulceration (Dahlin, Cohen, & Goldsmith, 2010). Long-term use of drying medicines may increase the risk of dental caries and periodontal disease, and may increase the risk of related systemic infections (de Conno, Sbanotto, Ripamonti, & Ventafidda, 2005).

This problem does not typically improve over time. Management of xerostomia includes the following:

- Sipping liquids frequently
- Chewing sugar-free gum
- Sucking on sugar-free lemon lozenges (if tolerated)
- Frequent oral care and toothbrushing
- Saliva substitute
- Xerostomia mouthwashes
- Regular dental checkups

Lightheadedness/Dizziness and Falls From Opioid and Other Pain Medications

Older, dehydrated, and deconditioned or weak patients are more susceptible to medication side effects of lightheadedness, dizziness (vertigo), and falls (Kragh, Emlstahl, & Atroshi, 2011). This problem typically improves over time, as the body becomes more tolerant to the side effects of the drug. However, some persons never fully accommodate. Management includes the following:

- Teach the patient how to safely stand up to prevent lightheadedness (see Table 6.3).
- Plan activities to avoid walking for 30 to 60 minutes after drug administration.
- Avoid and manage dehydration.
- Avoid taking multiple drugs that cause dizziness at the same time of day; these include the following:
  - Opioids, muscle relaxants, TCA antidepressants

Table 6.3 ■ *Patient Instructions: How to Safely Stand Up From Bed When You Feel Dizzy or Weak*

1. Get ready:
   a. Have someone nearby to help if you are significantly weak or dizzy.
   b. Turn on the light, and put on your distance glasses, if you use them.
2. First, sit up:
   a. Swing your legs off the bed.
   b. Sit on your bed for 30 to 60 seconds to make sure you are not feeling dizzy or lightheaded.
   c. Put on your shoes or sturdy slippers.
   d. Grab a cane or walker, if you use it.
3. Stand but don't walk yet:
   a. Stand up at the bedside, but don't start walking yet.
   b. Wait 30 to 60 seconds to make sure you feel alright before starting to walk. (If you start to fall, the bed will be right there.)
4. Walk!
   a. Be sure to use your cane or walker.
5. Safety in the home:
   a. Prevent falls by clearing away items that may cause a stumble, such as throw rugs, electrical cords, bedding, pets, or toys.
   b. Always turn on a light, even if you are taking a quick walk to the bathroom.

SERIOUS SIDE EFFECTS OF PAIN MEDICATIONS

The nurse must be vigilant for these less common, but potentially fatal, medication side effects. Patient and family education should include advising prudence and proper reporting of adverse effects, but should be balanced to avoid alarming the patient and family to the point they refuse to take a potentially helpful medicine.

Respiratory Depression

Respiratory depression is widely cited by medical professionals as a cause of great trepidation when initiating opioid therapy. Fear of creating a problem leads to underdosing of opioids, especially by inexperienced clinicians (Elliott & Opper, 2003). Inappropriate use of naloxone to reverse mild opioid-induced respiratory depression may lead to a pain crisis, which is difficult to manage.

Two key points must be kept in mind (De La Cruz & Bruera, 2010):
- Opioid-induced respiratory depression rarely occurs in the absence of sedation.
- Pain is an antagonist to opioid-induced respiratory depression.

However, respiratory depression may indeed be a concern in certain settings. Those who are at higher risk for opioid-induced respiratory depression include the following:

- Opioid-naïve patients (those who are not taking opioids) receiving rapidly escalating doses of opioids (e.g., in a postoperative setting)
- Experiencing sudden pain relief in a patient receiving moderate to high doses of opioids (e.g., neurolytic block for cancer pain with complete relief of pain)
- Intentional overuse of opioids with other sedating drugs (e.g., benzodiazepines, muscle relaxants, alcohol) while ignoring pain relief and sedating effect
- Sleep disrupted breathing, such as obstructive or central sleep apnea

Sleep Apnea and Opioid-Induced Respiratory Depression

Opioids increase the risk of problems from sleep disordered breathing. Many patients are unaware that they have sleep apnea, but brief questioning of the patient and their bed partner can screen for those at risk:
- Moderate to loud snoring
- Periods of apnea
- Awakening feeling unrefreshed
- Daytime sleepiness
- Morning headaches
- Obesity

There are two major types of sleep disordered breathing: obstructive sleep apnea (OSA) and central sleep apnea, or a mixture of the two. It is diagnosed by consultation with a sleep specialist and sleep study. *Obstructive sleep apnea* is caused by collapse of the upper airway during sleep. It is treated with continuous positive airway pressure (CPAP), oral mandibular devices, or nasopharyngeal surgery. *Central apnea* is disordered breathing initiated at the respiratory centers of the brainstem, and is typically worsened by respiratory depressants such as opioids, alcohol, or benzodiazepines. In severe cases of central apnea, it can become quite challenging to effectively manage cancer pain with opioid therapy without concern for worsening of the respiratory condition. Advice from sleep or respiratory specialists may be required for optimal management, and the treatment team may need to consider other opioid-sparing therapies for pain management.

The oncology nurse should assess the patient on opioid therapy with a comorbidity of OSA for compliance with the prescribed treatment plan, as 46% to 83% of patients are noncompliant with CPAP (Weaver & Grunstein, 2008). In addition, patients who have lost a significant amount of weight during the cancer treatment may need to have their CPAP mask refitted. If the bed partner reports new onset or worsening of nocturnal breathing issues in the patient without known OSA, the nurse should report this to the oncologist, primary care provider, or sleep specialist, especially if the breathing issues appear to be related to higher opioid doses.

MISCELLANEOUS SIDE EFFECTS OF PAIN MEDICATIONS

Several additional adverse effects occur from opioids and other pain medicines. Although these are not life threatening, they are bothersome to patients, and may result in discontinuation or underuse of the pain medicine.

Mood Changes

Euphoria (mood elevation) is a temporary side effect of opioids which occurs in some persons from opioids. Tolerance typically develops after a few weeks, and this response disappears (Elliott & Opper, 2003). However, euphoria may occasionally lead to inappropriate use of opioids, with ingestion of the medicine for the psychoactive effect, not the analgesic effect. Euphoria tends to be more pronounced with short-acting opioids, and less so with long-acting agents.

Dysphoria is a more problematic issue from opioid use. Some patients on long-term opioid therapy develop significant low mood, even clinical depression (Rowbotham et al., 2003). Dysphoria may improve over the course of a few weeks. If not, opioid rotation may be helpful. Patients who seem significantly depressed should be assessed for suicide risk, and referred to psychiatry or social work. Consideration should be given to starting an antidepressant if low mood does not improve.

Of course, a desired effect of antidepressants for pain management is therapeutic mood elevation. SNRIs, TCAs, and SSRIs are superb at treating depression and anxiety, and can have a profound positive impact on quality of life in the person with cancer. Some patients are reluctant to take antidepressants due to stigmatization of the drugs, but may agree to take SNRIs or TCAs to target cancer-related neuropathic pain. It is not uncommon for family members to notice the positive impact the antidepressants have on mood, coping skills, and ability to deal with stressors of cancer before the patient is aware of improvement. Anticonvulsants, such as gabapentin, are occasionally used off-label in psychiatry as mood stabilizers for bipolar disorder, and may provide unexpected improvement in mood (Yatham, 2004).

Urinary Retention

Urinary retention from opioids and TCAs (used for neuropathic pain) are not uncommon, especially in older men with benign prostatic hypertrophy (Verhamme, Sturkenboom, Stricker, & Bosch, 2008). It is more common with neuraxial (epidural, intrathecal) opioid therapy, and in the opioid naïve (De La Cruz & Bruera, 2010). This can become so problematic that a visit to the emergency department is required. Patients with chronic urinary retention are at risk for pyelonephritis and kidney damage. Older men started on opioids or TCAs should be instructed to call their health care provider, or seek urgent care if they are unable to void. Screening is done with a postvoid residual (PVR) bladder scan (ultrasound) performed in the clinic. A PVR greater than 50 cc warrants urinary catheterization for a diagnostic PVR assessment. If the catheterized PVR is greater than 100 cc, an indwelling catheter should be inserted, or instructions given for intermittent catheterization every 6 hours. Consultation with a urologist should be considered, and regular follow-up with the oncology team is required. Unfortunately, physiologic tolerance to urinary retention does not develop. If the problem persists, nonpharmacological and interventional management of cancer pain should be optimized, and the offending drug dose minimized as much as possible.

Endocrine Effects, Sexual Dysfunction, and Hypogonadism (Hypotestosterone, Cessation of Menses)

Sexual dysfunction is a bothersome side effect of opioid and antidepressants. A study in 2000 by Abs et al. found a decrease in libido in 95% of the men on chronic intrathecal opioid therapy for chronic pain. A 2007 review of sexual dysfunction from antidepressants estimates the rate to be approximately 49% (Haberfellner, 2007). This includes low libido, erectile dysfunction, anorgasmia and sexual pain. Patients typically will not discuss sexual problems unless specifically asked. This reluctance may be related to societal constraints to talk about sexuality, or perhaps to feeling a sense that they should be grateful for their health and not complain. The nurse can encourage discussion by creating an open and sensitive environment in which the patient feels free to express delicate concerns.

Long-term use of opioids in chronic pain patients frequently causes hypogonadism, with hypotestosteronism in men and cessation of menses in women (Abs et al., 2000). However, in the cancer patient, the cause and effect of hypogonadism is quite difficult to distinguish from other factors, such as long-term impact of chemotherapy and other cancer treatments.

Immune System Dysfunction

Clinical effects of opioids on the human immune system are unclear (Pergolizzi et al., 2008). Morphine is known to suppress the immune system in laboratory settings without pain, but in the presence of acute pain, opioid therapy may actually be protective (Page, 2005). The impact of long-term administration of opioids on immune function in the chronic noncancer pain setting is unknown. In the cancer setting, immune function would be quite difficult to study given the typical immune suppression from cancer treatment. In her excellent review of this topic, Page suggests that adequate treatment of pain most likely overcomes any negative effects that may occur to the immune system from opioid therapy (Page, 2005).

Opioid Withdrawal Syndrome

Withdrawal symptoms may occur in any patient who abruptly stops opioid intake after taking the drug regularly for more than a few days. This phenomenon is referred to as *opioid withdrawal syndrome*. It is manifested by the following (Farrell, 1994):

- Aches and pains
- Anxiety, agitation, restlessness, insomnia
- Rhinitis (runny nose)
- Runny eyes
- "Feeling sick"
- Stomach cramps
- Yawning

▓ Piloerection ("goose bumps," from which the phrase "stopping cold turkey" arises)
▓ Hypertension
▓ Craving the opioid

Patients must be reassured that experiencing opioid withdrawal syndrome does not reflect drug addiction, but rather, is a normal physiologic reaction to the sudden cessation of opioid after several days or weeks of therapy. This is referred to as "physiologic dependence," which occurs in laboratory animals as well as in humans. It is not the same as "psychological dependence," which defines "addiction." (See Chapter 12 for definitions.)

Patient education is the key to preventing opioid withdrawal syndrome. The nurse should explain the appropriate use of opioid analgesics, anticipated patterns of use, and the importance of avoiding sudden cessation of opioids. Using direct questioning, the nurse can address patient concerns regarding the risk of true addiction. Providing written patient education, such as the National Cancer Institute's (NCI) booklet, *Cancer Pain* (NIH, 2010), will assist the nurse with defining and properly using the terms "physiologic dependence" and "tolerance" as separate phenomena from "psychological dependence" ("addiction").

Cardiac Arrhythmias

Several cardiac arrhythmias are associated with medications used for pain, and may impact the choice of drug or dose prescribed. Methadone and TCAs may prolong the QT interval on the ECG. Clinically, the QT interval, which is corrected for heart rate, is referred to as the QTc. An abnormally prolonged QTc interval is defined differently depending on the reference. The typical designation is an interval greater than 450 milliseconds (ms) in men and greater than 470 ms in women (Straus et al., 2006); or, greater than 500 ms (Pickham et al., 2012). A prolonged QTc is associated with a two-fold increased risk of sudden cardiac death (Straus et al., 2006). This may be due to an associated serious cardiac rhythm called torsades de pointes. Should this arrhythmia occur, there is high risk for degeneration into ventricular fibrillation (VF) (Pickham et al., 2012). Torsades de pointes–associated VF is very difficult to defibrillate into a viable rhythm, and is usually fatal. Certain conditions are associated with prolonged QTc interval, such as hypocalcemia, hypothyroidism, high serum creatinine, hyperglycemia, and female gender. Drugs used in oncology that may prolong the QTc include ondansetron (Zofran), levofloxacin (Levaquin), haloperidol (Haldol), and tacrolimus (Prograf).

Before starting methadone or TCAs for cancer pain management, it is prudent to check an ECG. The QTc should be rechecked 4 to 6 weeks after drug initiation, and annually thereafter. A QTc of greater than 450 ms warrants caution, and a possible dose decrease. If the QTc is greater than 500 ms, there is increased risk of fatal arrhythmia, and the methadone or TCA should be tapered and discontinued.

Opioid-Induced Myoclonus

Myoclonus is brief, involuntary muscular jerking arising from the central nervous system. It is a common initial side effect of opioid therapy, but tolerance typically develops (Glare, Walsh, & Sheehan, 2006). Although myoclonus can occur from any opioid, oral morphine is oftentimes implicated due to the metabolites M-3-glucuronide and M-6-glucuronide (Cherny et al., 2001). The meperidine metabolite normeperidine causes significant myoclonus; however, meperidine use is not recommended in cancer pain (Miaskowski et al., 2008). Myoclonus occurs more commonly in end-of-life settings, in renal disease, dehydration, and at higher doses of opioids (De La Cruz & Bruera, 2010). Treatment depends on the patient's status and the severity of the myoclonus. If the condition is mild and not problematic to the patient, no treatment is needed. For the patient with moderate to severe myoclonus who is within hours to days of death, benzodiazepines (such as lorazepam 0.5 to 1 mg PO/SL TID) will control troublesome symptoms from myoclonus (Hanks, Cherny, & Fallon, 2005). Rotation to another opioid, or decreased opioid dose, is required for management of bothersome myoclonus (Mercadante & Portenoy, 2001).

Opioid-Induced Hyperalgesia

Opioid-induced hyperalgesia (OIH) refers to a rare and curious phenomenon in which the opioid appears to worsen pain (Mercadante & Arcuri, 2005). As pain worsens, the opioid dose is increased, but pain inexplicably continues to worsen despite higher and higher doses of opioids (Davis, 2005). OIH is difficult to diagnose, especially in cases of advanced disease with progressively worsening cancer-related pain from disease progression (Mercadante, Ferrera, Villari, & Arcuri, 2003). Experimental pain research shows that a cold pain test (immersion of the arm in ice water) is the most reliable test (Krishnan et al., 2012). However, in a clinical setting, significant unexpected whole-body skin sensitivity, along with paradoxical worsening of pain with opioid dose increases, are the best indicators. The nurse must maintain an index of suspicion for OIH, especially if there does not seem to be an appropriate analgesic response to higher doses of opioids. Consultation with a pain specialist, pharmacist, or hospice medical director is needed if OIH is suspected. In addition, other causes of uncontrolled pain should be assessed, such as neuropathic pain or existential crisis.

Management of suspected OIH includes trial opioid dose reduction with addition of adjuvant analgesics, or rotation to another opioid, especially a trial of methadone (Axelrod & Reville, 2007; Mercadante & Portenoy, 2001). In severe cases, transition to the NMDA receptor antagonist ketamine may be required, with concomitant opioid reduction. Palliative sedation is also an option for end-of-life pain management in the setting of severe OIH not managed by other options. Use of ketamine and palliative sedation requires specialist consultation (Quill et al., 2010).

Other Side Effects

The additional concerning side effects of NSAID-induced gastric bleeding and renal effects, and liver toxicity from acetaminophen are covered in Chapter 3.

SUMMARY

Medications are essential for optimal management of cancer pain. However, they have significant side effects, which can impact the tolerability and compliance with therapy. These problems may be mitigated by the old adage: "start low, go slow." This means to start the medication at a low dose, and titrate the dose over weeks instead of days. If this strategy is not practical or does not work, the addition of secondary medications, such as antiemetics may help. Nonpharmacologic therapy should always be utilized concurrently for optimal cancer pain management which may result in lower medication doses, and thus, fewer side effects.

Constipation is the primary concern in opioid side effect management, as this problem never improves over time. The nurse's role is essential in educating the patient in prevention and management of this troublesome issue. Additionally, fall prevention in the older frail patient and driving safety while taking sedating medications are two important topics that nurses should address with the patient.

Joe S. is a 56-year-old Caucasian male with recently diagnosed Stage III colorectal cancer. He was prompted to seek medical care when he noted progressive weight loss, changes in bowel habits, and vague abdominal and rectal pain. He underwent a colectomy and presents to the clinic 5 weeks postoperatively to meet the oncologist. He was discharged from the hospital on oxycodone CR (Oxycontin) 10 mg twice a day and oxycodone 5 mg tablets 1 to 2 tablets every 3 hours for breakthrough pain, as needed. He has been able to reduce the short-acting oxycodone from 20 tablets per day to 10 tablets per day, but does not feel he can further decrease the short-acting opioid, as it has helped improve his chronic back pain in addition to the surgical and cancer-related pain.

You meet with Joe and his wife after the oncologist's visit to provide patient education regarding chemotherapy, pain medications, and bowel regimen. Joe's oncologist has increased his oxycodone CR to 20 mg twice a day, with continued short-acting oxycodone on an as-needed basis.

Joe reports that he had diarrhea for many weeks after surgery, but is now starting to cross over toward constipation, and is worried he will get "bound up bad" from the increase in long-acting opioid dose.

You review the importance of a bowel regimen on a regularly scheduled basis (not "as needed") to prevent opioid-induced constipation. Per clinic protocol, you instruct him to take Senekot-S (senna 8.6 mg plus docusate 50 mg) 1 to 2 tablets once or twice daily. You provide written instructions, which include information on the importance of adequate fluid intake, as well as walking daily to encourage bowel peristalsis. You discuss a contingency plan with Joe should he become severely constipated. You check on Joe 1 week later before his first dose of chemotherapy. He reports that his pain is controlled and his bowel regimen is working well.

Joe starts on a chemotherapy regimen of FOLFOX (fluorouracil with oxaliplatin) every 3 weeks. After the second cycle, he calls to report that he developed profound diarrhea for a few days, then severe constipation. He reports worsening nausea. You ask Joe to gather all of his medications together, and have his wife join them on the phone call. His wife reports that she bought an over-the-counter antidiarrheal agent, loperamide, and told Joe to stop taking all laxatives several days ago. You discover that he is still taking the loperamide even though he is now severely constipated. In addition, he was taking the constipating antiemetic ondansetron 8 mg three times a day for the nausea. He restarted his routine bowel medications only that morning.

After consultation with the nurse practitioner, you call Joe and advise him to stop the loperamide. New bowel medications are called in to the pharmacy, and he is to start taking the medications that night: docusate 250 mg capsules twice a day; senna 8.6, 2 tablets at bedtime; and polyethylene glycol (MiraLax) 17 g daily. He was instructed to administer a Dulcolax suppository 10 mg that evening, and repeat the next evening if no bowel movement occurs the next day. You encourage him to increase his fluid intake by taking small sips every 15 minutes, and to take short 10 to 15 minute walks several times a day to encourage peristalsis. Lastly, you inform him that the worsening nausea was more likely caused by severe constipation than chemotherapy at this point in the cycle. You instruct Joe that ondansetron can be quite constipating, and ask him to try taking prochlorperazine for nausea first, before a trial of ondansetron.

You reinforce the importance of remaining on a daily bowel program while taking opioid medications. You instruct him that a "roller coaster" effect is common for persons on constipating medications such as opioids and 5-HT$_3$ antagonists who then develop diarrhea for a few days after chemotherapy. You instruct him to call before taking any antidiarrheal agents, as reducing the bowel medications for a few days will generally improve the diarrhea without leading to severe constipation. You also ask him to call if he stops his bowel medications for more than 2 to 3 days.

Questions to Consider

1. You request that Joe's wife gather all of the pill bottles together and join the phone conversation. How did that strategy assist you in understanding the problem?
2. What would you suggest if the above measures do not manage Joe's constipation?

REFERENCES

AAA Foundation for Traffic Safety. (2012). *The older and wiser driver.* Retrieved from http:// www.aaafoundation.org/pdf/older&wiser.pdf

Abs, R., Verhelst, J., Maeyaert, J., Van Buyten, J., Opsomer, F., Adriaensen, H., . . . Van Acker, K. (2000). Endocrine consequences of long-term intrathecal administration of opioids. *Journal of Clinical Endocrinology & Metabolism, 85*(6), 2215–2222.

Axelrod, D., & Reville, B. (2007). Using methadone to treat opioid-induced hyperalgesia and refractory pain. *Journal of Opioid Management, 3*(2), 113–114.

Beaver, K., Latif, S., Williamson, S., Procter, D., Sheridan, J., Heath, J., . . . Luker, K. (2010). An exploratory study of the follow-up care needs of patients treated for colorectal cancer. *Journal of Clinical Nursing, 19*(23–24), 3291–3300.

Bell, T., Panchal, S. J., Miaskowski, C., Bolge, S., Milanova, T., & Williamson, R. (2009). The prevalence, severity and impact of opioid-induced bowel dysfunction: Results of a US and European patient survey (PROBE 1). *Pain Medicine, 10*(1), 35–42.

Berger, S. L., & Berger, A. M. (2007). Nausea/vomiting, anorexia/cachexia and fatigue. In E. L. L., & S. L. Librach (Eds.), *Palliative care: Core skills and clinical competencies* (pp. 115–132). Philadelphia, PA: Saunders Elsevier.

Borgeat, A. (2010). Do opioids affect the ability to drive safely? *Journal of Pain & Palliative Care Pharmacotherapy, 24,* 167–169.

Brandman, J. (2005). Cancer patients, opioids, and driving. *The Journal of Supportive Oncology, 3*(4), 317–220.

Bruera, E., Miller, L., McCallion, J., Macmillan, K., Drefting, L., & Hanson, J. (1992). Cognitive failure in patients with terminal cancer: A prospective study. *Journal of Pain & Symptom Management, 7*(4), 192–195.

Byas-Smith, M., Chapman, S., Reed, B., & Cotsonis, G. (2005). The effect of opioids on driving and psychomotor performance in patients with chronic pain. *Clinical Journal of Pain, 21*(4), 345–352.

Cherny, N., Ripamonti, C., Pereira, J., Davis, C., Fallon, M., McQuay, H., . . . Ventafridda, V. (2001). Strategies to manage the adverse effects of oral morphine: An evidence-based report. *Journal of Clinical Oncology, 19*(9), 2542–2554.

Chi, D. S., Phaeton, R., Miner, T. J., Kardos, S. V., & Diaz, J. P. (2009). A prospective outcomes analysis of palliative procedures performed for malignant intestinal obstruction due to recurrent ovarian cancer. *The Oncologist, 14*(8), 835–839.

Clark, K., Urban, K., & Currow, D. C. (2010). Current approaches to diagnosing and managing constipation in advanced cancer and palliative care. *Journal of Palliative Medicine, 13*(4), 473–476.

Clemens, K., & Klaschik, E. (2008). Management of constipation in palliative care patients. *Current Opinion in Supportive and Palliative Care, 2,* 22–27.

Cook, S., Lanza, L., Zhou, X., Sweeney, C., Goss, D., Hollis, K., . . . Fehnel, S. E. (2008). Gastrointestinal side effects in chronic opioid users: Results from a population-based survey. *Alimentary Pharmacology and Therapeutics, 27*(12), 1224–1232.

Dahlin, C., Cohen, A., & Goldsmith, T. (2010). Dysphagia, xerostomia, and hiccups. In B. Ferrell, & N. Coyle (Eds.), *Oxford textbook of palliative nursing* (3rd ed., pp. 239–267). New York, NY: Oxford University Press.

Davis, M. P. (2005). Opioid-resistant pain. In M. Davis, P. Glare, & J. Hardy (Eds.), *Opioids in cancer pain* (pp. 307–330). Oxford, England: Oxford University Press.

de Conno, F., Sbanotto, A., Ripamonti, C., & Ventafidda, V. (2005). Mouth care. In D. Coyle, G. Hanks, N. Cherny, & K. Calman (Eds.), *Oxford textbook of palliative medicine* (3rd ed., pp. 673–687). Oxford, England: Oxford University Press.

De La Cruz, M., & Bruera, E. D. (2010). Opioid side effects and management. In E. D. Bruera, & R. K. Portenoy (Eds.), *Cancer pain: Assessment and management* (2nd ed., pp. 231–254). New York, NY: Cambridge University Press.

de Leon-Casasola, O. A. (Ed.). (2006). *Cancer pain: Pharmacologic, interventional, and palliative approaches.* Philadelphia, PA: Elsevier.

Downing, G. M., Kuziemsky, C., Lesperance, M., Lau, F., & Syme, A. (2007). Development and reliablity testing of the Victoria Bowel Performance Scale (BPS). *Journal of Pain and Symptom Management , 34*(5), 513–522.

Economou, D. C. (2010). Bowel management: Constipation, diarrhea, obstruction, and ascites. In B. R. Ferrell, & N. Coyle (Eds.), *Oxford textbook of palliative nursing* (3rd ed., pp. 269–289). New York, NY: Oxford University Press.

Elliott, J., & Opper, S. (2003). Opioids: Adverse effects and their management. In H. Smith (Ed.), *Drugs for pain* (pp. 133–151). Philadelphia, PA: Hanley & Belfus.

Emanuel, L. L., & Librach, S. L. (Eds.). (2007). *Palliative care: Core skills and clinical competencies.* Philadelphia, PA: Saunders Elsevier.

Entereg-Home. (n. d.). *Entereg-dosing and administration.* Retrieved from http://www.entereg.com/content/dosing/

Ersek, M., Cherrier, M. M., Overman, S., & Irving, G. (2004). The cognitive effects of opioids. *Pain Management Nursing, 5*(2), 75–93.

Farrell, M. (1994). Opiate withdrawal. *Addiction, 89*(11), 1471–1475.

Fitzgibbon, D. R., & Loeser, J. D. (2010). *Cancer pain: Assessment, diagnosis, and management.* Philadelphia, PA: Wolters Kluwer/Lippincott, Williams & Wilkins.

Fleming, V., & Wade, W. E. (2010). A review of laxative therapies for treatment of chronic constipation in older adults. *The American Journal of Geriatric Pharmacotherapy, 8*(6), 514–550.

Galski, T., Williams, B., & Ehle, H. (2000). Effects of opioids on driving ability. *Journal of Pain and Symptom Management , 19*(3), 200–208.

Glare, P., Walsh, D., & Sheehan, D. (2006). The adverse effects of morphine: A prospective survey of common symptoms during repeated dosing for chronic cancer pain. *American Journal of Hospice & Palliative Medicine, 23*(3), 229–235.

Haberfellner, E. (2007). A review of the assessment of antidepressant-induced sexual dysfunction used in randomized, controlled clinical trials. *Pharmacopsychiatry, 40*(5), 173–182.

Hanks, G., Cherny, N. I., & Fallon, M. (2005). Opioid analgesic therapy. In D. Doyle, G. Hanks, N. Cherny, & K. Calman (Eds.), *Oxford textbook of palliative medicine* (3rd ed., pp. 316–341). Oxford, England: Oxford University Press.

Harris, J. D., & Kotob, F. (2006). Management of opioid-related side effects. In O. A. De Leon-Casasola (Ed.), *Cancer pain: Pharmacologic, interventional, and palliative approaches* (pp. 207–230). Philadelphia, PA: Elsevier.

King, C., & Dana, T. (2010). Nausea and vomiting. In B. F. Ferrell & N. Coyle (Eds.), *Oxford textbook of palliative Nursing* (3rd ed., pp. 221–238). New York, NY: Oxford University Press.

Klaschik, E., Nauck, F., & Ostgathe, C. (2003). Constipation-modern laxative therapy. *Supportive Care in Cancer, 11*(11), 679–685.

Kragh, A., Emlstahl, S., & Atroshi, I. (2011). Older adults' medication use 6 months before and after hip fracture: A population-based cohort study. *Journal of the American Geriatrics Society, 59*, 863–868.

Krishnan, S., Salter, A., Sullivan, T., Gentgall, M., White, J., & Rolan, P. (2012). Comparison of pain models to detect opioid-induced hyperalgesia. *Journal of Pain Research*, 5, 99–106.

Kurita, G., Sjogren, P., Ekholm, O., Kaasa, S., Loge, J., Poviloniene, I., & Klepstad, P. (2011). Prevalence and predictors of cognitive dysfunction in opioid-treated patients with cancer: A multinational study. *Journal of Clinical Oncology, 29*(10), 1297–1303.

Lawlor, P. G. (2002). The panorama of opioid-related cognitive dysfunction in patients with cancer: A critical literature appraisal. *Cancer, 94*(6), 1836–1853.

Lewis, S. J., & Heaton, K. W. (1997). Stool form scale as a useful guide to intestinal transit time. *Scandinavian Journal of Gastroenterology, 32*(9), 920–924.

Lipman, A., Karver, S., Austin, G., Stambler, N., & Israel, R. (2011). Methylnaltrexone for opioid-induced constipation in patients with advanced illness: A 3-month open-label treatment extension study. *Journal of Pain and Palliative Care Pharmacotherapy, 25*(2), 136–145.

Mays, T. A. (2006). Tricyclic antidepressants. In O. A. de Leon-Casasola (Ed.), *Cancer pain: Pharmacologic, interventional, and palliative approaches* (pp. 303–316). Philadelphia, PA: Elsevier.

Mercadante, S., & Arcuri, E. (2005). Hyperalgesia and opioid switching. *American Journal of Hospice and Palliative Medicine, 22*(4), 291–294.

Mercadante, S., & Portenoy, R. (2001). Opioid poorly-responsive cancer pain. Part 3. Clinical strategies to improve opioid responsiveness. *Journal of Pain and Symptom Management, 21*(4), 338–354.

Mercadante, S., Ferrera, P., Villari, P., & Arcuri, E. (2003). Hyperalgesia: An emerging iatrogenic syndrome. *Journal of Pain and Symptom Management, 26*(2), 769–775.

Miaskowski, C., Bair, M., Chou, R., D'Arcy, Y., Hartwick, C., Huffman, L., . . . Manwarren, R. (2008). *Principles of analgesic use in the treatment of acute pain and cancer pain* (6th ed.). Glenview, IL: American Pain Society.

Miles, C., Fellowes, D., Goodman, M., & Wilkinson, S. (2009). Laxatives for the management of constipation in palliative care patients (Review). *Cochrane Database of Systematic Reviews 2006*, (4). doi: 10.1002/14651858.CD003448.pub2

Mugie, S. M., Benninga, M. A., & DiLorenzo, C. (2011). Epidemiology of constipation in children and adults: A systematic review. *Best Practice & Research Clinical Gastroenterology, 25*(1), 3–18.

National Cancer Institute (NCI). (2012). *Surveillance epidemiology and end results.* Posted to SEER website 2012. Retrieved from http://seer.cancer.gov/statfacts/html/all.html

National Comprehensive Cancer Network (NCCN). (2011). *Adult cancer pain.* Retrieved from http://www.nccn.org/professionals/physician_gls/pdf/pain.pdf

National Comprehensive Cancer Network (NCCN). (n.d.). *NCCN guidelines for supportive care: Palliative care.* Retrieved from http://www.nccn.org/professionals/physician_gls/pdf/palliative.pdf

National Institutes of Health (NIH). (2010, September). *Cancer pain: Support for people with cancer.* Retrieved from http://www.cancer.gov/cancertopics/coping/paincontrol.pdf

Page, G. (2005). Immunologic effects of opioids in the presence of absence of pain. *Journal of Pain & Symptom Management, 29*(5S), S25–S31.

Pasero, C., & McCaffery, M. (2011). *Pain assessment and pharmacologic management.* St. Louis, MO: Mosby Elsevier.

Pergolizzi, J., Böger, R., Budd, K., Dahan, A., Erdine, S., Hans, G., . . . Sacerdote, P. (2008). Opioids and management of chronic severe pain in the elderly: Consensus statement of an international expert panel with focus on the six clinically most often used WHO Step III opioids (buprenorphine, fentanyl, hydromorphone, methadone, morphine, oxycodone). *Pain Practice, 8*(4), 287–313.

Pickham, D., Helfenbein, E., Shinn, J., Chan, G., Funk, M., Weinacker, A., . . . Drew, B. J. (2012). High prevalence of corrected QT interval prolongation in acutely ill patients is associated with mortality: Results of the QT in practice (QTIP) study. *Critical Care Medicine, 40*(2), 394–9.

Quill, T. E., Holloway, R. G., Shah, M. S., Caprio, T. V., Olden, A. M., & Storey, J. C. (2010). *Primer of palliative care* (5th ed.). Glenview, IL: American Academy of Hospice and Palliative Medicine.

Rosti, G., Gatti, A., Costantini, A., Sabato, A., & Zucco, F. (2010). Opioid-related bowel dysfunction: Prevalence and identification of predictive factors in a large sample of Italian patients on chronic treatment. *European Review for Medical and Pharmacological Sciences, 14*(12), 1045–1050.

Rowbotham, M., Twilling, L., Davies, P., Reisner, L., Taylor, K., & Mohr, D. (2003). Oral opioid therapy for chronic peripheral and central neuropathic pain. *New England Journal of Medicine, 348*(13), 1223–1232.

Salix Pharmaceuticals. (n. d.). *Relistor package insert.* Retrieved from http://www.salix.com/products/relistor.aspx

Sjogren, P., Olsen, A., Thomsen, A., & Dalberg, J. (2000). Neuropsychological performance in cancer patients: the role of oral opioids, pain and performance status. *Pain, 86*(3), 237–245.

Stedman's Medical Dictionary (28th ed.). (2006). Philadelphia, PA: Lippincott Williams & Wilkins.

Straus, S., Kors, J., De Bruin, M., van der Hooft, C., Hofman, A., Heeringa, J., . . . Witteman, J. C. M. (2006). Prolonged QTc interval and risk of sudden cardiac death in a population of older adults. *Journal of the American College of Cardiology, 47*(2), 362–367.

Sykes, N. (2004). Constipation and diarrhoea. In N. Sykes, P. Edmonds, & J. Wiles (Eds.), *Management of advanced disease* (4th ed., pp. 94–100). London, England: Arnold.

Sykes, N. (2005). Constipation and diarrhoea. In D. Doyle, G. Hanks, & N. I. Cherny (Eds.), *Oxford textbook of palliative medicine* (3rd ed., pp. 483–496). New York, NY: Oxford University Press.

Sykes, N. P. (2006). The pathogenesis of constipation. *The Journal of Supportive Oncology,* *4*(5), 213–218.

Thomas, J. (2008). Opioid-induced bowel dysfunction. *Journal of Pain and Symptom Management, 35*(1), 103–113.

Verhamme, K., Sturkenboom, M., Stricker, H., & Bosch, R. (2008). Drug-induced urinary retention: Incidence, management and prevention. *Drug Safety, 31*(5), 373–388.

Weaver, T., & Grunstein, R. (2008). Adherence to continuous positive airway pressure therapy: the challenge of effective treatment. *Proceedings of the American Thoracic Society, 15*(2), 173–178.

World Health Organization (WHO). (1986). *Cancer pain relief.* Geneva, Switzerland: Author.

Yatham, L. (2004). Newer anticonvulsants in the treatment of bipolar disorder. *Journal of Clinical Psychiatry, 65*(Suppl. 10), 28–35.

7

Complementary and Alternative Medicine (CAM) Techniques for Managing Cancer Pain

Yvonne D'Arcy

OVERVIEW

Complementary/alternative medicine (CAM) and integrative techniques are attractive to patients with all types of pain, including cancer pain. The techniques do not require a prescription, the patient controls use, and many have no cost or have free classes that are offered in community centers or cancer treatment centers. The focus of this type of therapy is to enhance the quality of life for the cancer patient while helping to lessen pain and symptom burden. Some of the therapies provide relaxation while others help patients to fight fatigue and control pain.

Many patients do not think to tell their oncologist or primary care provider about their use of CAM therapies and many health care providers do not ask about them. Many patients are too shy to tell their physician that they are using something that he or she has not prescribed to lessen pain. This means that CAM is being used more widely than most health care providers know and there is very little discussion about the use of CAM therapies between health care providers and patients. In order to provide holistic care for patients with cancer pain, discussing the use of a variety of techniques and developing a multimodal plan of care can produce better outcomes and greater patient satisfaction.

For many cancer patients, the use of CAM seems very comfortable. The interventions are considered to be gentle, noninvasive, and most patients with cancer supplement their traditional treatments with one or more

117

CAM therapies. While using CAM therapies, the patient is in control of the option and can sense the improvement in physical and mental well-being provided by therapies such as massage, yoga, music, and relaxation therapy.

DIFFERENCES IN TYPES OF THERAPY

The National Center for Complementary and Alternative Medicine (NCCAM) located at the National Institutes of Health (NIH) has started to examine all of the techniques, therapies, and herbal supplements that are being used in CAM therapy. They have reviewed the literature for CAM and determined that in some cases there is not enough evidence to make a solid practice recommendation, while in other cases there is enough research support to recommend some of the CAM practices. More studies are being done to support the use of various CAM therapies since their positive effect on patient outcomes has become more evident.

CAM in general is defined as "a group of diverse medical and health care systems, practices, and products not presently considered to be a part of conventional medicine" (American Pain Society [APS], 2006; Stoney, Wallerstedt, Stagl, & Mansky, 2009; Yates et al., 2005). These nutritional supplements, techniques, and therapies are really meant to enhance curative therapy, not replace it. It does highlight the need for practitioners to ask patients about their use of CAM and educate patients about the appropriate use of the techniques.

Common definitions for CAM include:

Complementary: Techniques or additional therapies that are used in conjunction with recognized mainstream medical practices; an example is using yoga or music with medication to relieve nausea or provide distraction during chemotherapy.

Alternative: This is an approach that forgoes recognized medical therapy and substitutes another form of therapy as treatment for cancer; an example is a patient who forgoes chemotherapy in favor of nutritional supplements and vitamins. This type of therapy can be harmful either directly or indirectly when patients opt to delay or not choose recommended therapies with research support (Cassileth &Gubili, 2009).

Integrative: This is a more inclusive term that CAM practitioners understand as the use of pharmacotherapy and nonpharmacological methods to enhance medical treatment. The term was first used by Dr. Andrew Weil and seems to be the most common term used for CAM therapies (NCCAM, 2004) The inclusion of both sides of the treatment options would be a preferred practice for cancer patients (Bardia, Barton, Prokop, Bauer, & Moynihan, 2006).

The NCCAM has divided the CAM therapies into four divisions, as follows:

■ **Body-based therapies** that include the use of massage, yoga, exercise, and acupuncture
■ **Mind–body approaches** that include mind–body techniques such as cognitive–behavioral approaches, relaxation, biofeedback, meditation, distraction, imagery, and self-hypnosis
■ **Energy medicine**, which includes Reiki, therapeutic touch, and healing touch
■ **Diet and nutritional approaches**, which use diet, herbs, and vitamin supplements

Some of the techniques, such as relaxation, are simple and easy to use and require little cost and training. Others, such as self-hypnosis or yoga, require training and practice to be effective adjuncts for pain relief. And some of the more complex therapies require a trained practitioner to administer the treatment, such as Reiki or acupuncture.

PREVALENCE OF CAM USE IN CANCER PATIENTS

CAM is used more widely than most oncologists or primary care practitioners who see patients with chronic cancer pain suspect. Some studies indicate that the prevalence of CAM in the cancer population ranges from 54% to 77% (Smith, 2005). In a study of 752 newly diagnosed patients with cancer, 91% reported using at least one form of CAM for symptom management during their treatment period (Yates et al., 2005). The most commonly used CAM therapies in this study were prayer, relaxation, and exercise (Yates et al., 2005). Of the 752 patients, 57% had discussed the use of CAM therapies including diet, massage, and herbal medicine with their oncologist or primary care physician (Yates et al., 2005). Findings of studies indicate that the patients receiving active treatment who are most likely to use CAM are as follows:

■ Women
■ Patients with a high school diploma or some college education
■ Patients undergoing chemotherapy rather than radiation
■ Patients diagnosed with breast cancer over other types of cancer

Overall, the use of CAM therapies for adults and children with cancer pain is growing. Many patients feel that adding some form of CAM to their treatment regimen reduces anxiety and pain while providing a holistic approach to treating their pain.

There are practice barriers to using CAM as an adjunct for pain relief. Many physicians do not have enough accurate information about CAM therapies and do not understand how to use them (Bardia, Barton, Prokop et al., 2006). The research base for some of these therapies is not fully expanded and some research indicates that some therapies perform little better than placebo (Bardia et al., 2006; Caasileth & Gubili, 2009). Guidelines such as those published by the National Comprehensive Cancer Network mention the use of CAM but fail to provide evidence-based recommendations for clinical use.

Despite the lack of research support and lack of knowledge and information about these therapies, they continue to be popular with patients. Eighty-six percent of patients who used CAM indicated they were satisfied with the therapy and the outcomes of the therapy (Cassileth & Gubili, 2009). Hopefully, the NCCAM's research analysis will provide some concrete support for CAM and help define the best practices related to implementing CAM into the clinical setting. This research analysis may help provide patients with the ability to understand how to make better use of the holistic practices to achieve a better quality of life.

Clinical Pearl	Participation in some forms of CAM therapies is limited for patients with cancer and is dependent on the physical ability, energy level, and interest of the patient in any particular therapy.

BODY-BASED THERAPY

Body-based therapies are those that are focused on moving the body or providing a treatment physically. Some of the common body-based therapies that will be discussed in this chapter are:

- Acupuncture
- Massage
- Yoga
- Aromatherapy
- Magnets/laser therapy

Although this list does not address all physical therapies, it is a good representation of what patients are asking about and using. Some of the information will be for pain in general with specific recommendations for use with cancer patients. It can also be applied to the types of pain that these patients experience that is not directly related to their cancer, but may be a chronic condition that they have had for some time or pain they experience as a result of treatment.

Acupuncture

Acupuncture comes to modern medicine from ancient Chinese healers who used the placement of needles into a person's body at specific points to regulate and restore the proper function of *Qi* (pronounced "chi") or the body's vital energy. The needles are placed in specific locations along meridians on the body and are manipulated by hand or electrically stimulated, releasing neurotransmitters that can decrease pain (D'Arcy, 2011). The end point of the treatment is to open up the blocked energy points, called *chakras*, in the body and allow the body's natural energy to flow.

There are several different types of cancer conditions where acupuncture has proved useful, as follows:

- Pain and dysfunction after neck dissection
- Radiation-induced xerostomia in head and neck cancer
- Aromatase inhibitor–associated arthralgia in breast cancer
- Hot flashes in breast cancer and prostate cancer
- (Lu & Rosenthal, 2010)

Although the literature is not fully developed for this modality, there are some findings that indicate that using acupuncture for pain relief in cancer patients may be helpful. In a 43-patient sample of breast cancer patients with arthralgia from aromatase inhibitors, both real acupuncture and sham acupuncture were measured using pain intensity ratings prior to acupuncture and after 12 sessions. Pain ratings prior to the acupuncture sessions were a mean rating of 6.7 on a 10-point pain intensity scale. After the 12 sessions, the highest score in the treatment group was 3 out of 10, and in the sham group it was 5.5 (Crew et al., 2010).

In a study for neuropathic pain after cancer treatment, 79 patients received either auricular acupuncture, placebo auricular acupuncture, or placebo auricular seeds (Hollis, 2010). In the placebo groups pain scores were higher even at 30 and 60 days (Alimi et al., 2003), leading the researchers to the conclusion that auricular acupuncture was effective for pain relief even at 60 days. Other studies have used acupuncture for head and neck pain after dissection, stomach carcinoma pain, and chemotherapy-induced neuropathy (Hollis, 2010). Overall, the studies had small sample sizes and incomplete statistical data, so the findings had less strength.

Patients seem to like acupuncture as an adjunct for pain control with cancer pain. In a critical review article, the use of acupuncture for the relief of bone pain was cited as effective. Bone pain can be the result of chemical mediators such as cytokines from tumor cells, increased pressure within the bone, microfractures, periosteal stretching, muscle spasm, or nerve compression or infiltration (Paley, Bennett, & Johnson, 2011). Rationale for using acupuncture for relief of bone pain include the following:

- Acupuncture stimulates A-delta fibers in muscle and skin, which in turn results in the release of inhibitory enkephalins and reduced neuronal activity.
- Use of electrical currents during acupuncture has been shown to reduce sensitization of postsynaptic receptors and reduces neurotransmitter release (Paley et al., 2010).

Patients with cancer may need to be treated with acupuncture several times a week, initially with needles being inserted into innervations of the affected bonezs along with the adjoining levels of innervations for optimal effect. Cancer patients are encouraged to use oncology-specialized acupuncturists.

A Cochrane Review of the acupuncture research found insufficient evidence to determine if acupuncture was effective in treating cancer pain in adults and recommended that more high-quality studies be conducted (Paley, Johnson, Tashani, & Bagnall, 2011). Despite this finding, patients continue to use the techniques to relieve pain and other troublesome symptoms.

There is a low incidence of side effects reported with acupuncture and the rare serious side effects reported were infections, bloodborne diseases, and internal organ and tissue injury (Lu & Rosenthal, 2010). For immunosuppressed cancer patients, the risk of infection and bleeding is heightened. For these reasons, patients are discouraged from using acupuncture if they fall into the following categories:

- Patients actively receiving chemotherapy or radiation therapy
- Patients with severely impaired hematologic profiles such as neutropenia or thrombocytopenia
- Patients with advanced disease with major comorbidities
- Patients with brain metastasis with central nervous system involvement (Lu & Rosenthal, 2010)

Massage

Massage can take many forms—deep tissue, Swedish, Rolfing, reflexology, and so on. For pain management, massage has been used for low back pain, neck pain, headaches, and other chronic pain conditions. NCCAM defines massage as a form of manual therapy applied by a massage therapist using his or her hands to press, rub, and otherwise manipulate the muscles and soft tissue in multiple areas of the body (NCCAM, 2004; Stoney et al., 2009). The mechanism of action for massage is thought to be the stimulation of the endogenous opiate system as well as the release of oxytocin (Stoney et al., 2009). It can also increase oxygenation and blood flow in the area being massaged, which tends to lengthen and relax muscles (NCCAM, 2004). Massage not only relieves pain but it can promote relaxation, relieve tension and anxiety, and decrease nausea for cancer patients (Cassileth & Gubili, 2009).

The literature for the use of massage therapy with cancer patients is growing and results are still inconsistent. Study sizes are small, and pain relief seems to last only into the time period directly after the massage (Bardia et al., 2006). In one of the largest CAM studies, 1,290 patients were treated with massage for 3 years. Over time, patients reported a 50% reduction in symptoms, including pain (Vickers & Cassileth, 2006). For lung cancer patients, massage therapy given by a licensed massage therapist is recommended (1 C level evidence) as part of a multimodal treatment approach (Cassileth et al., 2007). Cancer populations where massage has proved effective for relieving pain include breast and lung cancer (Cassileth et al., 2007). Practitioners can combine aromatherapy with massage, which can enhance the effect and improve the patient's experience.

The safety profile for massage in cancer patients is very good. There are many good benefits with few drawbacks. The recommendations for use of massage with cancer patients include the following (Cassileth et al., 2007):

- Avoid deep or intense pressure.
- Patients with bleeding tendencies should receive only gentle pressure massage.
- Areas with lesions or surgically created anatomical distortions should be avoided.

Some massage therapists do lymph drainage on cancer patients, most commonly breast cancer patients. Lymphedema is the subcutaneous collection of edematous fluid and adipose tissue that can be very uncomfortable (Warren, Brorson, Borud, & Slavin, 2007). For the patient with breast cancer, the fluid collects on the operative side. The use of a compression sleeve can reduce the swelling but manually controlled compression of the fluid is performed by physical therapists or massage therapists. Lymphedema can also be an unwanted side effect of normal massage therapy. Avoiding the quadrants where treatment or surgery has occurred, using a lighter touch, and monitoring the patient for the beginning of swelling can avoid the unpleasant consequence of lymphedema for the patient with cancer.

Overall, massage can be both relaxing and beneficial for patients with cancer. It can also decrease pain from immobility and can decrease pain by increasing superficial circulation. For these reasons, the American Pain

Society's Cancer Pain Guidelines (2005) recommend the use of massage for patients with cancer.

Aromatherapy

Aromatherapy uses aromatic compounds to promote health and healing (Hirsch, 2008). The most common use of these substances is through inhalation. The olfactory sense is very unique and has a connection through the olfactory nerves to the cortex of the brain. Within the olfactory bulb are neurotransmitters such as glutamate, aspartate, cholecystokinin, luteinizing hormone releasing hormone (LHRH), and somatostatin (Hirsch, 2008). By the release of neurotransmitters that affect the action of the olfactory bulb, limbic system, and olfactory tracts affecting behavior and mood (Hirsch, 2008), pleasant odors can also provide a distraction to sensory input such as pain.

Aromatherapy odors that have been used for pain relief include the following:

- Combinations of geranium, lavender, and roman chamomile
- Lemon
- Mint
- Lavender
- Combination of lavender, bergamot, sweet orange, and marjoram
- Eucalyptus
- Clary sage
- Jasmine
- Chamomile (Hirsch, 2008)

These scents can be provided using the herbs themselves or the essential oils, which are more potent. Aromatherapy can be effectively combined with massage to enhance the overall effect for the patient. For some patients, such as asthmatics or patients with breathing disorders who have reactions to certain scents, aromatherapy would not be an option.

Magnets

The benefit of magnets is said to be the increased circulation into the area where the magnet is applied or used. There is, however, little research evidence on the technique and magnets are not recommended as an adjunct technique to relieve pain (D'Arcy, 2011). Electromagnetic therapy is also discouraged due to its lack of value for cancer patients (Vickers & Cassileth, 2006).

Mind–Body Approaches

Yoga

Yoga is a popular form of exercise in the United States. The term *yoga* is derived from the Sanskrit word *yug*, which means to yoke, bind, or join (Carlson & Bultz, 2008; DiStasio, 2008). This joining was felt to be a joining of the person with the larger universe. In reality, modern yoga is a combination of physical poses with meditation (Carlson & Bultz, 2008). To perform yoga, the patient uses movement, proper breathing, and posture. There is also an element of social support since most yoga is done in groups. There are at least five different forms of yoga and some are rigorous; other forms use more gentle posturing and movements.

In general, exercise is recommended for patients with cancer to fight fatigue and manage symptoms such as mood, stress, pain, anxiety, and to improve quality of life (DiStasio, 2008). There are no current contraindications for patients with cancer who wish to participate in yoga, but each patient needs to consider his or her ability to participate, which may be limited by physical weakness or impairment or uncontrolled side effects of treatment.

Studies on the use of yoga with cancer patients have the same limitations as many of the other CAM therapies: lack of studies, few replication studies, and study flaws such as small sample sizes. In a study with 10 breast cancer patients experiencing arthralgias, the group participated in a yoga program for 8 weeks. At the end of the time period, pain reduction was modest, with ratings reduced from 3.90 to 2.79 on a 0 to 10 pain intensity scale where 0 is no pain and 10 is the worst possible pain (Galantino et al., 2011). In this study, patients had both a significant improvement in functional ability as well as increased quality of life.

In another study with 20 breast cancer patients currently in therapy, the patients engaged in a structured yoga program for 8 weeks. The yoga program included breathing exercises, relaxation, and meditation. After the program, the participants had higher scores on their quality of life, decreased anxiety, were better able to perform activities of daily living, and had a high level of satisfaction with the yoga program (Ulger & Yagli, 2010). In another study with 39 lymphoma patients, yoga was provided for seven weekly sessions. The focus of the study was sleep. At the end of the study, participants reported improved sleep-related outcomes such as improved sleep quality, longer duration, and decreased use of sleep medications (Cohen, Warnecke, Fouladi, Rodriguez, & Choul-Reich, 2004). Although these studies do not directly use pain as an outcome, if the patient has not been sleeping or has high anxiety, it can negatively affect the way the patient copes with pain.

There are some safety concerns for patients with cancer who participate in yoga, as follows:

■ Poor balance would limit participation in yoga—props such as chairs can be used to enhance safe practice for these patients.

■ For patients who are febrile, neutropenic, or with significant thrombocytopenia, vigorous exercises should be avoided and crowded classes avoided.

■ Patients should buy their own yoga mats to avoid contamination from other students who are not cancer patients.

■ Patients should listen to their own bodies; if they note any increased pain, shortness of breath, dizziness, lightheadedness, or numbness, they should come out of their yoga posture and rest and modifications should be discussed with the yoga teacher (DiStasio, 2008).

There are many positive outcomes for patients with cancer that can be achieved with the use of yoga. Nurses should be aware of the availability of yoga classes in their area and offer patients information on how to join local yoga programs.

Mind–Body Therapies/ Cognitive Behavioral Therapy (CBT)

About 75% to 90% of patients with cancer pain who implemented psychological therapies as adjunct pain relief had benefit (APS, 2005). The techniques that they used ranged from imagery, hypnosis, and coping skills to a combination of the techniques. Some of the techniques were especially helpful for procedure-related pain. A meta-analysis of the cognitive–behavioral therapies indicated that these therapies performed as good as, if not better than, placebo or no treatment (APS, 2005).

Not all patients are open to trying these techniques. For those patients who are willing to invest the time and energy in learning how to use these methods, a good outcome can be expected. For cancer patients, having the time and energy to invest in using these techniques may vary. For more compromised patients with less energy, using relaxation tapes or music might be a better fit for their particular stage of disease.

Relaxation

There are several different types of relaxation techniques that can be used to help control pain. There are various levels and types of relaxation techniques, such as the following:

■ Regulating breathing to decrease respiratory efforts

■ Relaxation tapes for progressive relaxation

■ Relaxation exercises

Relaxation techniques have been effective for decreasing pain in patients with cancer (APS, 2005). These techniques result in the reduction of physical tension, muscle relaxation, and the promotion of emotional well-being (NCCAM, 2004). Relaxation is beneficial for patients with cancer since it results in a lessening of the symptom burden, eliminates physical tension, decreases emotional stressors, and can aid sleep (Elkins, Fischer, & Johnson, 2010). Major benefits of relaxation include an improved sense of well-being and higher scores on quality-of-life scales (Dillard & Knapp, 2005).

When patients use relaxation, they are asked to either progressively relax their muscles starting from the top of the body and progressing to the lower extremities, or they can focus on one process such as controlling breathing. There are prerecorded tapes with relaxation exercises on them that patients can purchase to use at certain times of the day such as when they feel stress building or as a help for relaxing to fall asleep. The patient can keep track of progress with a pain diary or journal.

In a study comparing progressive relaxation and massage for reducing pain, the progressive muscle relaxation demonstrated greater benefit and pain relief (Anderson, Cohen, & Mendoz, 2006). Other studies had mixed results, but there was a positive correlation between relaxation techniques and improved quality of sleep for some patients with cancer (Elkins et al., 2010).

Imagery

Imagery is a form of relaxation using a mental image. It involves the use of the mind to achieve a clinical goal such as a slowed heart rate (Carlson & Bultz, 2008). When using imagery, the patient is encouraged to create a peaceful or soothing image. The patient can enjoy the feeling of comfort that the scenario provides. Images can be created by the patient or provided by tapes if the patient has difficulty developing the mental images. For example, a patient could be asked to picture a lovely warm beach. The patient is asked to hear the ocean and feel the sun on his face. He can smell the sea and feel the breeze. Sea birds can be heard in the background as the surf washes up on the beach. The patient becomes more relaxed as the scene takes over the conscious being. This image is peaceful and pleasant. The patient should choose an image that can be easily called up from memory when needed for pain relief or stress reduction.

Using imagery for pain relief can also include the use of an image that locates the area of pain, such as the abdomen. The patient can picture the abdominal pain as a red or dark color when pain is present. Working with the image, the patient can use relaxation and cognitive restructuring to see the pain leaving the abdomen, getting smaller in size, or see the color turning to a more peaceful, restful blue tone. This type of imagery is a little more complex, but patients can learn to use it effectively to help decrease pain.

For patients with cancer, using imagery coupled with other cognitive–behavioral methods will produce better results (APS, 2005). To use imagery effectively, the patient can practice in a quiet place where recalling the image is an easier task. Learning to focus on the image can help the patient relax and it will distract the patient from the pain stimulus.

Meditation or Mindfulness-Based Stress Reduction

Meditation, or focusing the mind, is a part of several different cognitive–behavioral therapies such as relaxation. It can also be combined with yoga, where a more contemplative approach is used. The definition of meditation is to focus the mind on a single target or perception (Carlson & Bultz, 2008). Although it is hard to isolate the effect of meditation, mindfulness-based stress reduction has shown positive results in decreasing the symptom burden of cancer (Carlson & Bultz, 2008).

Studies with cancer patients have shown that meditation can positively affect the following:

- Improve sleep
- Improve quality of life
- Reduce stress
- Create a spirit of appreciation for life as a meaningful process
- Improve immune function
- Relieve anxiety (Carlson & Bultz, 2008)

Although these studies were not all the result of rigorous research, they do provide insight into the benefits of using a cognitive–behavioral technique such as meditation or mindfulness-based stress reduction to add to the patient's medication regimen.

Self-Hypnosis

Self-hypnosis is a technique that requires training and practice for the patient with cancer to use it effectively. It is defined as a natural state of aroused, attentive focused concentration coupled with a relative suspension of peripheral awareness and aimed clinically at symptom relief (Carlson & Bultz, 2008). Clinically, it is defined as an altered state of consciousness, awareness, and perception (Elkins et al., 2010). The relaxed state induced by hypnosis is very beneficial for aiding in pain relief. In a randomized study with advanced stage cancer patients, hypnosis demonstrated a pain-relieving effect and allowed patients to feel more control over their environment (Elkins et al., 2010).

Not only has hypnosis been used for acute symptom control in cancer patients, it has also been found to be effective for patients with chronic cancer pain. In other studies, hypnosis has shown a good effect for controlling procedural pain in cancer patients and reducing anxiety (Carlson & Bultz, 2008). In a study of patients undergoing breast biopsy, patients who were placed into the intervention group of hypnosis had less pain and distress (Montgomery, Weltz, & Seltz, 2002). In a review of all studies on hypnosis from 1999 to 2006, hypnosis was found to reduce pain and anxiety without side effects while allowing patients to become active participants in their own comfort and well-being (Carlson & Bultz, 2008). For patients who are interested in hypnosis or self-hypnosis, a referral to a local psychologist who works with cancer patients may be beneficial and may add a strong element to the plan of care.

Music/Humor

Many patients listen to music to relax or block out noise so they can rest better. To use music as a therapy, the first question should be what type of music the patient prefers. The patient's selections can be offered using CDs or radio broadcasts.

In a randomized controlled study of music to relieve pain in cancer patients, two groups were used, one with the intervention and one control group. The study was done in China with 126 hospitalized cancer patients. In the study group, findings indicate that there was significantly less pain and distress in the group offered music (Huang, Good, & Zauszniewski, 2010). In the study group, more patients selected Taiwanese music (71%) over American music (29%) but both types were appreciated and provided reduced pain and distress (Huang et al., 2010).

Humor is also appreciated by cancer patients. Both music and humor can serve as a form of distraction for pain. Laughter can make people feel good and stimulate a feeling of general well-being (Christie & Moore, 2004). Laughter can serve as a coping mechanism, promote relaxation, and stimulate healing (Christie & Moore, 2004).

To use humor effectively, it is important to know how the patient responds to humor and what the patient finds humorous. Once preferences have been determined, providing funny videos or tapes, recalling funny incidents, looking at a funny card or picture, or just being around happy people can provide benefit.

In a study where patients either watched a humorous video or a nonhumorous video while an extremity was submerged in an ice water bath, the patients who watched the humorous video showed increased pain thresholds for 30 minutes after viewing the humorous video (Carroll et al., 2000). If the patient is open to using music or humor for relaxing and coping, it is a good way to provide a noninvasive form of therapy that most patients enjoy.

Energy Therapies

Oriental cultures have used energy healing for many centuries. The idea of channeling energy from the universe through the patient to open blocked chakras is derived from the concept of Qigong, an external and internal energy life force. In order to use these therapies with patients in modern days, several newer energy therapies were developed to include Reiki, therapeutic touch, and healing touch (Pierce, 2009). There are some differences in the practices but the overall concepts have a similar intent, as follows:

- The human body has an energy field that is generated from within the body to the outer world.
- There is a universal energy that flows through all living things and it is available to them.
- Self-healing is promoted through the free-flowing energy field.
- Disease and illness may be felt in the energy field and can be felt and changed by the healing intent of the practitioner (Pierce, 2009).

These energy therapies are effective for pain relief and relaxation. Two of the most commonly practiced are therapeutic touch and Reiki.

Reiki

The Reiki practitioner who is performing a therapeutic session on a patient uses the natural energy of the universe and channels it through the patient's body to unblock chakras, or energy points. The techniques used by Reiki practitioners were developed and taught by the Buddhist monk Mikao Usui from Japan beginning in 1914 (Pierce, 2009). In basic Reiki, the Reiki practitioner places his or her hands in specific configurations on the patient's body to channel the universal energy through the chakras, opening up blocked points. In more advanced levels of practice, a Reiki practitioner transmits energy long distances to benefit a specific person (NCCAM, 2004).

Reiki has been used in Eastern cultures to ease both the mind and body. There are three levels of Reiki practice. Each level includes some additional form of energy transfer. Even with the basic level, the patient feels relaxed and experiences emotional and physical healing. The

Reiki practitioner who channels the energy for the patient also receives benefit: The practitioner may feel more relaxed and in tune with his or her own body energy after the session is completed.

Studies to determine the benefit of Reiki have focused on patients with cancer. In a study with 24 cancer patients using Reiki or rest periods, the Reiki patients had a significant decrease in pain (Pierce, 2009).

Therapeutic Touch

Therapeutic touch originated in the 1970s as a collaboration between two women, Dolores Krieger and Dora Kunz. The practice was based on similar concepts as Reiki. Although the two originators hoped that therapeutic touch would become a part of standard patient care, it has proved to be more difficult to operationalize than anticipated (Pierce, 2009). At this time, the practice remains a nonstandard addition to patient care, although it is popular in some areas of the country.

Therapeutic touch is a form of energy medicine where the practitioner does not touch the patient receiving the therapy, but rather focuses the energy on the patient's aura. Smoothing the aura by the energy transfer from the practitioner to the patient can help provide healing energy. It is often mistakenly referred to as "laying on of hands," which has a more religious connotation. The premise of therapeutic touch is that the practitioner's healing force transfers or channels energy, thereby positively affecting the patient's recovery (NCCAM, 2004). As the therapeutic touch practitioner allows his or her hands to move over the patient, blocked energy is identified and, through the practitioner's hands, healing forces are directed to the area to promote healing and pain relief.

There are some studies that indicate greater pain relief with the use of therapeutic touch in patients with chronic pain and fibromyalgia when compared to patient groups not receiving the energy treatment option (Pierce, 2009). It is difficult to conduct randomized placebo-controlled studies with therapeutic touch, and therefore is hard to measure the true effect of the practice.

Nutritional Therapy

Most American homes have some type of home remedy or homeopathic treatment that they use to treat minor pain and aches. Most patients do not think about telling their physician that they use it. The reasons for nondisclosure include thinking it is just an over-the-counter herbal or supplement, not "true medicine," and a potential embarrassment.

For the patients with cancer, it is important to explore the use of these substances; therefore, questioning the patient about their use of herbals, supplements, and homeopathic remedies should be a part of the interview and follow-up process. Research indicates that only 40% of patients who are using these substances discuss it with their physicians or health care providers (Micozzi, 2008). For cancer patients, up to 60% of patients use herbal supplements during or after therapy (Cassileth & Gubili, 2008). For this patient population, however, the risk of medication interaction becomes an extremely serious issue. A study of anesthesiologists in the United Kingdom indicated that 65% felt that there was potential for harmful effects with surgical patients and 82% of them felt that they had inadequate knowledge of herbal remedies (Micozzi, 2008). It has also become a bigger issue since reliable resources for information on medication interactions and effects on cancer treatments are limited.

In a qualitative study with six focus groups with six to eight patients each already taking herbal remedies, researchers explored the use of herbal preparations, sources for information on the use of these supplements, and what information would be helpful for these patients (Gratus et al., 2009). Findings indicated the following:

- Support groups and family and friends are the most common sources of advice on herbal medication.
- Very few patients trust the Internet as a source of information or support.
- Accessible, interpretable, and reliable information materials need to be developed for patients, use in critical decision making regarding the use of herbal medicines (Gratus et al., 2009).

Herbal Supplements

The use of herbal supplements by patients with cancer is driven by the need for symptom control, quality of life, and fears of cancer recurrence (Cassileth et al., 2008). To use a botanical agent in an herbal supplement, either raw ingredients, juices, resins, or oils are mixed potentially with other materials with questionable quality control. There is also a high reliance on the quality of the plant itself. There are also questions as to where it was grown and what was applied to the plant (e.g., herbicides). One interaction that was problematic for patients with cancer undergoing chemotherapy was the use of St. John's wort for depression while on chemotherapy. St. John's wort induces the cytochrome p450 3A4, which is the enzyme responsible for metabolism of many different drugs, including chemotherapy (Cassileth et al., 2008).

Other herbal supplements without value to patients with cancer include the following:

- Essiac: An herbal compound developed by a native healer and promoted by a Canadian nurse. It contains four herbs—burdock, turkey rhubarb, sorrel, and slippery elm. The NCAAM research group found no cancer benefits for the compound and that an adverse effect was the stimulation of breast cancer cells.
- Kava: Although shown to be more effective in treating anxiety, stress, and insomnia, it also had the unwanted effect of fatal hepatotoxicity.
- Dong quai and licorice: These have phytoestrogen activity, which adversely affects the chemotherapeutic action of aromatase inhibitors and tamoxifen.
- Iscador (mistletoe extract): Despite frequent use in Europe, there have been no definitive studies that show positive effect with the use of the botanical (Cassileth & Gubili, 2008; Vickers & Cassileth, 2006).

There is one botanical that is commonly used for pain that cancer patients could use for chemotherapy- or treatment-induced neuropathy. Topical capsaicin is an over-the-counter drug that comes in two strengths: 0.025% and 0.075%. The amount of the active ingredient in the cream is very small because the cream can have an intense burning sensation when applied.

Capsaicin is the active ingredient in cayenne peppers (Khatta, 2007). It can be made into plasters or applied as a cream over the painful area. The patient needs to use the cream four times a day for 2 weeks to expect any change in the pain (D'Arcy, 2011). Patients should use gloves when applying the cream to avoid any contact with other areas of the body.

The use of capsaicin is recommended for neuropathic pain of all types. This includes the following:

- Painful diabetic neuropathy
- Postherpetic neuralgia
- Fibromyalgia
- Cluster headaches
- Postmastectomy pain syndrome
- Cutaneous pain associated with skin tumors
- Postamputation stump pain (Micozzi, 2008)

Vitamins

The use of vitamins in patients with cancer also can be controversial. Riboflavin, magnesium, vitamin E, and thiamine are all used for a variety of noncancer pain types. However, when the patient has cancer, there are more considerations about adding a benign-looking substance that can have unwanted adverse effect on therapy and outcome.

For patients with breast cancer, vitamin D deficiency can be associated with bone loss, arthralgias, and falls (Peppone et al., 2011). Research data also suggest that vitamin D deficiency is associated with an increased incidence of breast cancer (Abbas et al., 2008). In a retrospective study with 224 women diagnosed with breast cancer, baseline vitamin D levels were obtained for all patients. Approximately 66.5% had vitamin D deficiencies at baseline. Those patients with low vitamin D levels had an increased rate of low spinal bone mineral density. Findings indicate that patients with breast cancer should receive careful supplementation of vitamin D to avoid arthralgias, injury from falls, and bone loss (Peppone et al., 2011).

Dangers with the use of vitamins and supplements include the following:

- Metabolic interactions affecting the action of the cytochrome P450 3A4 pathways
- Antioxidant action that occurs with ingestion of antioxidants such as grape seed extract can have the effect of suppressing chemotherapy-induced apoptosis
- Hormonal effects such as those seen with soy products that affect antiestrogen therapies such as tamoxifen or raloxifene (Vickers & Cassileth, 2006)

Herbal supplements can upregulate unwanted substances: pgp-170, which is a multidrug-resistant transporter in several recognized cancer cell lines and for patients having surgery; and garlic and vitamin E, which increase the potential for bleeding (Vickers & Cassileth, 2006). It is for this reason that for patients undergoing active treatment, it is suggested that they avoid supplements and vitamins. For lung cancer patients, it is specifically recommended that use of botanical agents occurs solely within clinical trials (Cassileth et al., 2007). All patients with cancer who are interested in botanicals or vitamins should discuss this carefully with their oncologist or other physician to avoid counterproductive and harmful effects.

One of the strongest recommendations for patients is to exercise and eat a healthy diet as a means of helping to control symptoms and reduce adverse effects of therapy (APS, 2005).

SUMMARY

Cancer patients can benefit from the adjunctive use of CAM therapies if the patient has fully discussed their use with their physician. Herbals and vitamins should never be used without consulting the physician to determine what adverse effects are possible, while other therapies like yoga or exercise can be helpful and are noninvasive. Since so many patients admit that they use these techniques, health care providers should always include a discussion about these techniques in their patient interactions to determine just what types of therapy the patient is interested in using. Combining these techniques into a multimodal plan of care can help the patient better manage pain, increase quality of life, and relieve stress and anxiety.

Case Study

Susan J. is a 50-year-old patient who is undergoing chemotherapy for breast cancer. She finds the treatment very hard to tolerate and hopes there is something she can use for both treatment and symptom control that is not so hard on her body. She comes in to her usual appointment and asks about some complementary therapies she learned about over the Internet. She wants to know about the use of relaxation techniques and replacing the chemotherapy with natural cancer-fighting agents such as mistletoe extracts. She likes music but has no interest in acupuncture. Her pain is always in the moderate level 4 to 6/10 at the surgical site of her lumpectomy and she has recurrent nausea. What kinds of therapies can you suggest and what kind of information does Susan need to know?

Questions to Consider

1. As with any addition to the treatment regimen, doing a risk–benefit analysis is a good start. What would you say about Susan's requests?
2. What are some positive forms of CAM therapy that you could suggest to Susan?
3. How will you educate Susan about CAM therapies and how to use them effectively?

REFERENCES

Abbas, S. Lineseisen, J., Slanger, T., Kropp, S., Mutschelknauss, E., Flesch-Janys, D., & Chang-Claude J. (2008). Serum 25-hydroxyvitamin D and risk of post-menopausal breast cancer—Results of a large case-control study. *Carcinogenesis, 29*, 93–99.

Alimi, D., Rubino, C., Pichard-Leandri, E., Fermand-Brulee, S., Dubreuil-Lemarie, M., & Hill, C. (2003). Analgesic effect of auricular acupuncture for cancer patients: A randomized blinded controlled trial. *Journal of Clinical Oncology, 21*, 4120–4126.

American Pain Society (APS). (2006). *Pain control in the primary care setting.* Glenview, IL: Author.

Anderson, K., Cohen, M., & Mendoz, T. (2006). Brief cognitive behavioral audiotape interventions for cancer related pain. *Cancer, 107*, 207–214.

Bardia, A., Barton, D., Prokop, L., Bauer, B., & Moynihan T. (2006). Efficacy of complementary and alternative medicine therapies in reliving cancer pain: A systematic review. *Journal of Clinical Oncology, 24*(34), 5457–5464.

Carlson, L., & Bultz, B. (2008). Mind-body interventions in oncology. *Current Treatment Options in Oncology, 9*, 127–134.

Carroll, J., Gray, R., Orr, V., Chart, P., Fitch, M., & Greenberg, M. (2000). Changing physicians' attitudes toward self-help groups: An educational intervention. *Journal of Cancer Education, 15*, 14–18.

Cassileth, B., Deng, G., Gomez, G., Johnstone, P., Kumar, N., & Vickers A. (2007). Complementary therapies and integrative oncology in lung cancer: The ACCP evidence based clinical practice guidelines. *Chest, 132*, 340S–S345.

Cassileth, B., & Gubili, J. (2009). Integrative oncology: Complementary therapies in cancer care. In *Cancer and drug discovery development: Supportive care in cancer therapy* (pp. 269–277). Totowa, NJ: Humana Press.

Christie, W., & Moore, C. (2005). The impact of humor on patients with cancer. *Clinical Journal of Oncology Nursing, 9*(2), 211–218.

Cohen, L., Warnecke, C., Fouladi, R., Rodriguez, M., & Choul-Reich, A. (2004). A psychological adjustment and sleep quality in a randomized trial of the effects of a Tibetan yoga intervention in patients with lymphoma. *Cancer, 100*(10), 2253–2260.

Crew, K., Capodice, J., Greenlee H., Brafman, L., Fuentes, D., Awad, D., . . . Hershman, D. L. (2010). Randomized, blinded, sham-controlled trial of acupuncture for the management of aromatase inhibitor-associated joint symptoms in women with early stage breast cancer. *Journal of Clinical Oncology, 28*(7), 1154–1160.

D'Arcy, Y. (2011). *Compact clinical guide to chronic pain.* New York, NY: Springer Publishing.

Dillard, J., & Knapp, S. (2005). Complementary and alternative pain therapy in the emergency department. *Emergency Medical Clinics of North America, 23*, 529–549.

DiStasio, S. (2008). Integrating yoga into cancer care. *Clinical Journal of Oncology Nursing, 12*(1), 125–130.

Elkins, G., Fisher, W., & Johnson, A. (2010). Mind-body therapies for integrative oncology. *Current Treatment Options in Oncology, 11*, 128–140.

Galantino, M., Desai, K., Greene, L., DeMichele, A., Stricker, C. T., & Mao, J. J. (2011). Impact of yoga on functional outcomes in breast cancer survivors with aromatase çinhibitor-associated arthralgia. *Integrative Cancer Therapies.* doi:10.1177/1534735411413270

Gratus, C., Wilson, S., Greenfield, S., Damery, S., Warmington, S., Greive, R., & Routledge, P. (2009). The use of herbal medicines by people with cancer: A qualitative study. *BMC Complementary and Alternative Medicine, 9*(14), 1–7.

Hirsch, A. (2008). Aromatherapy. In M. Weintraub, R. Mamtani, & M. Micozzi., *Complementary and integrative medicine in pain management.* Philadelphia, PA: Springer Publishing.

Hollis, A. (2010). Acupuncture as a treatment modality for the management of cancer pain: The state of the science. *Oncology Nursing Forum, 37*(5), E344–348.

Huang, S. T., Good, M., & Zauszniewski, J. A. (2010). The effectiveness of music in relieving pain in cancer patients: A randomized controlled trial. *International Journal of Nursing Studies, 47.* 1354–1362.

Khatta, M. (2007). A complementary approach to pain management. *Topics in Advanced Practice Nursing e-Journal, 7*(1). Retrieved from http://www.medscape.com/viewarticle/556408

Lu, W., & Rosenthal, D. (2010). Recent advances in acupuncture and safety considerations in practice. *Current Treatment Options in Oncology, 11,* 141–146.

Micozzi, M. (2008). Herbal remedies and micronutrients. In M. Weintraub, R. Mamtani, & M. Micozzi., *Complementary and integrative medicine in pain management.* Philadelphia, PA: Springer Publishing.

Montgomery, G., Weltz, C., & Seltz, M. (2002). Brief presurgery hypnosis reduces distress and pain in excisional biopsy patients. *International Journal of Clinical Experiments in Hypnosis, 50,* 17–32.

National Center for Complementary and Alternative Medicine (NCCAM). (2004). *NCCAM-funded research for 2003.* Retrieved from http://nccam.nih.gov/research

Paley, C., Johnson, M., Tashani, O., & Bagnall, A. (2011). Acupuncture for cancer pain in adults. *The Cochrane Database of Systematic Reviews 2011,* Volume 1.

Paley, C., Bennett, M., & Johnson, M. (2010). Acupuncture for cancer induced bone pain. *Evidence-Based Complementary and Alternative Medicine.* doi: 10.1093/ecam/neq020

Peppone, L., Huston, A., Reid, M., Rosier, R., Zakharia, Y., Trump D., . . . Morrow, G. (2011). The effect of various vitamin D supplementation regimens in breast cancer patients. *Breast Cancer Research and Treatment, 127,* 171–177.

Pierce, B. (2009). A non-pharmacologic adjunct for pain management. *The Nurse Practitioner, 34*(2), 10–13.

Smith, A. (2005). Opening the dialogue: Herbal supplementation and chemotherapy. *Clinical Journal of Oncology Nursing, 9*(4), 447–450.

Stoney, C., Wallerstedt, D., Stagl, J., & Mansky, P. (2009). The use of complementary and alternative medicine for pain. In *Biobehavioral approaches to pain* (pp. 381–408). New York, NY: Springer Science and Business Media.

Ulger, O., & Yagh, N. (2010). Effects of yoga on the quality of life in cancer patients. *Complementary Therapies in Clinical Practice, 16,* 60–63.

Vickers, A., & Cassileth, B. (2006). Principles of complementary and alternative medicine for cancer. *Oncology,* section one, 194–203.

Warren, A., Brorson, H., Borud, L., & Slavin, S. (2007). Lymphedema: A comprehensive review. *Annals of Plastic Surgery, 59*(4), 464–472.

Yates, J., Mustian, K., Morrow, G., Gilles, L., Padmanabhan, D., Atkins, J., . . . Colman, L. (2005). Prevalence of complementary and alternative medicine use in cancer patients during treatment. *Supportive Care in Cancer, 13,* 806–811.

Infusions and Regional Techniques

Yvonne D'Arcy

RATIONALE FOR USE OF REGIONAL ANALGESIA

For some patients with cancer, there is a need for more aggressive types of pain management because oral medications alone do not provide the desired analgesic level. Regional techniques can be used at the beginning of pain therapy during a surgical procedure, or with cancer survivors who have chronic pain. These techniques would include both epidural injections, local anesthetic infusions, blockade, and implanted techniques. (Information on blocks and implanted therapies is given in Chapter 9.) Most of these techniques are used by anesthesia providers either in hospitals for acute care or in pain clinics for outpatient treatment. Using multiple techniques to control pain can have synergistic effects that single therapies cannot provide.

Cancer pain can come from a variety of sources—tumor growth, nerve impingement, or treatments such as chemotherapy. Some patients with cancer have surgery and pain control is important during that period of time; while a cancer survivor may have residual pain from the disease or treatments that can be more effectively treated with combination medication and interventional options.

The use of regional anesthesia has been recommended by the American Society of Anesthesiologists (ASA, 2004) as a means of extending the superior pain management of the operating room. There are several techniques that are used: intraoperative neural blockade (a one-time procedure), epidural catheters, and continuous peripheral nerve or wound catheters. Patients with cancer who have tumor resections, thoracotomies for lung cancer, or amputations for bone cancer can all benefit from using a combination of techniques to provide analgesia.

139

By using a block with local anesthetic, or a continuous local anesthetic infusion, opioid use can be minimized in the postoperative setting, resulting in fewer adverse effects such as nausea and vomiting. The level of pain relief with a regional analgesia technique is superior to opioids alone and reduces opioid-related side effects such as nausea, vomiting, sedation, and pruritis (LeWendling & Enneking, 2008; Liu & Salinas, 2003; Richman et al., 2006). Pain relief and functionality are improved with the use of peripheral catheters (PCs) with local anesthetic and functionality has been reported as improved with PCs (Rosenquist & Rosenberg, 2003). There is also some indication that the use of regional anesthesia, epidurals, and regional analgesia (via PCs) has a positive impact on mortality and morbidity with high-risk patients (Hanna, Murphy, Kumar, & Wu, 2009).

The current-day anesthesia provider has many more options for increasing the effectiveness of postoperative analgesia by extending the controlled anesthetic and analgesic techniques of the operating room into the postoperative time period. Using single injections for regional blockade and inserting PCs that can provide extended adjunct pain relief can help the surgical patient recover faster with fewer side effects.

Intraoperative Blockade

For patients with cancer, having adequate pain relief after surgery can be an effective means of providing a better quality of life and relieving fears of pain that cannot be controlled. Postoperative one-time blocks can last for up to 24 hours, but tend to wear off in that relatively short period of time (Hurley, Cohen, & Wu, 2010). The use of epinephrine in the block solution can help extend the action of the block.

Solutions that are used for blocks are local anesthetics. For example, 2% lidocaine and 1.5% mepivacaine have a rapid onset combined with a short duration of action (Wallace & Staats, 2005). Another example is 0.5% bupivacaine, 0.75% ropivacaine, and 0.5% levobupivacaine, which have extended action but a slower onset time (Wallace & Staats, 2005).

These single-dose intraoperative blocks can be placed in a wide variety of surgical locations. The blocks are designed to provide lack of sensation in the surgical area and they are done with a local anesthesic such as bupivacaine that can have an extended action if epinephrine is included in the block solution.

Areas that commonly are used for blockade include those in the following section.

Axillary

This block is used for upper extremity surgery such as procedures of the forearm, wrist, hand, chronic pain syndromes, and vascular diseases. It blocks the terminal branches of the brachial plexus.

Interscalene

This block is commonly used for open shoulder surgery, rotator cuff repair, acromioplasty, shoulder arthroplasty, and proximal upper limb surgery (May & DeRuyter, 2009). The block performed is a brachial plexus block. When performed as a surgical adjunct, this block may not produce analgesia for the ulnar nerve and the loading bolus may produce phrenic nerve block. The patient can develop hoarseness from laryngeal blockade as well as Horner's syndrome as a result of sympathetic blockade.

Femoral

The femoral block is commonly used for surgeries of the knee and femur. Anesthesia of the anterior thigh, femur, and most of the knee joint is produced with blockade. It can be combined with a sciatic block, which effectively blocks both the anterior and posterior aspects of the knee. These blocks have been most effective when a continuous local anesthetic infusion is used, leading to improved patient outcomes and fewer side effects in the postoperative time period. Careful assessment is needed to determine if there is muscle weakness in the lower extremity, primarily quadriceps muscle weakness, from the block before getting the patient out of bed, to avoid buckling of the extremity. Some of the more important patient outcomes when this block is used are increased ability to move the surgical joint, opioid sparing, decreased side effects such as postoperative nausea and vomiting, and increased patient satisfaction.

Sciatic

Sciatic blocks provide anesthesia to the skin of the posterior thigh, hamstring, biceps muscle and part of the hip and knee joint, and the entire leg below the knee with the exception of the skin of the lower leg. It can be combined with a femoral block for knee surgery or lumbar plexus block for hip and femur surgery (Indelli, Grant, Neilsen, & Parker, 2005).

Thoracic Paravertebral

The thoracic paravertebral block is commonly used for surgeries of the breast, chest wall, and abdominal surgeries. For patients with cancer, using this type of technique intraoperatively for mastectomy or thoracotomy can decrease the severity of postoperative pain. Other uses for this type of block include anesthesia and/or analgesia for herniorrhaphy, iliac crest bone grafts, soft tissue mass excisions and analgesic adjunct for laparoscopic surgery, cholecystectomy, nephrectomy, appendectomy, thoracotomy, obstetric analgesia, minimally invasive cardiac surgery, and hip surgery. Positive patient outcomes with this type of block include reduction in pain scores, opioid-sparing effect, decreased postoperative nausea and vomiting, and decreased length of stay (May & DeRuyter, 2009; Melton & Liu, 2010; Wallace & Staats, 2005).

Peripheral Catheters (PCs) for Postoperative Analgesia

In certain patient populations such as orthopedic patients where high levels of pain are expected, using opioid medications in the PC infusion has become accepted practice. Patients with cancer requiring orthopedic surgery can benefit from using this technique to reduce pain after the surgery. PCs can also be placed as a *soaker hose* configuration along large incisions such as thoracotomy and large abdominal surgeries. During surgery, the catheter is inserted into the area where blockade is desired. The additional option of a patient-controlled button device can allow the patient to provide a bolus dose of medication when needed.

Most PCs use some type of infusion device to provide continuous flow. One example is the On-Q pump, an elastomeric device that can be configured to deliver a preset rate of continuous flow but also allows the patient to self-administer a bolus dose (see Figure 8.1).

Placement of PCs

In order to place a PC, the anesthesia provider uses a hollow Touhy-type needle connected to a nerve stimulator or an ultrasound. Once placement has been confirmed, the provider threads the catheter down the hollow center of the needle to the area that needs analgesia. To test placement, the provider confirms location with one of two techniques.

■ Nerve stimulator (NS): To locate the correct site for placement using a nerve stimulator, the anesthesia provider uses a short, beveled, Teflon-coated needle inserted into the area for blockade attached to a nerve stimulator with a pulse duration of 0.15 ms. The correct nerves are located by the twitches elicited by the stimulation. The stimulation intensity is reduced after the block is injected, then the catheter is inserted and the needle is removed.

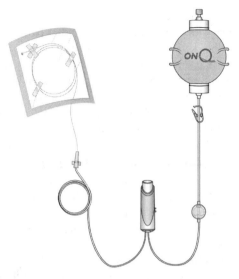

Figure 8.1 ■ ON-Q pump. *Source:* Used
by permission of I-Flow Corp.

■ Ultrasound (US) guided peripheral nerve block: To locate the correct
site for placement with US, a short, beveled, Teflon-coated needle is
inserted into the area for blockade so that the entire shaft of the needle is in the US beam and both the shaft and the tip of the needle
are visualized. Once the site is located, the injection is completed and
the catheter is threaded through the needle. Spread of local anesthetic
is confirmed with continuous sonography (Fingerman, Benonis, &
Martin, 2009).

The onset of blockade with US has been reported as faster compared
with the older nerve stimulation technique. The use of ultrasound is a
grade A recommendation, with level 1b evidence, because it improves onset and success of sensory blockade, decreases local anesthetic needs, and
decreases time to achieve lower extremity blockade (Salinas, 2010). Ultrasound imaging may not be reliable if there is tissue damage in the neigh-
boring structures, resulting in inadequate analgesia in a small number of
patients (LeWendling & Enneking, 2008). Nerves that can be blocked
using continuous local anesthetic infusion after surgery include those that
were described earlier for block locations.

The risk of using a PC is very low. Nerve injury with blocks is estimated to be 0% to 10% with upper extremity single-shot blocks and 0.5% with lower extremity blocks (Melton & Liu, 2010). Systemic local anesthetic toxicity is reported as rare (Bleckner et al., 2010). Pneumothorax rates are reported as low with both interscalene and paravertebral blocks. Infections with blocks and catheters are rare. The American Society of Regional Anesthesia and Pain Management (ASRA) has recommended the use of aseptic technique for catheter placements with monitoring for infections (2002).

Patient-Controlled Analgesia (PCA) and Infusions

Some patients need intravenous opioids after cancer surgery. In some cases, the patient has breakthrough pain with such rapid onset that PCA is preferred for opioid analgesia. In other cases, the patient with cancer may not have an oral route available and using a PCA can provide analgesia. In some instances, end-stage patients with cancer will need continuous infusions of opioids to control pain and PCAs are used either through an intravenous access or placed subcutaneously. Home health or hospice agencies provide medications and technical support at home so that the patient can receive medications via a PCA. For end-stage patients who need large amounts of medication, using higher concentrations of medications such as morphine 5 mg/mL or morphine 20 mg/mL can help control the pain despite increased need.

Epidural Catheters

Although epidural catheters are used for analgesia in the postoperative setting, they can also be useful for specific types of pain that are more long term. Rectal pain is particularly difficult to treat in some patients and using a epidural catheter placed very low in the spine can provide a blockade that can reduce the pain to a tolerable level. Combinations of preservative free morphine or hydromorphone along with local anesthetic are most commonly used for this technique. For some of these patients, the unremitting pain urge to defecate can destroy quality of life. Using an epidural catheter for pain relief in these patients can improve the quality of analgesia and allow the patient to have a higher level of overall functioning.

For some patients, a tunneled epidural catheter can be placed to provide extended pain relief and improve quality of life. The epidural catheter is tunneled away from the spine several inches, and a clear occlusive dressing is placed over the insertion site. The medication is given via a small patient controlled delivery device. This type of catheter placement can last for up to thirty days.

Case Study

Casey J., 42, has been diagnosed with a sarcoma in his left lower extremity that will need below-knee amputation. He is concerned about his pain relief after surgery. He has read about phantom limb syndrome and wonders if there is something that can be done to minimize the potential for this. He discusses the analgesic treatment options with the anesthesiologist and they decide to use a continuous infusion of local anesthetic to reduce the potential for the occurrence of phantom limb syndrome. However when you see him 2 weeks after his surgery, he tells you, "I can still feel the foot on the leg that was amputated. It feels funny and tingly sometimes and other times it feels like I can move it. Overall though, the pain was really not as bad as I expected."

Questions to Consider

1. Amputation is an aggressive measure to remove the cancer and surrounding tissue. There is nociceptive pain at the surgical site and often neuropathic pain. What type of pain is Casey experiencing?
2. Would opioids alone have relieved the pain to the extent that the patient experienced after his surgery?
3. Would the use of intraoperative blockade or PC have made any difference in the outcome of Casey's surgery?
4. Could you combine an epidural catheter with a PC?

REFERENCES

American Society of Anesthesiologists Task Force on Acute Pain Management. (2004). Practice guidelines for acute pain management in the perioperative setting. *Anesthesiology, 100*(6), 1573–1581.

American Society of Regional Anesthesia and Pain Management (ASRA). (2002). *Consensus statement: Regional anesthesia in the anticoagulated patient: Defining the risks.* Retrieved from http://www.asra.com/consensus-statement/2.html

Bleckner, L., Bina, S., Kwon, K., McKnight, G., Dragovich, A., & Buckenmaier, C. (2010). Serum ropivacaine concentrations and systemic local anesthetic toxicity in trauma patients receiving long-term continuous peripheral nerve block catheters. *Regional Anesthesia, 110*(2), 630–634.

Capdevila, X., Bringuier, S., & Borgeat, A. (2009). Infectious risk of continuous peripheral nerve blocks. *Anesthesiology, 100*, 182–188.

Casati, A., Danelli, G., Baciarello, M., Corradi, M., Leone, S., DiCianni, S., & Fanelli, G. (2009). A prospective, randomized comparison between ultrasound and nerve stimulation guidance for multiple injection axillary brachial plexus block. *Survey of Anesthesiology, 53*(4), 186–189.

Fingerman, M., Benonis, J., & Martin, G. (2009). A practical guide to commonly performed ultrasound-guided peripheral-nerve blocks. *Current Opinion in Anesthesiology, 22*, 600–607.

Hanna, M., Murphy, J., Kumar, K., & Wu, C. (2009). Regional techniques and outcome: What is the evidence? *Current Opinion in Anesthesiology, 22*, 672–677.

Hurley, W., Cohen, S., & Wu, C. (2010). *Acute pain in adults in Bonica's management of pain* (pp. 699–751). Philadelphia, PA: Lippincott Williams & Wilkins.

Ilfeld, B., Le, L., Ramjohn, J., Loland, V., Wadhwa, A., Gerancher, J., . . . Mariano, E. (2009). The effects of local anesthetic concentration and dose on continuous intraclavicular nerve blocks: A multicenter, randomized, observer-masked, controlled study. *Regional Anesthesia, 108*(1), 345–350.

Indelli, P. F., Grant, S., Neilsen, K., & Parker, T. (2005). Regional anesthesia for hip surgery. *Clinical Orthopedic and Related Research, 441*, 250–255.

LeWendling, L., & Enneking, F. K. (2008). Continuous peripheral nerve blockade for postoperative analgesia. *Current Opinion in Anesthesiology, 21*, 602–609.

Liu, S., & Salinas, F. (2003). Continuous plexus and peripheral nerve blocks for postoperative analgesia. *Anesthesia & Analgesia, 96*(1), 263–272.

Liu, S., Richman, J., Thirlby, R., & Wu, C. (2006). Efficacy of continuous wound catheters delivering local anesthetic for postoperative analgesia: A quantitative and qualitative systematic review of randomized controlled trial. *Journal of the American College of Surgeons, 203*(6), 914–932.

May, M., & Deruyter, M. (2009). Continuous peripheral nerve catheter techniques. In H. Smith (Ed.), *Current therapy in pain* (pp. 84–92). New York, NY: Saunders Pub.

McGough, R. (2006, June 13). Pain pump tested in battle. *The Wall Street Journal.*

Melton, S., & Liu, S. (2010). Regional anesthesia techniques. In S. Fishman, J. Ballantyne, & J. Rathmell (Eds.), *Bonica's management of pain* (5th ed., pp. 92–106). Philadelphia, PA: Lippincott Williams & Wilkins.

Richman, J., Liu, S., Courpas, G., Wong, R., Rowlingsen, A., McGready, J., . . . Wu, C. (2006). Does continuous peripheral nerve block provide superior pain control to opioids? A meta-analysis. *Anesthesia & Analgesia, 102*(1), 248–257.

Rosenquist, R., & Rosenberg, J. (2003). Postoperative pain guidelines. *Regional Anesthesia, 28*(4), 279–288.

Salinas, F. (2010). Ultrasound and review of evidence for lower extremity peripheral nerve blocks. *Regional Anesthesia and Pain Medicine, 35*(2, Suppl. 1), S16–S24.

Wallace, M., & Staats, P. (2005). *Pain medicine and management.* New York, NY: McGraw-Hill.

9

Specialty Blocks and Implanted Techniques for Cancer Pain Management

Yvonne D'Arcy

OVERVIEW

When patients with cancer pain require outpatient blocks or implanted techniques, they are often referred to a pain clinic specializing in this type of care, most often an anesthesiology-based clinic. Although 80% to 90% of cancer pain can be relieved using the World Health Organization's (WHO) analgesic ladder, there are still patients who require more aggressive measures to treat their pain (Meuser et al., 2001). Using both medications and interventional treatments can provide a higher level of pain relief than either option used alone.

Because some pain clinics specialize in using only one or two types of therapy—such as injections, nonpharmacological rehabilitation, or medication management for complex patients—it is important to select a clinic that has experience with treating oncology patients. For example, for patients with visceral pain radiating to the upper abdomen related to pancreatic cancer, a neurolytic celiac plexus block can provide a high quality of pain relief and offer a better quality of life with opioid-sparing effect (Brogan, 2010).

In general, a pain clinic referral is indicated when:

▪ The patient has had a number of medications that have failed to relieve the pain even though doses have been titrated and other medications have been tried.
▪ The patient continues to complain of severe pain or cannot comply with the expected treatment regimen.

147

■ The health care provider is unsure about continuing a treatment regimen or needs confirmation that a certain treatment regimen is the correct approach to treating the patient's pain.

■ The patient seems to have a condition that persists and may be helped by an interventional pain management technique such as an implanted pump or specialized block.

PAIN CLINIC INTERVENTIONS

Pain clinics can offer a wide variety of treatments for pain. For patients with chronic low back pain, epidural steroid injections are routinely performed. For patients with cancer, more specialized blocks and infusions along with implanted pumps may be recommended.

There is a wide variety of interventional methods for cancer pain relief that include the following:

■ Injections such as epidural steroid injections and facet joint injections (Figure 9.1)
■ Neurolytic blocks
■ Specialized intrathecal infusions
■ Implanted intrathecal pumps

Depending on the pain complaint and the patient's condition, the pain specialist will select an option that will provide the greatest benefit to the patient. More information on specific interventions will be provided in the later sections of the chapter.

EVALUATION BY A PAIN SPECIALIST FOR INTERVENTIONAL PAIN MANAGEMENT

All patients who are seen for evaluation in a pain clinic or by a pain specialist undergo a panel of tests and assessments that are designed to help determine the best approach to the pain problem. Patients with cancer pain have been seen by any number of surgeons, oncologists, radiation therapists, and primary care physicians. They are usually very familiar with pain medications, the type of pain they are experiencing, and what will make the pain better or worse. What they fear most is that the pain will not be controlled or that it signals progression of the disease. In order to get a comprehensive picture of the pain, a detailed medical history will be taken that may include some or all of the following components:

■ Past pain experiences
■ Current or past chemical use, illicit or prescription substance abuse, or a history of a substance abuse disorder

- Medical history including oncology records
- Surgical history of any debunking or tumor resections
- Psychiatric history, especially if an implanted technique is being considered
- Medication use history, current opioids and doses
- Laboratory findings
- Imaging results, such as CT scans or MRIs
- Other pertinent workup results, such as electromyography (EMG) (American Society for Pain Management Nursing [ASPMN], 2002, 2009)

Since most of these patients will have been through many examinations, they may feel like this is one more time where they will be told that there is little that can be done. Encouraging the patient to be very open to the experience will help set a positive tone for the patient's visit. Taking the time to listen to patients describe their pain and what has worked and what has not been beneficial will pay a large dividend. Establishing a positive relationship with patients from the beginning of the process will help ensure that the best outcomes will be achieved at the end of the treatment period.

Patient education about pain and pain treatment options is essential to any pain clinic visit. These patients may have been seen by a variety of practices and specialists. Cancer pain can be a complex phenomenon and teaching the patient about treatment options, medications uses, and combinations of therapy will help patients to understand their role in the process. Creating a reachable goal and realistic expectation about the result of any interventional options can help patients feel they are getting maximum benefit from an injection, implanted device, or other type of interventional modality such as neurolytic blocks.

Clinical Pearl

Using a pain diary is one way to track progress with pain control and emotions. Patients should keep a daily diary to track their best and worst pain levels during the day, and what made the pain increase. They should also record the feeling they have about their pain on that day—their emotional response to the pain. When they bring the diary into the pain clinic, the pain specialist or pain nurse can have a discussion with patients about the pain intensities that were recorded and see what activities intensified the pain. They can also determine what type of emotional response the patients had and look for signs of anger, depression, fears of prognosis, or sadness over lost functionality or relationships.

SPINAL INJECTIONS

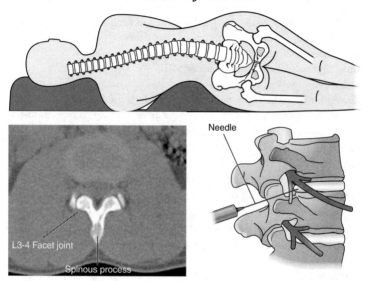

Figure 9.1 ■ Facet injection.

Spinal injection therapy is commonly performed by pain clinic practitioners, usually anesthesiologists. There is a variety of reasons that spinal injection therapy can provide pain relief for the cancer survivor with chronic pain, as follows:

■ Age-related changes in the spine can cause bone spurs and facet arthropathy that can cause nerve impingement, or degenerative disc disease, in which the associated nerve can be compressed by the vertebral body as the disc dries out.

■ Some patients who have back surgery do not get the expected result of pain relief. These patients are said to have "failed back syndrome." Injections can help relieve the pain of the nerve damage or impingement.

■ In herniated nucleus pulposus (HNP) (e.g., herniated disc), the disc may press on the adjacent nerve root, causing pain. If this occurs at the lower lumbar or sacral nerve roots, it can cause pain and weakness in the leg, called *sciatica*.

■ Conditions such as spinal stenosis are caused by the thickening of the spinal bones as they age, with spinal canal narrowing that is extremely painful and limits mobility.

■ Chronic neck pain is the result of aging, trauma, surgery, or facet joint arthropathy.

For patients with cancer, a block with local anesthetic can serve a dual function: pain relief and diagnostic function. Some patients with spinal nerve impingement or radicular pain can benefit from a local anesthetic block. Patients who would be considered good candidates for epidural, selective nerve root, or facet injections include the following:

■ Patients who have a specific nerve being impinged or compressed by a tumor, creating pain in a specific dermatome; for example, intercostal (rib) block from lung cancer

■ Patients where arthritis has narrowed the spinal facet and the nerves that run through the opening are being compressed

■ Patients who have tumor-associated low back pain with a radicular component to the pain, causing pain radiating down one or both legs (D'Arcy, 2007)

Some injections are performed as a treatment, while others may be used as a diagnostic tool to determine the source of the pain, to differentiate types of pain (e.g., visceral or somatic thoracoabdominal pain), and to determine if a neurolytic block would be beneficial (American Pain Society [APS], 2005). Neurolytic or neuroablative blocks provide the interruption of pain pathways either surgically, chemically, or thermally (Thapa, Rastogi, & Ahuja, 2011). There is a variety of neurolytic blocks, but two of the most common are described in the following.

Celiac Plexus Block

One of the most successful neurolytic blocks is performed as an injection of alcohol or phenol into the celiac plexus. This destroys the neural pathway that create the pain. A diagnostic block with local anesthetic is performed after the celiac plexus is visualized under fluoroscopy and, if pain relief is achieved with the injection of local anesthetic, a neurolytic block is performed. There are two approaches for a celiac plexus block: percutaneous or endoscopic. The percutaneous route is typically performed by a specialized anesthesiologist under CT guidance and/or fluoroscopy. The celiac plexus is accessed posteriorly (transcrural) or anteriorly (transaortic) with unilateral or bilateral needles. Endoscopic blocks are performed by gastrointestinal proceduralists, often at the same time as a pancreatic biopsy or common bile duct stent placement.

It is difficult to predict the amount of pain relief until the block is performed, but tumors located at the head of the pancreas have a better chance for success than the tail or body of the pancreas. Tumor infiltration into surrounding areas can also reduce the efficacy of the block

(Brogan, 2010). Opioids may need to be tapered if adequate pain relief is achieved from the celiac plexus block. If this is done rapidly, the patient will need to be monitored carefully for possible opioid withdrawal syndrome (Thapa et al., 2011). The block may be repeated once or twice if necessary.

In a meta-analysis of 1,145 patients, 89% of the patients reported good to excellent pain relief within 2 weeks (Eisenberg, 1995). Partial or complete pain relief was reported by 90% of the patients at 3 months and 70% to 80% until death (Eisenberg, 1995).

Side effects of celiac plexus block include transient orthostatic hypotension, lower extremity sensory changes, or diarrhea. Less common, but more serious, complications are permanent lower extremity sensory loss or motor weakness, paraplegia, aortic dissection, or death (Fitzgibbon & Loeser, 2010).

Superior Hypogastric Plexus Block

For patients with visceral pain from advanced cervical, bladder, rectal, and prostate cancer, a superior hypogastric plexus block may provide pain relief. This block is performed either percutaneously by an anesthesiologist, or intraoperatively by a surgeon. Under CT guidance, the percutaneous block is performed with unilateral or bilateral needles, usually with an anterior approach, but may be done posteriorly depending on tumor location. A local anesthetic diagnostic block is performed and, if successful, the neurolytic block is performed. Although not as common as the celiac plexus block, outcomes have shown good to excellent pain relief in 70% of the patients (Brogan, 2010). It has been shown to reduce opioid usage by up to 43% in 72% of the patients (Thapa et al., 2011). Serious side effects are uncommon if done by a skilled technician. They include bladder puncture, retroperitoneal hematoma, and urinary or fecal incontinence. The success of the block is limited in cases of retroperitoneal or pelvic side wall disease (Fitzgibbon & Loeser, 2010).

Saddle Block

For uncontrolled pain of the perineum, scrotum, penis, or anus, a more caudal block may be required. Saddle blocks are performed in the sitting position with a hyperbaric neurolytic agent, which sinks down to the sacral roots, resulting in numbness of the saddle area. The needle is placed at L5/S1 or L4/5. Complications may include loss of bladder and rectal function, and lower extremity weakness (Fitzgibbon & Loeser, 2010).

INTRATHECAL (IT) INFUSIONS

For patients who are opioid tolerant and are still having significant pain, intrathecal infusions can deliver small amounts of medication, about 1/100th of the systematic dose, to the cerebrospinal fluid (CSF) and provide high-level pain relief. Because the medication is infused into the CSF, it can act directly on the central nervous system effector sites (Brogan, 2010). It is felt that IT infusions can provide a better level of relief for cancer pain as many cancer pain presentations can have a neuropathic element that responds well to clonidine and local anesthetics in IT infusions (Brogan, 2010). All solutions used for IT medication delivery need to be preservative free.

To trial IT therapy, a simple lumbar puncture is performed and a percutaneous catheter is inserted at the lumbar level of the spine and IT opioids are infused at doses consistent with the patient's opioid doses. Medications that can be used for IT delivery to treat cancer pain include the following (Deer et al., 2011):

- Opioids: First-line therapy for nociceptive pain, second-line therapy for neuropathic pain; the most common drugs used are fentanyl, morphine, and hydromorphone. Morphine and hydromorphone recommended as first line. Fentanyl is second line.
- Ziconotide: First-line therapy when used as monotherapy. May be added to second-, third-, and fourth-line therapies
- Local anesthetics: Fifth-line therapy when used as monotherapy. However, commonly combined with opioids in second and third line therapy. For nociceptive and neuropathic pain, examples include lidocaine and bupivacaine
- Clonidine: Third line therapy when used as monotherapy. Commonly used in combination with second and third line local anaesthetic and opioid therapy for neuropathic and nociceptive pain
- Other drugs: ropivacaine, buprenorphine, midazolam, ketorolac; fifth line therapy for pain
- Experimental agents: gabapentin, octreotide, conpeptide, neostigmine, adenosine, and others; sixth line therapies

For patients who cannot tolerate a procedure such as an implanted pump or who have a short life expectancy, a tunneled IT catheter can be placed for short infusions. If this method is used, antimicrobial filters are needed along with meticulous site care. For end-of-life patients, hospice nurses or even well-trained family members can deliver IT boluses to control pain, if needed. If the patient has a 6-month life expectancy and is physically able to tolerate a surgical procedure, the pain specialist may consider placing an implanted IT delivery device.

IMPLANTED MODALITIES

Implanted IT Pumps

IT drug delivery systems can be used to help control cancer pain in patients with at least a 6-month prognosis and who have exhausted all other medication management techniques and have maximized medication doses. The technique consists of an implanted computerized pump that automatically delivers a prescribed doseof medication at a set rate (see Figure 9.2). The medication is delivered from the pump into the intrathecal space by a flexible catheter that is tunneled from the spinal insertion point along the lateral aspect of the patient's body and connected to the pump. The pump itself is placed by creating a pocket in theabdominal or other subcutaneous tissue close to the skin's surface to make refilling the pump easier. Pump refills are done by a pain clinic nurse approximately once a month according to the medication concentration and the infusion rate of the medication. A special refill kit is used to withdraw any leftover medication in the pump reservoir and new medication is inserted into the pump reservoir. The pump refill date is then reset to a new date determined by the concentration of the medication and medication delivery rate.

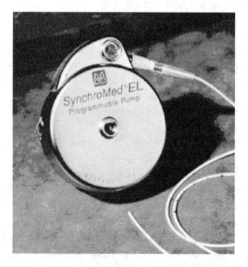

Figure 9.2 ■ Intrathecal pump. *Source:* Used with permission of Medtronic, Inc.

Medications that are FDA approved for use in implanted IT pumps are as follows:

- Morphine
- Baclofen
- Ziconotide (Prialt)

All medications used in implanted IT pumps should be preservative free since preservatives will cause damage to the spinal cord. Morphine is the most common medication and using IT medication delivery can provide morphine doses that are 300 times as potent as oral morphine (Wallace & Staats, 2005). Before the pump is permanently implanted, a 2-week trial is performed with the anticipated medication, generally morphine. During the trial period, the drug selection is based on the following:

- History of opioid tolerance
- Side effect history
- Pain-afferent spinal cord level compared with catheter tip location (Wallace & Staats, 2005)

The lipophilicity of the selected pain medication, the available lipid supply of the spinal cord, the accessibility of the cerebrospinal fluid, and the blood supply can directly affect the analgesic action of the medication being used (Wallace & Staats, 2005).

Ziconotide (Prialt)

Prialt is a one-of-a-kind medication classified as a neuronal-type (N-type) calcium channel blocker. It is derived from the venom of the cone snail, a marine snail. It must be administered intrathecally using a continuous infusion (Lynch, Cheng, & Yee, 2006). It can be used to treat both chronic nociceptive and neuropathic pain (Schroeder, Doering, Zamponi, & Lewis, 2006). There are some specific side effects, mainly neuropsychiatric, that can be significant. These include the following:

- Depression
- Cognitive impairment
- Depressed levels of consciousness
- Hallucinations
- Elevated creatinine kinase levels (Lynch et al., 2006)

Prialt use should be reserved for patients for whom all other more conventional medications and interventions have failed.

Practitioners are using other medications in implanted pumps, such as hydromorphone or bupivacaine, when pain is not controlled with the standard FDA-approved medications. However, the risk of pump dysfunction increases when unapproved medications are used in these pumps.

Clinical Pearl

Following is the procedure for selecting a candidate for IT medication delivery:
- Ineffective oral analgesia with multiple oral or transcutaneous trials, including dose titration
- Intolerable side effects despite opioid rotation
- Functional analgesia during temporary trial infusion
- Psychologic stability and reasonable goals
- Access to care—the patient will return to the pain clinic for pump refills and dose adjustments
- Patient acceptance
- For baclofen—intractable spasticity unrelieved by oral antispasmodics, with improved spasticity with baclofen test dosing (Wallace & Staats, 1005, p. 342)

The use of an IT medication delivery system can have a variety of problems, such as infection, pump failure, or catheter dislodgement. In addition, IT pumps are a costly option. The patient risk–benefit ratio should be carefully weighed and all other reasonable options should be tried before the pump implantation is tried. If the patient does not have a 50% reduction in pain levels with the pre-pump implantation trial, the final implantation should be reconsidered. There are some risks that the patient should be aware of before the catheter is placed.

Clinical Pearl

Following are risks and considerations with IT medication administration (Wallace & Staats, 2005):
- Does the patient have any placement issues such as spinal deformity, past spinal surgery, or abdominal surgery that would make placement difficult?
- All patients are at risk for infection, meningitis, arachnoiditis, and catheter-related granuloma formation.
- Anticoagulation can cause a compressive hematoma when the catheter is being placed or removed.
- Pump malfunction can cause a withdrawal syndrome.
- Low pressure spinal headaches.
- Need for dose escalation and the development of tolerance.

SUMMARY

For patients with intractable pain or for whom medications have had poor effect, using an interventional option may provide pain relief that cannot be achieved in any other way. Referring a patient to a pain specialist may provide pain relief that can help the patient and family enjoy final days in comfort.

Case Study

Sarita is a 57-year-old patient who has had intractable pain from her pancreatic cancer for several weeks. She complains about abdominal pain and some back pain that feels like it goes straight through her torso "like someone stuck a sword in me!" She has tried many different types of pain medication but she gets nauseated at the higher doses. She is afraid that this pain cannot be managed. She asks you to please help her, she cannot stand the pain. Her family is hopeful that the pain clinic visit will produce a solution to the awful pain. It is very hard for the family to see Sarita suffering so much. Sarita has been taking oxycodone for over 3 months with trials of extended-release opioids and other short-acting medications such as hydrocodone. Even with regular medication, Sarita cannot sleep and has been nauseated.

Questions to Consider

1. Sarita has a somewhat typical presentation for a pancreatic cancer patient. Would changing her medication or increasing the dose make any difference at this point?
2. What type of interventional technique could benefit Sarita and greatly reduce both her her pain and medication need?
3. Given the type of cancer Sarita has and her pain, would using an implanted device be a good option? Would her physical condition be a factor when considering implantation?
4. What will you do about Sarita's opioid medication if she has an interventional treatment that provides adequate analgesia?

REFERENCES

American Pain Society (APS). (2005). *Cancer pain in adults and children.* Glenview, IL: Author.

American Society of Pain Management Nurses. (2009). *Core curriculum for pain management nursing.* Dubuque, IA: Kendall Hunt Pub.

Brogan, S. (2010). Interventional pain therapies. In *Bonica's management of pain* (pp. 605–618). Philadelphia, PA: Lippincott Williams & Wilkins.

D'Arcy, Y. (2007). *Pain management: Tools and techniques for nursing professionals.* Marblehead, MA: HcPro.

Deer, T., Smith, H., Burton, A., Pope, J., Doleys, D., Levy, R., . . . Cousins, M. (2011). Comprehensive consensus based guidelines on intrathecal drug delivery systems in the treatment of pain caused by cancer pain. *Pain Physician, 14*, E283–E312.

Eisenberg, E., Carr, D., & Chalmers, T. C. (1995). Neurolytic celiac plexus block for treatment of cancer pain: A meta analysis. *Anesthesia & Analgesia, 80*(2), 290–295.

Fitzgibbon, D. R., & Loeser, J. D. (2010). *Cancer pain: Assessment, diagnosis, and management.* Philadelphia, PA: Wolters Kluwer.

Lynch, S. S., Cheng, C. M., & Yee, J. L. (2006). Intrathecal ziconotide for refractory chronic pain. *Annals of Pharmacotherapy, 40*(7–8), 1293–1200.

Meuser, T., Pietruck, C., Radbruch, L., Stute, P., Lehmann, K. A., & Grond, S. (2001). Symptoms during cancer pain treatment following WHO guidelines: A longitudinal follow-up study of symptom prevalence, severity, and etiology. *Pain, 93*(3), 247–257.

Schroeder, C. I., Doering, C. J., Zamponi, G. W., & Lewis, R. J. (2006). N-type calcium channel blockers: Novel therapeutics for the treatment of pain. *Medicinal Chemistry, 2*(5), 535–543.

Stearns, L., Boortz-Marx, R., & DuPen, S. (2005). Intrathecal drug delivery for the management of cancer pain: A multidisciplinary consensus of best clinical practices. *Journal of Supportive Oncology, 3*(6), 399–409.

Thapa, A., Rastogi, S., & Ahuja, A. (2011). Cancer pain management-current status. *Journal of Anesthesiology Clinical Pharmacology, 27*(2), 162–168.

Wallace, M., & Staats, P. (2005). *Pain medicine and management.* New York, NY: McGraw-Hill.

10

Palliative Chemotherapy, Radiotherapy, and Surgery for Pain Control

Pamela Stitzlein Davies

Chemotherapy, endocrine therapy, radiation therapy and surgery can be quite useful to control cancer pain, even in advanced disease settings. While these treatments are the mainstay of cancer therapy when the goal is cure or remission, they may also have a role in a palliative care setting, when the intent is to reduce pain and improve quality of life. In some instances, they may help to extend life. Effective palliation can have an opioid-sparing effect, reducing the total dose of analgesics needed to control pain. This chapter will focus on the use of palliative chemotherapy, radiotherapy, and surgery for pain control in the setting of *advanced disease*. Management of oral mucositis is also covered.

CHEMOTHERAPY FOR PAIN CONTROL IN ADVANCED CANCER

"Palliative chemotherapy" refers to use of antineoplastic agents to treat the symptoms associated with advanced cancer (Sun, 2010). It is used to reduce pain, improve quality of life, and in some cases, to extend survival. Pain and other physical symptoms in cancer are typically highly correlated to tumor burden. Therefore, chemotherapy that does not stall tumor growth will have little impact on pain (Weissman, 2009). Patients with advanced disease from breast, ovarian, and colon cancer are more likely to have improved symptoms with palliative chemotherapy, whereas those with relatively chemo-resistant tumors, such as pancreatic, hepatocellular, and melanoma, are less likely to benefit (Sun, 2010).

The choice of chemotherapy agent depends on the type of cancer, and previous treatments received. For example, a patient with recurrent metastatic ovarian cancer received the following chemotherapy regimens to help control abdominal pain and ascites: carboplatinum, gemcitabine, and bevacizumab (Avastin). When her disease progressed, she was changed to single-agent doxorubicin (Doxil) for several months. She was then rotated to topotecan and bevacizumab after further disease progression. After a total of 11 months of "palliative chemotherapy," the disease progressed to the point that she was too weak to tolerate any further therapy. She was enrolled in hospice and died 3 weeks later. Ultimately, these palliative chemotherapies proved to slow the tumor growth, resulting in better pain and symptom control, improved quality and length of life, all at a "reasonable" burden for this particular patient.

Although the goal of palliative chemotherapy is improved overall quality of life, patients will still struggle with the chemotherapy side effects, most commonly fatigue. Depending on the agent used, nausea, anemia, rashes, hot flashes, and immunosuppression may also be problematic, leading to more frequent clinic visits for lab work, hydration; granulocyte colony stimulating factor (G-CSF, such as filgrastim) injections; additionally, hospitalization for severe toxicity reactions may be required. Therefore, the benefit-to-toxicity ratio must be assessed carefully when utilizing chemotherapy in advanced disease (Desai, Kim, Fall, & Wang, 2007; McIllmurray, 2005).

It is important to remember that chemotherapy administration may lead to painful conditions. Examples include mucositis from methotrexate, or chemotherapy-induced painful peripheral neuropathy from paclitaxel (Cawley & Benson, 2005). A unique drug side effect is palmar–plantar erythrodysesthesia (PPE; hand-foot syndrome) from agents such as capecitabine (Xeloda). PPE causes painful burning from dry, cracked skin on the palms and feet. Prevention includes liberal use of emollients, and protection of hands and feet from injury and from temperature extremes (Webster-Gandy, How, & Harrold, 2007).

What Is the Role of Palliative Chemotherapy in "Best Supportive Care" in Advanced Cancer?

There are very few studies of "best supportive care" versus palliative chemotherapy with "best supportive care," which makes the choice for palliative chemotherapy challenging (Sun, 2010). There is no guideline for appropriateness of therapy in advanced cancer, and treatment types and duration vary widely (Best et al., 2008). Ideally, treatment with a given regimen continues if there is ongoing clinical benefit, but the toxicities of treatment may limit its use (Barrios, Sampaio, Vinholes, & Caponero, 2009). In some tumor types, patients have the option of taking a break from therapy, or using a lower toxicity treatment, such as the immune therapy trastuzumab (Herceptin) or endocrine therapy (Amar, Roy, & Perez, 2009). It is important for clinicians in the palliative and oncology spheres to work closely together and integrate their specialties in order to provide the most advantageous disease-modifying therapy, along with optimal symptom control and psychosocial support (Bruera & Hui, 2010; Ferris et al., 2009; MacDonald, 2005).

A 2008 Cochrane Database meta-analysis of palliative chemotherapy for advanced or metastatic colorectal cancer found that treatment produced a significant improvement of 3.7 months in median survival and tumor response was approximately 25% (Best et al., 2008). Data relating to treatment toxicity and quality of life were "inadequately addressed" in the majority of the trials, despite this being one of the primary goals of utilizing chemotherapy in the advanced disease setting. Inconsistent tools were utilized for measurement of symptoms, quality of life, and toxicities, making comparisons between trials difficult.

A prospective study from South Korea assessed the quality of life, anxiety, and depression in 146 patients with advanced cancer (most common types were gastric, nonsmall cell lung, and colorectal) while on palliative chemotherapy (Bang et al., 2005). They noted a "short-lived" improvement in functional scores, pain, sleep, quality of life, and anxiety while on chemotherapy. However, the high drop-out rate of 33% (most were lost to follow up) makes these interesting findings underpowered.

Halting Palliative Chemotherapy: A Difficult Decision

The decision to halt chemotherapy may be very difficult for both the patient and the oncology team on many levels (Harrington & Smith, 2008). It is not unusual for chemotherapy to be continued, even if it does not appear to be providing significant improvement in pain, symptoms, or quality of life (MacDonald, 2005). The reasons for this are multiple. Ongoing treatment with chemotherapy may engender a false sense of hope, as many patients fail to understand that the purpose of therapy is *palliative*, not *curative*. In addition, patients or family members may be desperately seeking to "do something" to treat the cancer in the face of eventual death. Lastly, patients often appreciate the focus and attention they receive while on treatment, even if continuation of therapy requires frequent and tiresome clinic visits.

Oncologists may find themselves avoiding conversations about the futility of therapy, as these conversations are difficult, time consuming, and require special communication skills that oncologists may not have mastered (Back, Arnold, & Tulsky, 2009). Physicians may fear that patients will think the team is "giving up" on them, and the patient may indeed feel abandoned when treatment is stopped (Sun, 2010). For these reasons, nurses may observe that antineoplastic treatments are continued in the advanced cancer patient even though the patient's performance status is very poor, and the treatment appears to be making quality of life worse. This difficult situation is the ideal time to call a meeting with the patient and family and the oncologist, nurse, and other team members such as social work, chaplaincy, or palliative care, to discuss the goals of care and probable outcomes from chemotherapy (MacDonald, 2005).

Hospice "Open Access" or "Dual Enrollment"

Some hospice agencies, in an effort to encourage earlier enrollment, have "open access" or "dual enrollment" programs which allow hospice enrollment while receiving palliative chemotherapy (Wright & Katz, 2007). This is a "best of both worlds" situation, utilizing disease-modifying therapies and optimal symptom management to promote quality of life. However, due to the capitated reimbursement rates in hospice (in the range of $150 per day per patient), only lower-cost chemotherapy agents can be considered. Additional supportive therapies, such as blood product support (e.g., platelets), or colony-stimulating factor injections (e.g., filgrastim [Neupogen]), may drive the cost of care to over $10,000 per month (Wright & Katz, 2007). This becomes too costly for the hospice to cover and ultimately may prevent enrollment. "Open-access" enrollment is determined on a case-by-case basis by the hospice medical director.

Phase 1: Clinical Trials

Patients with advanced cancer may be asked to participate in Phase 1 clinical trials, which are essential for development of new anticancer therapies. Traditional Phase 1 studies are unique, as they are designed to determine the maximum tolerated *dose* and *toxicity* of the novel drug in humans; treatment of the disease is not the primary goal. It is common for patients to misunderstand the purpose of a Phase 1 study, sometimes believing they are receiving a new "miracle cure" for the cancer. When this "last chance" chemotherapy does not work, and the cure is not realized, the emotional consequences can be devastating.

There is a concern that optimum pain management in the advanced cancer patient may be impacted by participation in a Phase 1 trial (Sun,

2010). Unfortunately, these trials generally preclude enrollment in hospice, and may limit the types of analgesic therapies allowed (especially NSAIDs and acetaminophen, occasionally allowing for use of only specific opioids). Palliative care services should be mobilized in "hospice-eligible" patients in Phase 1 studies to focus on pain and symptom management until the patient enrolls in hospice. Such care can be given in coordination with the study protocol requirements to optimize symptoms.

Casarett, Karlawish, Henry, and Hirschman studied the feasibility of having patients with limited prognosis have dual enrollment in Phase 1 trials and home hospice care (2002). Forty-five Phase 1 Principle Investigators (PIs) and 92 hospices were surveyed. While 91% of PIs agreed with hospice dual enrollment, only 67% of hospice centers agreed with this model, most of them citing cost concerns or other issues.

RADIATION THERAPY FOR PAIN CONTROL IN ADVANCED CANCER

Radiation is a key therapy for pain control in advanced cancer. By shrinking the tumor size, radiotherapy relieves pressure in the bone or organs, thereby relieving pain (Rutter & Weissman, 2004). Treatment of painful metastasis to bone is one of the primary uses of radiation therapy. Radiation is also used to decrease tumor-associated bleeding and management of fungating wounds (malignant wounds from tumor infiltration of the skin, discussed in the next section). Radiation is delivered in different forms, as follows (Fairchild & Chow, 2010; Miaskowski et al., 2008):

- External beam radiation
  - Photon beams (x-rays or gamma rays). This is the "standard" radiation therapy administered via a linear accelerator.
  - Electrons (for superficial tumors)
  - Proton therapy, which is a specialized form of radiotherapy that releases energy at precise depths to decrease damage to surrounding tissues, is used primarily for tumors in the head, neck, spine, lung, and gastrointestinal tract. It is available in only a few centers nationally.
- Radiopharmaceutical
  - Injectable strontium-89 or samarium-153, for widespread metastatic bone cancer, generally used when no further chemotherapy is planned
- Brachytherapy
  - Radioactive sources precisely delivered on the surface or inside tissue or a body cavity. It is used in cervical, prostate, or breast cancers

External beam radiotherapy is useful for pain control in many situations, including the following (Kirkbride & Barton, 1999; Quill et al., 2010; Sainsbury, Vaizey, Pastorino, Mould, & Emberton, 2005):

- Painful bony metastatic lesions
- Impending fracture from bony metastasis causing pain, especially with weight bearing
- Chest pain and dyspnea from advanced lung cancer
- Pain from obstructive symptoms or bleeding from metastatic pelvic masses or local recurrence of colon cancer
- Malignant fungating wounds from cutaneous tumors
- Control of bleeding from superficial tumors
- Spinal cord compression
- Headache from brain metastasis (whole-brain radiation or stereotactic radiosurgery)

Metastasis to the Bone

Metastatic cancer to bone occurs in up to 80% to 85% of patients with breast, lung, and prostate cancer, and up to 30% of bladder and thyroid cancers (Finlay, Mason, & Shelley, 2005; Roqué i Figuls, Martinez-Zapata, Scott-Brown, & Alonso-Coello, 2011). It may cause severe pain, pathologic fractures, impending fractures, and the potentially emergent condition of spinal cord compression (the latter is discussed in Chapter 14). Pain from bone metastasis is believed to be caused by nerve damage and destruction in the bones from excessive stretch, mechanical pressure, inflammation, and cytokines caused by the tumor. Bone pain from metastasis is a major problem, since lung, breast, and prostate cancers account for about 45% of all cancers in the United States (Hoskin, 2005).

Response rates to radiotherapy for pain associated with bony metastasis are high. Fairchild and Chow (2010) report that 90% of patients experience some pain relief, and 54% achieved complete relief after radiation therapy, with maximum pain relief reached within 4 to 6 weeks, and the median duration of pain relief 12 to 15 weeks. The 2008 Cochrane Review by McQuay, Collins, Carroll, and Moore report that 25% of patients will achieve complete relief of pain at 1 month, and an additional 35% will have at least half of their pain resolved (2008). Efficacy was the same regardless of dose and fractionation schedule (number of treatments given.)

Pain Flare After Radiation Therapy

Patients should be warned that they may experience *worsening* pain starting 3 to 7 days after initiation of radiation. This is a temporary condition occurring in 10% to 44% of patients receiving palliative radiation for bone metastasis, and is caused by inflammatory response of the bone and tissues. The pain flare typically lasts 1 to 6 days, and then improves. It is treated with increased doses of breakthrough opioid analgesics, NSAIDs, or short-term use of steroids such as dexamethasone (Fairchild & Chow, 2010).

Radioisotopes for Metastatic Bone Pain

Radioisotopes, such as strontium-89 or samarium-153, are used to manage pain when the bony metastatic disease is widespread. These beta-emitting agents are injected intravenously, and have an affinity for areas of high bone turnover. A 2011 Cochrane Review found "moderate" quality evidence supporting a beneficial effect of radioisotopes for management of pain from metastatic bone disease at 1 to 6 months (Roqué i Figuls et al., 2011). However, the major adverse effects of leukocytopenia, thrombocytopenia, and anemia are significant limitations to use of this route. Radiopharmaceuticals do not appear to reduce the incidence of spinal cord compression or affect mortality, and data are lacking on the impact on quality of life, hypercalcemia, and prevention of pathologic fractures. For this reason, the Cochrane Review indicated it is a "secondary option" when other treatments for pain from bony metastasis have failed. In addition, many oncologists will consider this option only when no further chemotherapy will be considered due to the long-term effect on blood counts.

SURGERY AND PROCEDURES FOR PAIN CONTROL IN ADVANCED CANCER

In carefully selected patients with advanced disease, palliative surgery and procedures may provide significant improvement in pain, symptoms, and quality of life (Sainsbury et al., 2005). Surgical resection of locally advanced or metastatic lesions may, in some cases, also prolong survival (Cummins, Vick, & Poole, 2004; Kaufman et al., 2008).

Procedures with palliative intent are performed to improve pain, symptoms, and quality of life, but, depending on the circumstances, frequently leave local or metastatic residual disease (Ronnekleiv-Kelly & Kennedy, 2011). Examples of palliative procedures include the following (Koh & Portenoy, 2010; Oida et al., 2009; Sainsbury et al., 2005; Shah et al., 2006):

- Colostomy to relieve tumor obstruction of the colon or rectum, or for rectovaginal fistula
- Ileostomy for distal small bowel obstruction
- Ileal conduit for vesicovaginal fistula

- Gastroenterostomy (gastric bypass) for gastroduodenal outflow obstruction in advanced gastric and pancreatic cancer
- Hepatectomy (liver resection) of metastatic lesions from colon or breast cancer causing pain from capsule distension, jaundice, and inferior vena cava obstruction
- Pulmonary wedge resection via open thoracotomy or VATS (video-assisted thoracic surgery) to resect metastatic tumors or perform pleurodesis for repeated pleural effusions
- Nephrostomy tubes to relieve tumor-induced ureteral obstruction causing hydronephrosis

The primary literature base for palliative surgery in advanced cancer is found on metastatic colorectal cancer. Twenty percent of patients with colorectal cancer have metastases at the time of diagnosis, and 70% undergo tumor resection (Eisenberger, Whelan, & Neugut, 2008). Surgery is performed to relieve obstruction, perforation, fistulas, or tenesmus (painful bowel spasms), or to treat anemia from intractable gastrointestinal bleeding (Eisenberger et al., 2008). Surgery may profoundly improve pain, symptoms, quality of life, and possibly survival, for symptomatic conditions such as bowel perforation.

Patients who are considered reasonable surgical risks for management of malignant bowel obstruction are those with the following (Davis & Hinshaw, 2006):

- A single site of bowel obstruction
- Absence of palpable abdominal tumors
- Less than 3 L of ascites fluid
- Preoperative weight loss less than 9 kg
- Anticipated prognosis of 2 to 3 months or more

Patients at poor risk for surgery are those with the following:

- Carcinomatosis (spread of tumor throughout the abdomen)
- Multiple sites of tumor causing obstruction
- Massive ascites
- Extensive tumor burden outside the abdomen
- Cachexia with significant weight loss
- Frailty
- Limited prognosis (less than 2 months)

For inoperable malignant obstructions, a venting gastrostomy or jejunostomy may reduce abdominal discomfort and intractable nausea and vomiting for those with limited life expectancy. A percutaneous endoscopic gastrostomy (PEG) tube for gastric venting can be performed under conscious sedation as an outpatient procedure (Ronnekleiv-Kelly & Kennedy, 2011).

Two points must be remembered when palliative surgery is done for pain and symptom management of malignant bowel obstruction. First, the overall pain will likely *worsen* for a week or two while the patient copes with postoperative incisional pain. Second, although the patency of the bowel lumen may be re-established, bowel motility may continue to be impaired due to tumor compression of the mesentery, and functional bowel syndrome caused by carcinomatosis; therefore, surgery may result in minimal overall improvement in bowel function (Davis & Hinshaw, 2006).

Stents

Stents are temporary plastic or permanent expandable metal tubes that are inserted into a lumen by endoscope to maintain patency, thereby improving pain and symptoms from tumor obstruction of ducts or bowel. They are inserted via endoscopy, and typically have a low complication rate. Stent procedures are performed for the following (Koh & Portenoy, 2010):

- Biliary (bile duct) obstruction
- Pancreatic duct obstruction
- Duodenal obstruction
- Gastric outlet tumor obstructions
- Tracheoesophageal perforations
- Colon or rectal stents

Stents inserted into lumens obstructed by tumor are at high risk of eventually becoming obstructed again, sometimes in just a few weeks.

OTHER THERAPIES FOR PAIN CONTROL IN ADVANCED CANCER

There are several additional therapies for palliative management of pain in advanced cancer, which are currently established or emerging treatments.

Bisphosphonates and Other Bone-Stabilizing Agents for Pain From Bone Metastasis

Bisphosphonates, such as pamidronate (Aredia) and zoledronic acid (Zometa); and the newer RANK-ligand bone-stabilizing agent denosumab (Xgeva) are used to treat pain from metastatic disease to the bone in breast cancer, prostate cancer, and multiple myeloma (Smith, 2011). These drugs inhibit osteoclast-mediated bone resorption (Costa & Major, 2009). Bisphosphonates are used to prevent fractures in women with metastatic breast cancer and to treat hypercalcemia, and have been shown to improve overall quality of life (Pavlakis, Schmidt, & Stockler, 2005). Van Poznak et al. (2011) recommends that all patients receive a dental examination prior to initiation of bone-stabilizing therapy, due to the rare—but potentially serious—adverse effect called *osteonecrosis of the jaw*(Van Poznak et al., 2011). Zoledronic acid requires dose adjustment for moderate to severe renal impairment (von Moos, 2006).

A 2009 Cochrane Review found evidence of a modest benefit from bisphosphonates in treating the pain of bone metastasis, stating that it should be considered a second-line therapy after other standard treatments, such as analgesics and radiation. Maximum effect was noted at 4 weeks. Side effects were mild, typically nausea and vomiting (Wong & Wiffen, 2009).

Vertebroplasty, Kyphoplasty, and Radiofrequency Ablation of Painful Metastatic Lesions to Vertebral Bodies

The 2011 National Comprehensive Cancer Network (NCCN) Cancer Pain Guidelines recommend consideration of percutaneous vertebroplasty, kyphoplasty, or radiofrequency ablation to painful vertebral metastatic lesions. Vertebroplasty is an established therapy that involves injection of cement into the vertebral fracture. The goal is to reduce pain and stabilize the spine. It is theorized that the cement also provides additional benefit by exerting a direct toxic effects on tumor cells (Katonis et al., 2009). Kyphoplasty is similar to vertebroplasty, but utilizes a balloon to create a space for cement injection as well as to partially restore vertebral height (Katonis et al., 2009).

Radiofrequency ablation of painful bone lesions is a newer approach to metastatic vertebral fractures. Using local anesthesia or conscious sedation, a high-energy radiofrequency electrode tip is inserted into the necrotic bone via CT guidance. The ablation process takes about 8 minutes (Katonis et al., 2009). Pain relief may start as early as 24 hours, but typically at 1 week postprocedure (Thanos et al., 2008).

OTHER PAINFUL CONDITIONS ASSOCIATED WITH ADVANCED CANCER OR CANCER TREATMENT

There are several painful conditions associated with advanced cancer, or cancer treatment that are not addressed elsewhere in this text. These include mucositis, acute chemotherapy-induced neuropathy, and pain from malignant cutaneous wounds.

Mucositis

Oral mucositis is a complication of chemotherapy, as well as radiation to the head and neck, with an overall incidence of 40%, and a range of 10–100% (Raber-Durlacher, Elad, & Barasch, 2010). It is most commonly associated with high-dose chemotherapy for hematologic malignancies and conditioning for hematopoietic stem cell transplant (HSCT), occuring in 76% of cases (Naidu et al., 2004). When aggressive myelosuppressive chemotherapy is combined with concurrent head and neck radiation, the incidence of mucositis increases to 90% to 100% (Cawley & Benson, 2005).

Mucositis may be seen in the palliative setting, especially with "salvage" chemotherapy for lung cancer, leukemia, or lymphoma. The chemotherapy agents most commonly associated with mucositis include: bleomycin, cyclophosphamide, cytarabine, doxirubicin, etoposide, fluorouracil, melphalan, methotrexate, paclitaxel, and vincristine (Cawley & Benson, 2005). Other risk factors include poor oral hygiene, smoking, alcohol intake, and younger age (Naidu et al., 2004).

Severe toxicity results in oral pain, diminished quality of life, and decreased oral intake resulting in weight loss and poor nutritional status. It may lead to modification of antineoplastic therapy, requiring reduced doses or treatment breaks (Clarkson et al., 2010). The pain of mucositis may be so intense that inpatient management is required for symptom control. Wong and colleagues reports that patients with severe mucositis "avoided swallowing at all cost" (2006, p. 34).

Measures to prevent or minimize mucositis include: a pretreatment dental exam, regular toothbrushing and flossing, sips of water to keep the mucosa moist, eating of only soft, bland foods, and frequent oral rinses with saline or sodium bicarbonate solution (Cawley & Benson, 2005). Spicy, acidic, or coarse foods should be avoided, as well as mouthwashs containing alcohol.

A wide variety of therapies have been studied for mucositis including rinses with Magic Mouthwash (lidocaine, diphenhydramine, and magnesium or aluminum hydroxide), allopurinol, amifostine, and tetracaine, but the effectiveness of these therapies is not established (Clarkson et al., 2010; Harris et al., 2008). Use of benzydamine rinses (a nonsteroidal available in Europe and Canada) and zinc appear promising, but larger studies are needed (Harris et al., 2008). Therapies that appear to be effective, but only in specific populations, include cryotherapy (holding ice water in the mouth for 30 minutes after chemotherapy with short half-life, such as bolus 5-fluorouricil and melphalan), palifermin (a recombinant growth factor for use in HSCT) and low-level laser therapy, also for HCT. In all settings, oral care protocols for prevention and opioid therapy for pain control remain the cornerstone of treatment (Cawley & Benson, 2005).

Acute Neuropathy From Chemotherapy

While it is not the intent of this text to review all chemotherapy reactions that may occur, acute neuropathy reactions are an interesting phenomenon that deserve a brief mention. Chronic chemotherapy-induced peripheral neuropathy (CIPN) is addressed in Chapter 17.

Oxaliplatin, a pro-drug of 5-fluorouracil, is used for treatment in advanced colorectal cancer. Nearly all patients will develop an acute transient neurotoxicity, which starts during or within a few hours of the infusion (Cruciani, Strada, & Knotkova, 2010). It is triggered by cold, such as drinking ice water, or holding a cold cup in the hand. Sensory symptoms include paresthesias and dysesthesias in the fingers and perioral area. More severe, and frightening, are motor reactions which include muscle spasms, jaw spasms, and pseudolaryngospasm. Acute symptoms typically resolve after hours to days. Dose modification may be needed for symptoms that are severe, painful, or persist between cycles. A variety of agents are being assessed for prevention or management of the symptoms, and the most promising appears to be intravenous calcium and magnesium infusions (Saif & Reardon, 2005). It is unclear if development of the acute neurotoxicity predisposes a patient to development of chronic oxaliplatin-induced peripheral neuropathy (Park et al., 2009). Patient education is the key to prevention and management of this condition, with an emphasis on avoiding eating or drinking cold food or fluids and using gloves to handle any cold items, including taking items out of the refrigerator or freezer (Saif & Reardon, 2005).

Management of Pain in Malignant Fungating Wounds

Malignant wounds occur in 10% of patients with metastatic disease, most commonly in breast cancer. Other tumors types include melanoma, lung, and colorectal cancers (Seaman, 2006). The term *fungating* refers to the tumor penetrating the skin causing ulceration with proliferation (Pearson & Mortimer, 2005; Cochran & Jakubek, 2010). These wounds cause physical and emotional suffering due to pain, odor, exudate, bleeding, and disfigurement. Serious complications include hemorrhage if the tumor invades a large vessel, or compression of a major vessel or airway (Seaman, 2006). Management is a challenge, especially as patients are typically in a state of advanced illness (Seaman & Bates-Jensen, 2010).

Strategies to control pain associated with malignant fungating wounds depend on the pain source: nociceptive (either deep or superficial) or neuropathic pain (Doughty, 2010). Systemic opioids are used for deep nociceptive pain, either continuously or as a premedication 60 minutes prior to dressing changes or debridement. Topical agents are useful for superficial pain associated with these procedures, including local anesthetics, such as EMLA (eutectic mixture of local anesthetics), or compounded topical opioids (Bates-Jensen, 2010).

A neuropathic source should always be considered as a cause of wound pain, as many fungating wounds cause pressure on surrounding nerves (Grocott & Dealey, 2005). This is treated with standard systemic adjuvant agents, such as anticonvulsants (e.g., gabapentin) or antidepressants (e.g., duloxetine). Consideration can be given to topical application of these agents, but there is no evidence to support this route; a compounding pharmacist should be consulted for additional information (Coyne, Hansen, & Watson, 2006).

A short course of palliative radiation may be used to control wound bleeding and pain, especially if other measures are not helpful (Cochran & Jakubek, 2010). Palliative chemotherapy may stall tumor growth somewhat, therefore assisting in pain management.

Controlling exudate and regular wound cleansing will reduce the pain associated with dressing removal (Doughty, 2010). Cleansing can be done in the shower if the patient is ambulatory, or with warmed normal saline or Dakin's solution (Cochran & Jakubek, 2010). Gentle removal of dressings will reduce pain by preventing excess tissue trauma (Doughty, 2010). Strategies to control odor include regular cleansing, followed by application of topical metronidazole 0.75% gel (MetroGel) or 250 mg or 500 mg tablets (Flagyl) crushed and sprinkled on the wound (Cochran & Jakubek, 2010). Systemic metronidazole is not recommended.

SUMMARY

Radiation therapy, surgery, chemotherapy, endocrine therapy, and other supportive treatments can have a significant role for pain management, even in the setting of advanced disease. The challenge for the treatment team is to find the proper balance between therapies that improves pain, symptoms, and quality of life, versus those that do not. Patients with advanced cancer typically struggle with profound fatigue, which may be worsened with frequent clinic visits for treatments and tests that simply wear them down without improving overall quality of life. The old adage is useful here: "Just because you *can* give a treatment, doesn't mean you *should* give it." The role of the oncology nurse is to assist the patient and family with navigating the various treatment options, help clarify the patient's goals, and communicate those goals to the entire team. The overall purpose is to help keep the patient with advanced cancer as comfortable as possible, reducing pain and symptoms, while minimizing unnecessary clinic visits. Mackillop (1996) emphasizes this goal in his *Ten Rules for the Practice of Palliative Radiotherapy*, stating: "Time is precious when life is short" (p. 7).

Case Study

Esmeralda is an 82-year-old Spanish-speaking Hispanic woman with recurrent breast cancer to the chest wall. She presents to the clinic with her son, having recently arrived from Mexico. She has a grapefruit-sized tumor on the right anterior upper lateral chest, which is causing severe pain. She is right-handed, and the tumor location makes it difficult for her to use her right arm. She is in severe distress, crying and anxious, and complaining of unbearable pain despite hydrocodone/acetaminophen 5/500 1 tablet every 6 hours.

The oncologist refers her to the radiation oncologist for urgent radiotherapy to control pain. She is started on a fentanyl patch at 12 mg/hr every 72 hours, and the hydrocodone/acetaminophen is changed to oxycodone 5 mg tablet, 1 to 2 tablets every 3 hours as needed. She is urged to use the oxycodone if her pain is severe. Over the next week, she starts radiation therapy in 15 fractions (3 weeks of treatment), and her fentanyl patch is increased to 25 mcg/hr every 72 hours.

Two weeks into therapy, the tumor is markedly reduced in size, and three weeks after completing radiation, the chest wall tumor has nearly disappeared. The patient says her pain is nearly gone. Her son notes she seems to be more sleepy than usual lately.

Questions to Consider

1. What is the most likely cause of Esmeralda's new sedation?
2. What opioid taper schedule would you recommend?

REFERENCES

Amar, S., Roy, V., & Perez, E. (2009). Treatment of metastatic breast cancer: Looking towards the future. *Breast Cancer Research and Treatment, 114*(3), 413–422.

Back, A., Arnold, R., & Tulsky, J. (2009). *Mastering communication with seriously ill patients: Balancing honesty with empathy and hope.* New York, NY: Cambridge University Press.

Barrios, C., Sampaio, C., Vinholes, J., & Caponero, R. (2009). What is the role of chemotherapy in estrogen receptor-positive, advanced breast cancer? *Annals of Oncology, 20*(7), 1157–1162.

Bang, S., Park, S., Kang, H., Jue, J., Cho, I., Yun, Y., Cho, E. K., Shin, D. B., & Lee, J. H. (2005). Changes in quality of life during palliative chemotherapy for solid cancer. *Supportive Care in Cancer, 13*(7), 515–521.

Bates-Jensen, B. (2010). Skin disorders: Pressure ulcers-prevention and management. In B. Ferrell, & N. Coyle (Eds.), *Oxford textbook of palliative nursing* (3rd ed., pp. 359–386). New York, NY: Oxford University Press.

Best, L., Simmonds, P., Baughan, C., Buchanan, R., Davis, C., Fentiman, I., . . . Williams, C. (2008). *Palliative chemotherapy for advanced or metastatic colorectal cancer. Cochrane Database of Systematic Reviews 2000.* doi: 10.1002/14651858.CD001545

Bruera, E., & Hui, D. (2010). Integrating supportive and palliative care in the trajectory of cancer: Establishing goals and models of care. *Journal of Clinical Oncology, 28*(25), 4013–4017.

Casarett, D., Karlawish, J. H., Henry, M., & Hirschman, K. (2002). Must patients with advanced cancer choose between a phase 1 trial and hospice? *Cancer, 95*, 1601–1604.

Cawley, M., & Benson, L. (2005). Current trends in managing oral mucositis. *Clinical Journal of Oncology Nursing, 9*(5), 584–592.

Clarkson, J., Worthington, H., Furness, S., McCabe, M., Khalid, T., & Meyer, S. (2010). Interventions for treating oral mucositis for patients with cancer receiving treatment (Review). *Cochrane Database of Systematic Reviews* (8); Art. No.: CD001973.

Cochran, S., & Jakubek, P. (2010). Malignant cutaneous diseases. In M. Haas, & G. Moore-Higgs (Eds.), *Principles of skin care and the oncology patient* (pp. 77–100). Pittsburgh, PA: Oncology Nursing Society.

Costa, L., & Major, P. (2009). Effect of bisphosphonates on pain and quality of life in patients with bone metastases. *Nature Clinical Practice. Oncology, 6*(3), 163–174.

Coyne, P., Hansen, L., & Watson, A. (2006). Compounded drugs: Are customized prescription drugs a salvation, snake oil, or both? *Journal of Hospice & Palliative Nursing, 8*(4), 222–226.

Cruciani, R., Strada, E., & Knotkova, H. (2010). Neuropathic pain. In E. Bruera & R. Portenoy (Eds.), *Cancer pain: Assessment and management* (pp. 478–505). New York, NY: Cambridge University Press.

Cummins, E., Vick, K., & Poole, G. (2004). Incurable colorectal carcinoma: The role of surgical palliation. *American Surgeon, 70*(5), 433–437.

Davis, M., & Hinshaw, D. (2006). Management of visceral pain due to cancer-related intestinal obstruction. In O. de Leon-Casasola (Ed.), *Cancer pain: Pharmacological, interventional and palliative care approaches* (pp. 481–495). Philadelphia, PA: Saunders Elsevier.

Desai, M., Kim, A., Fall, P., & Wang, D. (2007). Optimizing quality of lifethrough palliative care. *Journal of the American Osteopath Association, 107*(Suppl. 7), ES9–ES14.

Doughty, D. (2010). Skin and wound pain: Assessment and management. In M. Haas, & G. Moore-Higgs (Eds.), *Principles of skin care and the oncology paitent* (pp. 237–255). Pittsburgh, PA: Oncology Nursing Society.

Eisenberger, A., Whelan, R., & Neugut, A. (2008). Survival and symptomatic benefit from palliative primary tumor resection in patients with metastatic colorectal cancer: A review. *International Journal of Colorectal Disease, 23*(6), 559–568.

Fairchild, A., & Chow, E. (2010). Palliative radiotherapy. In E. Bruera & R. Portenoy (Eds.), *Cancer pain: Assessment and management* (2nd ed., pp. 379–398). New York, NY: Cambridge University Press.

Ferris, F., Bruera, E., Cherny, N., Cummings, C., Currow, D., Dudgeon, D.,... Von Roenn, J. H. (2009). Palliative cancer care a decade later: Accomplishments, the need, next steps— From the American Society of Clinical Oncology. *Journal of Clinical Oncology, 27*(18), 3052–3058.

Finlay, I., Mason, M., & Shelley, M. (2005). Radioisotopes for the palliation of metastatic bone cancer: A systematic review. *Lancet Oncology, 6*(6), 392–400.

Grocott, P., & Dealey, C. (2005). Nursing aspects. In D. Doyle, G. Hanks, N. Cherny, & K. Calman (Eds.), *Oxford textbook of palliative medicine* (3rd ed., pp. 628–640). New York, NY: Oxford University Press.

Harrington, S., & Smith, T. (2008). The role of chemotherapy at the end of life: "When is enough, enough?". *Journal of the American Medical Association, 299*, 2667–2678.

Harris, D., Eilers, J., Harriman, A., Cashavelly, B., & Maxwell, C. (2008). Putting evidence into practice: Evidence-based interventions for the management of oral mucositis. *Clinical Journal of Oncology Nursing, 12*(1), 141–152.

Hoskin, P. (2005). Radiotherapy in symptom management. In D. Doyle, G. Hanks, N. Cherny, & K. Calman (Eds.), *Oxford textbook of palliative medicine* (3rd ed., pp. 239–255). New York, NY: Oxford University Press.

Katonis, P., Pasku, D., Alpantaki, K., Bano, A., Tzanakakis, G., & Karantanas, A. (2009). Treatment of pathologic spinal fractures with combined radiofrequency ablation and balloon kyphoplasty. *World Journal of Surgical Oncology, 7*(90), 1–8.

Kaufman, M., Radhakrishnan, N., Roy, R., Gecelter, G., Tsang, J., Thomas, A., . . . Mehrotra, B. (2008). Influence of palliative surgical resection on overall survival in patients with advanced colorectal cancer: a retrospective single institutional study. *Colorectal Disease, 10*(5), 498–502.

Kirkbride, P., & Barton, R. (1999). Palliative radiation therapy. *Journal of Palliative Medicine, 2*(1), 87–97.

Koh, M., & Portenoy, R. (2010). Cancer pain syndromes. In E. Bruera & R. Portenoy (Eds.), *Cancer pain: Assessment and management* (2nd ed., pp. 53–85). New York, NY: Cambridge University Press.

MacDonald, N. (2005). Palliative medicine and modern cancer care. In D. Doyle, G. Hanks, N. Cherny, & K. Calman (Eds.), *Oxford textbook of palliative medicine* (3rd. ed., pp. 24–28). New York, NY: Oxford University Press.

Mackillop, W. J. (1996). The principles of palliative radiotherapy: A radiation oncologist's perspective. *Canadian Journal of Oncology, 6*(1), 5–11.

McIllmurray, M. (2005). Palliative medicine and the treatment of cancer. In D. Doyle, G. Hanks, N. Cherny, & K. Calman (Eds.), *Oxford textbook of palliative medicine* (3rd ed., pp. 229–239). New York, NY: Oxford University Press.

McQuay, H., Collins, S., Carroll, D., & Moore, R. (2008). Radiotherapy for the palliation of painful bone metastases. *Cochrane Database of Systematic Reviews* (4). Art. No.:
CD001793.

Miaskowski, C., Bair, M., Chou, R., D'Arcy, Y., Hartwick, C., Huffman, L., . . .
Manwarren, R. (2008). *Principles of analgesic use in the treatment of acute pain and cancer
pain* (6th ed.). Glenview, IL: American Pain Society.

Naidu, M., Ramana, G., Rani, P., Mohan, I., Suman, A., & Roy, P. (2004). Chemotherapy-
induced and/or radiation therapy–induced oral mucositis—Complicating the treatment of cancer. *Neoplasia, 6*(5), 423–431.

Oida, T., Mimatsu, K., Kawasaki, A., Kano, H., Kuboi, Y., & Amano, S. (2009). Modified
Devine exclusion with vertical stomach reconstruction for gastric outlet obstruction:
A novel technique. *Journal of Gastrointestinal Surgery, 13*(7), 1226–1232.

Park, S., Lin, C., Krishnan, A., Goldstein, D., Friedlander, M., & Kiernan, M. (2009).
Oxaliplatin-induced neurotoxicity: Changes in axonal excitability precede development of neuropathy. *Brain, 132*, 2712–2723.

Pavlakis, N., Schmidt, R., & Stockler, M. (2005). Bisphosphonates for breast cancer.
Cochrane Database of Systematic Reviews (3). Art. No.: CD003474.

Pearson, I., & Mortimer, P. (2005). Skin problems in palliative medicine. In D. Doyle,
G. Hanks, N. Cherny, & K. Calman (Eds.), *Oxford textbook of palliative medicine*
(3rd ed., pp. 618–628). New York, NY: Oxford University Press.

Quill, T. E., Holloway, R. G., Shah, M. S., Caprio, T. V., Olden, A. M., & Storey, J. C. (2010).
Primer of palliative care (5th ed.). Glenview, IL: American Academy of Hospice and
Palliative Medicine.

Raber-Durlacher, J. E., Elad, S., & Barasch, A. (2010). Oral mucositis. *Oral Oncology, 46*,
452–456.

Ronnekleiv-Kelly, S., & Kennedy, G. (2011). Management of stage IV rectal cancer:
Palliative options. *World Journal of Gastroenterology, 17*(7), 835–847.

Roqué i Figuls, M., Martinez-Zapata, M., Scott-Brown, M., & Alonso-Coello, P. (2011).
Radioisotopes for metastatic bone pain. *Cochrane Database of Systematic Reviews* (7).
Art. No.: CD003347.

Rutter, C., & Weissman, D. (2004). Radiation for palliation-Part 1 & Part 2; Fast Facts
#65 & #66. *Journal of Palliative Medicine, 7*(6), 865–867.

Saif, M., & Reardon, J. (2005). Management of oxaliplatin-induced peripheral neuropathy.
Therapeutics and Clinical Risk Management , 1(4), 249–258.

Sainsbury, R., Vaizey, C., Pastorino, U., Mould, T., & Emberton, M. (2005). Surgical palliation. In D. Doyle, G. Hanks, N. Cherny, & K. Calman (Eds.), *Oxford textbook of
palliative medicine* (3rd ed., pp. 255–266). New York, NY: Oxford University Press.

Seaman, S. (2006). Management of malignant fungating wounds in advanced cancer.
Seminars in Oncology Nursing, 22(3), 185–193.

Seaman, S., & Bates-Jensen, B. (2010). Skin disorders: Malignant wounds, fistulas, and sto-
mas. In B. Ferrell, & N. Coyle (Eds.), *Oxford textbook of palliative nursing* (3rd ed.,
pp. 387–404). New York, NY: Oxford University Press.

Shah, S., Haddad, R., Al-Sukhni, W., Kim, R., Greig, P., Grant, D., . . . Wei, A. C. (2006).
Surgical resection of hepatic and pulmonary metastases from colorectal carcinoma.
Journal of the American College of Surgeons, 202(3), 468–475.

Smith, H. (2011). Painful osseous metastases. *Pain Physician, 14*, E373–E405.

Sun, V. (2010). Palliative chemotherapy and clinical trials in advanced cancer: The nurse's role. In B. Ferrell & N. Coyle (Eds.), *Oxford textbook of palliative nursing* (3rd ed., pp. 969–980). New York, NY: Oxford University Press.

Thanos, L., Galani, P., Tzavoulis, D., Kalioras, V., Tanteles, S., & Pomoni, M. (2008). Radiofrequency ablation of osseous metastases for the palliation of pain. *Skeletal Radiology, 37*(3), 189–194.

Van Poznak, C., Temin, S., Yee, G., Janjan, N., Barlow, W., Biermann, J., . . . Von Roenn, J. H. (2011). American Society of Clinical Oncology executive summary of the clinical practice guideline update on the role of bone-modifying agents in metastatic breast cancer. *Journal of Clinical Oncology, 29*(9), 1221–1227.

von Moos, R. (2006). Bisphosphonate treatment recommendations for oncologists. *Oncologist, 10*, 19–24.

Webster-Gandy, J., How, C., & Harrold, K. (2007). Palmar–plantar erythrodysesthesia (PPE): A literature review with commentary on experience in a cancer centre. *European Journal of Oncology Nursing, 11*(3), 238–246.

Weissman, D. (2009). *Palliative chemotherapy, Fast facts #14.* Retrieved from http://www.eperc.mcw.edu/fastFact/ff_14.htm

Wong, P., Dodd, M., Miaskowski, C., Paul, S., Bank, K., Shiba, G., & Facione, N. (2006). Mucositis pain induced by radiation therapy: Prevalence, severity, and use of self-care behaviors. *Journal of Pain & Symptom Management, 32*(1), 27–37.

Wong, R., & Wiffen, P. (2009). Bisphosphonates for the relief of pain secondary to bone metastases. *Cochrane Database of Systematic Reviews* (4). Art. No.: CD002068.

Wright, A., & Katz, I. (2007). Letting go of the rope—Aggressive treatment, hospice care, and open access. *New England Journal of Medicine, 357*(4), 324–327.

11

The Effect of Opioid Polymorphisms and Other Physiologic Factors on Treating Cancer Pain

Yvonne D'Arcy

OVERVIEW

Opioids have long been considered the mainstay for treating cancer pain as part of a multimodal approach to pain management (American Pain Society [APS], 2005; Droney & Riley, 2009; Hanks & Reid, 2005; Mercadante & Bruera, 2006; Slatkin, 2009; Vadalouca, Moka, Argyra, Sikioti, & Sifaka, 2008; World Health Organization [WHO], 1996). However, not all patients respond to the opioids prescribed for treating their pain in the same way. All opioids bind to an area of the cell called the mu receptor found in many areas of the body such as peripheral nerves, pre- and postsynaptic neural junctions, and even in the colon, which is considered to be the major mechanism for opioid-induced constipation (Inturrisi & Lipman, 2010). Recent research has shown that there may be 45 or more different variations in the makeup and action of the mu receptor sites (Pasternak, 2005) and many more variations in the proteins required to allow cellular binding of the opioid to the receptor site (Pasternak, 2010). We know that individual variations such neuronal plasticity and wind-up, gender, metabolism rates, race, and familial tendencies also affect the way the patient responds to both pain stimulus and opioid medication (APS, 2005; D'Arcy, 2011b; Fillingim, 2010).

For many years, the use of morphine was considered to be the best and most effective method for treating patients who were having significant pain from cancer. Today we know that there are any number of opioid and nonopioid combinations that are effective for pain relief and many different types of interventions such as regional anesthesia that can help provide analgesia for patients with cancer pain. The current trend reflects the need to tailor the pain management strategies to each individual and utilizing those that provide the best level of relief for the patient.

What we also have come to understand is the large number of individual factors that can affect the speed that the patient metabolizes opioids and the way the patient is genetically programmed to utilize opioids. For years clinicians noted that not all patients having certain procedures such as abdominal surgery responded in the same way to pain medications even though the surgical procedure was the same. In the past, nurses might tell patients, "most people with this surgery are out of bed by day two," while patients with poor pain control or significant adverse effects were still in bed, hoping to stay there all day. Today, we look at the patient as an individual who brings a large number of factors to the pain management process. Hopefully, the choices we make for controlling pain produce an optimal outcome.

Phamacogenomics is the study of variations in the human genome and how these variations affect the response to drugs (Janetto & Bratanow, 2011). Factors that can affect the way the patient responds to a given drug are as follows:

- Age
- Sex
- Race
- Comorbidities
- Drug–drug interactions
- Hepatic/renal function
- Genetics, especially the differences in disposition and metabolism of the drugs (Fillingim, 2010; Jannetto & Bratanow, 2011)

Today, we know these variations in response could be a reflection of the individual patient's genetic configuration for a particular opioid to provide pain relief. Patients who are rapid metabolizers of opioids have a very different response to opioids when compared to patients who are ultra-slow metabolizers. For the first type of patient, there may not be enough opioid prescribed to control the pain, pain intensity ratings will continue to be high, and the patient may continue to ask for more medication when all prescribed doses have been given. The ultra-slow opioid metabolizers may need only very small amounts of medication to achieve adequate pain control, and the medication that is given can remain in the patient's system for longer than other patients. These patients may not know that they are not the same genetically, but both types of patients know that pain relief for them is difficult. Nurses are not aware of how any individual patient metabolizes medication or if the patient cannot respond to certain opioids. This makes finding the right combination of medications and doses for any individual patient a challenge.

Cancer treatments are also affected by genetic differences. In some breast cancer patients, the cancer is estrogen sensitive. This in turn affects what type of chemotherapy is most effective for treating the cancer. Genetically engineered viruses that express specific neurotrophins are being studied to see if they can control neuropathic pain, while specially coded herpes simplex virus is being studied as a means of controlling metastatic bone pain, inflammatory pain, and neuropathic pain in animal models (Thapa, Rastogi, & Ahuja, 2011). We are beginning to understand that genetics plays a big role in how medications for pain work in patients and how to determine what those differences mean clinically. For patients with cancer, choosing the right treatment plan for their disease can mean a big difference in prognosis and quality of life.

This chapter will discuss the sources of opioid polymorphisms. It will cover the topics of opioid rotation or switching, effects of metabolism on opioid activity, the role of the mu receptor, and the occurrence of opioid hyperalgesia. In order to fully understand how to rotate opioids for best effect, the concept of equianalgesia will also be reviewed.

THE ROLE OF THE MU RECEPTOR

Opioids in general bind to a section of the cellular membrane called the mu receptor site. The opioid molecule locates the opioid receptor site and binds with the site, creating an analgesic effect (see Figure 11.1).

In the past, the opioid binding mechanism was considered to be a lock-and-key effect, but now we know the action is highly complex and dependent on a large number of factors such as sex, genetics, protein type, and metabolism rates. These differences are considered to be important factors and, when applied to mu activity, are called *opioid polymorphisms*.

There are three major types of binding sites for pain medications, as follows:

■ *Mu:* Primary binding site for pure mu opioid agonists, such as morphine, hydromorphone, and fentanyl. The mu receptor is responsible for not only analgesia but several other related effects such as respiratory depression and tolerance.

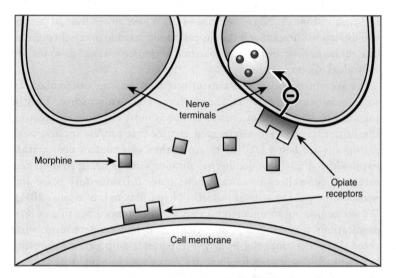

Figure 11.1 ■ Opioid binding mechanism.

■ *Kappa:* A secondary binding site for mixed agonist–antagonist medications such as nalbuphine and buprenorphine. They bind as agonists at the kappa site and antagonists at the mu site and since they are located lower on the spinal cord have less potential for respiratory depression.

■ *Delta:* A less well-known binding site whose action has not been fully explored (Gourlay, 2005; Inturissi & Lipman, 2010)

The mu receptor sites are located throughout the body in many areas of the brain, in the periphery, and on some circulating immune cells (Shi, Cleeland, Klepstad, Miaskowski, & Pedersen, 2010). Receptor genes that are associated with these receptor sites include the mu receptor gene *MOR-1*, a delta receptor site called *DOR-1*, and a kappa receptor site called *KOR-1* (Gourlay, 2005). Of particular interest is that these receptor sites may be expressed in overlapping configurations, making it difficult to determine the most effective binding potential. Currently, there are thought to be as many as 100 polymorphisms of the *OPRM1* gene (Nagashima et al., 2007).

There are three findings that are salient when considering the effect of genetic polymorphisms of pain, as follows:

1. Nearly all naturally occurring and manufactured opioids as well as endogenous (naturally produced by the body) opioids bind to the high-affinity, naloxone-sensitive mu1 receptor with similar affinity as the source of analgesia.

2. Agonist binding affinities create the analgesic response.

3. Splice variants called *heterodynes* or *homodimers* are also thought to be responsible for analgesic response (Gourlay, 2005).

As our knowledge of the genetic effects on opioid binding and affinity expands, new information on gene splice variants has provided additional insight on the topic. Some of these variants like the MOR/KOR heterodimers are affected by estrogen levels and are only seen in females (Chakbarati, Liu, & Gintzler, 2010), while splice variants can occur at either end of the gene, causing wider variation in the makeup of the binding sites, affecting the dose requirement of opioids for pain control.

Clinical Pearl	Why do we need pain? Pain can serve a protective function. In a rare occurrence in nature, there is one genetic variation that does not allow the person to experience pain, referred to as *congenital insensitivity to pain.* These non-sense mutations in genes are rarely expressed but when they do occur it can be very serious for the person with the condition, causing painless injuries, chronic skin ulcers, and distal amputations (Miaskowski, 2009; Trembaly & Hamet, 2010).

The genetic profile for a patient is as individual as a fingerprint or iris pattern. Genetically, there are innumerable combinations of genes that can produce any one human being. For opioids, the gene that encodes for morphine activity, called mu-opioid receptor gene (*OPRM1*), is the key to the response of patients to the mu agonist morphine. The catechol-O-methyltransferase (*COMT*) gene is also a highly likely candidate for influencing the efficacy and side effects of morphine in patients with cancer (Shi et al., 2010). The combined action of these two genes can affect the ability of morphine to control pain, affect morphine consumption, and produce side effects. In a study of 207 hospital inpatients who had been using morphine for pain control for at least 3 days, carriers of the Met/Met and AA genotype in the *OPRM1* and *COMT* genes needed less morphine for pain relief (Reyes-Gibby et al., 2007). More specifically, carriers of the *OPRM1 GG* genotypes needed 93% higher morphine doses when compared to the *AA* variant of the genotype. For the *COMT* genotypes, the *Val/VAL* and *Val/Met* genotypes required 63% and 23% higher morphine doses, respectively, when compared to the *Met/Met* genotype of the *COMT* gene (Reyes et al., 2007).

SEX, GENDER, AND RACE

As research has expanded into the area of differences in response to pain and pain medications, the idea of differences in sex, gender, and race have become integral issues to explore. In a review of animal research studies from 1996 to 2005, 79% of the studies used male subjects only on their research (Mogil, 2009). Even in early studies of breast cancer research, they were conducted using only male participants. At that point, women were felt to be emotional responders to pain and the effect of estrogen was poorly understood, causing researchers to eliminate them from studies to avoid trying to control for the variables.

In the mid-1990s, publications started appearing in reputable journals that highlighted the need to study the pain response of women and determine if there was a difference that made women's pain a unique experience for them. At the same time, the National Institutes of Health (NIH) developed several initiatives on pain in women that generated significant interest in the topic. After this initiative, researchers began to explore the various areas of pain in women and tried to determine if there was an overall difference in pain in women or if there were only a difference in some of the pain syndromes that were more common in women than men such as fibromyalgia and osteoarthritis pain.

Do men and women experience pain differently? Yes, they do, as a result of their hormonal variation and differences in pain pathway activation when a pain stimulus is presented for interpretation. Are there differences in the way that men and women respond to pain medications? Again the answer is yes, for a variety of reasons. Some of these reasons include the following:

- Kappa specific pain pathways found only in women
- Differences in the way pain is processed
- Effect of sex hormones
- Differences in response to opioid medications
- Lower threshold and tolerance for pain (Wilson, 2006)

There are some pain syndromes that are more specific to women than men. Examples of these syndromes include the following:

- Fibromyalgia
- Temporomandibular joint (TMJ) pain
- Phantom breast pain
- Postmastectomy pain syndrome
- Menstrual-related migraine
- Irritable bowel syndrome
- Interstitial cystitis
- Vulvodynia

In a study to compare the analgesic effect of morphine in both men and women, three important conclusions were derived, as follows (Dahan, Kest, Waxman, & Sarton, 2008):

1. Morphine is more potent in women than in men.
2. The onset and offset of morphine is slower in women than in men.
3. Plasma concentrations of both the active drug and two metabolites were identical for both sexes.

These findings are particularly important for acute pain and postoperative pain management. Since morphine is considered the gold standard for pain management medication comparison and commonly used in postoperative pain relief, these differences in potency and onset are important considerations when pain relief is assessed. As an interesting addendum, the sex effect with morphine disappears with older patients, leading to the speculation that hormones have an effect on morphine's ability to pass through the blood–brain barrier (Dahan et al., 2008).

In addition to the differences in morphine with men and women, the side effects from opioid medications tend to have some sex-related relationships. The most common are nausea/vomiting, sedation, cardiovascular effects, and respiratory depression. These differences include the following:

- There is more nausea/vomiting in women using opioids for postoperative pain control.
- There is increased risk for opioid-induced respiratory depression in women.
- Morphine is associated with a lower heart rate in women but the development of hypertension in men.
- With opioid use, women reported more feelings of euphoria (a high feeling) and reported more instances of dry mouth (Dahan et al., 2008).

Other differences with pain medications were related to differences seen with kappa agonist medications such as nalbuphine, butorphanol, and pentazocine.

The melanocortin-1 receptor gene, *Mc1r*, has a specific role in modulating a pain pathway that exists only in women. This gene is commonly associated with people who have red hair, fair skin, freckles, and a high predisposition to melanoma (Dahan et al., 2008):

- This was tested by giving pentazocine to both men and women
- There was pain relief in redheaded, fair-skinned women, but no pain relief in men
- The hypothesis is that men and women have separate pain modulation pathways that are created by different genes and neurochemicals (Mogil & Max, 2006)

The study of differences in pain response both physiologically and in men and women is a very new area of research. Much more research is needed to confirm these early findings. The early research is promising and points the way to finding the true differences between men and women in both pain response and medication efficacy.

THE GENETIC EFFECT

Variations in genetics have been identified that affect the major mechanisms of medication management. These variations in medication use affect medication:

- Absorption
- Distribution
- Metabolism
- Elimination (Janetto & Bratanow, 2011)

The genetic effect on pain relief is starting to be an area of great interest in pain management practices. Since each patient comes to us as a genetic unknown, we need to look at the research to determine what pieces of information we can use to help maximize pain relief. Research in this area is by no means complete but there are some studies that illustrate how genetics affects pain relief. Studying the single-nucleotide polymorphism of the *MOR* gene, responsible for mu-opioid receptor activity, has provided some interesting findings.

In a study of 74 patients who were having total knee replacements, genetic profiling revealed three separate groups of patients. To determine how much medication provided pain relief for each group, morphine via patient-controlled analgesia (PCA) was used for postoperative pain management. Analgesia reports and opioid consumption were tracked for 48 hours postsurgery.

- *AA*-homozygous patients with an efficient morphine metabolism: This group used 25 mg of morphine and had good pain relief.
- *AG*-heterozygous variant patients: Used 25 mg of morphine and had good pain relief.
- *GG*-homozygous nonsensitive genetic variant patients with reduced or impaired morphine sensitivity: These patients had very different results. They used 40 mg of morphine, and had many more attempts on the PCA trying to get a better level of pain control (Chou et al., 2006)

Specifically for pain in cancer patients, research has identified eight single-nucleotide polymorphisms (SNPs) that were significantly involved in opioid therapy outcomes for at least 570 patients (Galvan, Skorpen, et al., 2011). Inflammatory markers were also identified in lung cancer patients where *CC* genotypes were at lower risk for severe pain, while *NFKBIA*, a specific genetic substance, was identified as allowing for severe pain (Reyes-Gibby et al., 2009).

As far as ethnic origins, a study comparing ethnicity with pain in 2,294 patients with cancer found four genetic profiles that spanned country of origin and affected pain relief (Galvan, Fladvad, et al., 2011). As research in these areas develops, more information will be available to determine just what type of patient response can be expected with specific genotypes and how the role of genetics affects pain management outcomes in patients with cancer.

NEURONAL PLASTICITY, WIND-UP, ALLODYNIA, OPIOID HYPERALGESIA, AND OTHER FACTORS

One of the factors that has an obvious effect on opioids is the rate of medication metabolism. Patients are now classified as ultra-rapid or rapid metabolizers, moderate metabolizers, or ultra-slow medication metabolizers. For the clinician, the ultra-rapid or rapid metabolizer uses up the medication and continues to complain of pain well before the next dose of medication is due. There is currently a black box warning on the use of acetaminophen and codeine with breastfeeding mothers for rapid medication metabolizers since the active metabolite, morphine, was being passed to the infants through breast milk (D'Arcy, 2011a). The ultra-slow metabolizer needs just a small amount of medication and may become oversedated or have side effects such as nausea. These patients may report that they are sensitive to opioids or that many opioids tend to make them nauseated.

Both rapid or slow metabolizers will report difficulty with pain medications. Listening to the patients explain their past experience will provide insight into the complexities of managing pain in these individuals.

Drug–drug interaction can also affect the quality of pain relief for the patients with cancer pain. Since most medications are activated in the liver through the CYP 450 system, any drug that inactivates or potentiates opioids can affect the quality of pain relief.

Plasticity

When pain becomes a chronic condition as with many patients with neuropathic pain, the repeated pain stimulus can cause changes in the patient's body and the way it responds to and processes the pain. With repeated pain stimuli, the body changes its function to respond more globally and the neurons have the ability to change function called *neuronal plasticity*.

Pain-facilitating substances such as Substance P and other cytokines are recruited at the site of pain, creating a heightened sensation of pain over a larger area, and inflammation is created. Peripheral sensitization is the result with resultant *hyperalgesia* and/or *allodynia*. Long-term use of high-dose opioids is implicated in the creation of a specific hyperalgesic condition called *opioid-induced hyperalgesia*. The treatment for this condition is as follows:

▨ Opioid rotation
▨ Dose reduction of opioids, which requires the implementation of alternate sources of pain relief

---

Clinical Pearl Hyperalgesia: A heightened response to a normally mild pain such as a pinprick.

Allodynia: A pain response when the sensation is normally not painful, such as being stroked with a wisp of cotton or cotton swab.

With prolonged pain from the periphery, the central nervous system changes its processing of the pain signals, causing increased pain intensity and pain duration. This phenomenon is called *wind-up*. Once the pain begins to be activated by the central nervous system, receptors called N-methyl-d-aspartate (NMDA) are activated causing further intensification and progression of the pain. The whole process becomes a vicious cycle and is much more difficult to treat. Examples of conditions where this type of pain is found are osteoarthritis and complex regional pain syndrome (CRPS).

EQUIANALGESIA AND OPIOID ROTATION

Equianalgesia is the conversion of one opioid to the equivalent analgesic dose of another opioid based on equivalency charts. These equianalgesic charts are designed to provide guidance for practitioners who are prescribing or treating patients who are on opioid therapy. Although it seems like a simple process to take one medication, look to see what an equivalent dose is, and then start the new medication, there are pitfalls and risks that make the process challenging.

One of the major pitfalls for the use of equianalgesic tables is the variability from one individual to another and from one medication to the next. There are outside factors that can influence how potent a medication is for the patient, which can skew the results of a comparison.

Equianalgesic tables are based on single-dose trials in healthy volunteers (usually young adult males). Equianalgesic doses have been determined in the past by expert opinion, single-dose studies, and studies in noncancer patients (Shaheen, Walsh, Lasheen, Davis, & Lagman, 2009). This makes using these tables an estimation only. The best use of equianalgesic tables is to use the doses as a guide rather than an absolute. In a study comparing equianalgesic tables, findings indicate that in some tables the conversion for oral to parenteral morphine ranged from 2:1 to 6:1; and ranges for oral to parenteral hydromorphone were from 2:1 to 5:1 (Shaheen et al., 2009).

For the clinician, this lack of concrete applicability is problematic. Here is where the art and science of pain management meet. The science of pain management provides the structure for an equianalgesic conversion, while the art allows the clinician to interpret the best dose for the patient. Knowing the patient is an important part of a successful conversion. Allowing for additional breakthrough medication can also provide for adequate pain relief if the conversion falls a bit short of what is needed to maintain sufficient pain relief.

Clinical Pearl	Equianalgesia is defined as the dose at which two opioids provide approximately the same pain relief. The gold standard is 10 mg of parenteral morphine (Shaheen et al., 2009).

There are many sources for equianalgesic conversion tables. Appendix B provides an example of a conversion table. Other sources that can be accessed include the following:

- American Pain Society's *Principles of Analgesic Use in the Treatment of Acute Pain and Cancer Pain*, available at www.ampainsoc.org
- Online opioid analgesic converter available at www.globalrph.com/narcoticcanv.htm
- American Academy of Hospice and Palliative Medicine's (AAHPM) *Primer of Palliative Care* (2010, 5th ed.), available at http://www.aahpm.org/
- Dosing equivalencies from the *Physicians' Desk Reference*
- Prescribing information from the package inserts

There are pros and cons of using any equianalgesic table. One of the biggest pros is that it simplifies the mathematical conversion from one medication to another. The list is usually a conversion of the most commonly used medications. The cons, however, are still very significant and include the following:

- There is a failure to standardize a reference opioid.
- Many tables are the product of a single-dose conversion in a laboratory setting with volunteers using artificially produced acute pain.
- There is a wide range of doses in the table.
- Equianalgesia is compared with short- and long-acting medications, not at steady state; therefore, the dose needed may be lower than estimated.
- Computations are used instead of a clinical trial to determine equianalgesic doses (Shaheen et al., 2009).

Opioid rotation is needed for about 40% of patients with cancer who have advanced disease (Shaheen et al., 2009). For those patients who do require an opioid switch, about 70% to 80% have an improvement in the balance between analgesia and adverse effects (Mercadante & Bruera, 2006). The rationale for using an opioid rotation is to increase the pain relief being provided by the patient and/or lessen intolerable side effects such as nausea. Patients who complain of the following are candidates for opioid rotation:

- Decreased efficacy of the opioids
- Lack of improved analgesia with increased doses
- Intolerable side effects but with remaining significant pain

A Cochrane Review of the literature on opioid rotation reports that the evidence for opioid switching is largely anecdotal or based on lower-level studies (Quigley, 2010). However, the practice is established in the cancer pain population where high-dose opioids are used routinely to control pain.

For cancer patients, opioid switching offers an option for improved pain relief, increased opioid response, and decreased unwanted side effects. In a review of the literature on opioid switching, Mercadante and Bruera (2006) reported that clinical improvement is seen in approximately 50% of patients with chronic pain who have a poor response to a specific opioid. It can be very anxiety producing for a patient with cancer who does not have decreased pain relief with dose escalations. Providing the patient with an opioid rotation may improve pain control and decrease fears of having pain that cannot be controlled.

To perform an opioid rotation, the clinician first reviews an equianalgesic chart to determine equivalencies. Then the clinician needs to evaluate the following:

- Level of pain
- Effect of the adverse effects

■ Any comorbidities that affect medication choice (such as renal or hepatic impairment, or QTc prolongation)
■ Concomitant medications

Extreme care must be used when converting patients from high-dose opioids to another medication to avoid overdosing or underdosing the patient and preserving patient safety throughout the process.

Data on conversions from morphine to hydromorphone or hydrocodone are more available and the result is more predictable. Converting patients from long-acting medications such as methadone or morphine requires a careful and measured response. Data for the success of such conversions are scant and using a pharmacist for assistance should be considered.

Clinical Pearl	Opioid rotation is defined as a therapeutic maneuver aimed at increasing analgesia while decreasing opioid side effects. It is a change in opioid drug or route of administration with the goal of improving outcomes (Fine & Portenoy, 2009). This includes changing medications using the same route or maintaining the current medication but changing the route of administration or both (Knotkova et al., 2009; Vadalouca et al., 2008).

Issues that should be considered when performing an opioid rotation in order to avoid an error include the following (Shaheen et al., 2009):
■ Knowledge of opioid pharmacology
■ Awareness of the limitation of equianalgesic tables
■ Application of the conversion/rotation guidelines
■ Tailoring opioid doses to the individual patients and monitoring the response

Because the patient may be more responsive to the new opioid dose, there are some considerations that should be used before completing the conversion. Before implementing an opioid rotation, best practice guidelines indicate the following:
■ Use an equianalgesic table to calculate the new opioid dose.
■ For most opioids other than fentanyl or methadone, use an automatic dose reduction of 25% to 50%. If methadone is the new opioid, reduce the dose by 75% to 90%.
■ Use caution with high-dose conversions (greater than 1,000 mg per day of oral morphine equivalent). Expert consultation is recommended. These conversions may require inpatient monitoring, including serial electrocardiograms.

■ Reduce the dose by 50% if the patient is on high-dose opioids, is not Caucasian, or the patient is elderly or frail.

■ Reduce the dose by 25% if the patient is on a low to moderate dose of opioids, is Caucasian, under age 60, and reasonably robust, or if the change is from one route to another with the same medication.

■ Assess the patient for the severity of the pain or other medical characteristics that would point to a need for higher or lower doses and decrease or increase the dose by an additional 15% to 30% to reduce side effects, improve analgesia, or to avoid withdrawal.

■ Maintain a schedule of frequent reassessment and monitoring and titrate the dose to maximize outcomes.

■ Provide adequate rescue or breakthrough pain doses for titration at 5% to 15% of the total 24 hour opioid dose (Fine & Portenoy, 2009).

Knowing the patient well and understanding how he or she has reacted to opioid medications in the past is part of a comprehensive evaluation to performing an opioid rotation. Since there is the potential for opioid cross-tolerance, a conservative approach and the use of frequent breakthrough medication can help reduce the risk during the period of rotation. Monitoring the effect of the new medication is essential. In the following box an example of a simple opioid rotation is provided.

EXAMPLE OF AN OPIOID ROTATION CONVERSION OF MS CONTIN TO OXYCONTIN

Original Medication: MS Contin

Dose: MS Contin 120 mg twice per day with MSIR 30 mg every 4 hours as needed for pain (using an average of 4 tablets per day = 120 mg/day)

New Medication: Oxycontin

Equianalgesic conversion: MS Contin 120 mg twice per day (240 mg/day) is equal to Oxycontin 80 mg twice per day (160 mg/day)

MSIR 30 mg is equal to oxycodone 20 mg every 4 hours

Decrease the new dose by 25% to 50%

25% = Oxycontin 60 mg twice per day with 15 mg of oxycodone every 4 hours for breakthrough pain

50% = Oxycontin 40 mg twice per day with 10 mg of oxycodone every 4 hours for breakthrough pain

Source: D'Arcy, 2011a.

For patients who need opioid rotation, converting from one problematic opioid to another, more successful opioid can provide patients with cancer pain the relief they need.

Case Study

Sally B. is a 45-year-old patient who just had a colon resection related to a malignancy. She reports a high level of pain at 8/10 consistently, no matter what type of opioid is tried. She is taking nothing by mouth yet and she is having nausea and vomiting. She has had a morphine PCA discontinued because it provided little pain relief and the surgeon is trying a fentanyl PCA to see if it will provide better pain relief and reduce the side effects. She has had trouble with anesthesia before and she has related that to her red hair and fair-skinned physiology. She keeps asking the nurse, "Are you sure that machine is working? No matter how many times I push the button, I still have all this pain."

Sally has a history of poor pain relief from her oral pain medications prescribed prior to her surgery, Percocet. Her physician tried to increase the dose of her oral opioids, but Sally reported that the pain was still just about as intense as with the lower doses. What do you suspect is the cause of Sally's poor analgesia?

Questions to Consider

1. Does the fact that Sally is a woman, fair-skinned, and red-headed play into the poor response to the opioid medications?
2. What actions could you take to make Sally's analgesia better? Should you consider adding additional types of medications or interventions?
3. Does Sally need an opioid rotation?

REFERENCES

American Pain Society (APS). (2005). *Guideline for the management of cancer pain in adults and children.* Glenview, IL: Author.

Chakrabati, S., Liu, N., & Gintzler, A. (2010). Formation of u-/k-opioid receptor heterodimer is sex-dependent and medicates female-specific opioid analgesia. *Proceedings of the National Academy of Sciences, 107*(46), 20115–20119.

Chou, W. Y., Yang, L. C., Lu, H. F., Ko, J. Y., Wang, C. H., Lin, S. H., & Hsu, C. J. (2006). Association of mu-opioid receptor gene polymorphism (A118G) with variation in morphine consumption for analgesia after total knee arthroplasty. *Acta Anaesthesiologica Scandinavica, 50*(7), 787–792.

Dahan, A., Kest, B., Waxman, A., & Sarton, E. (2008). Sex-specific response to opiates: Animal and human studies. *Anesthesia & Analgesia, 107*(1), 83–95.

D'Arcy, Y. (2011a). *Compact clinical guide to chronic pain management.* New York, NY: Springer Publishing.

D'Arcy, Y. (2011b). Women's pain management issues. *Pain Management Nursing, 12*(1), S1–S3.

Droney, J., & Riley, J. (2009). Recent advances in the use of opioids for cancer. *Journal of Pain Research, 2*, 135–155.

Fillingim, R. (2010). Individual differences in pain: The roles of genetics, ethnicity, and genetics. In *Bonica's management of pain* (pp. 86–98). Philadelphia, PA: Lippincott Williams & Wilkins.

Fine, P., & Portenoy, R. (2009). Establishing "best practices" for opioid rotation: Conclusions of an expert panel. *Journal of Pain & Symptom Management, 38*(3), 418–425.

Galvan, A., Fladvad, T., Skorpen, F., Gao, X., Klepstad, P., Kaasa, S., & Dragani, T. (2011). Genetic clustering of European cancer patients indicates that opioid-mediated pain relief is independent of ancestry. *The Pharmacogenomics Journal,* 1–5.

Galvan, A., Skorpen, F., Klepstad, P., Knudsen, A., Fladvad, T., Falvella, F., . . . Dragani, T. (2011). Multiple loci modulate opioid therapy response for cancer pain. *Clinical Cancer Research, 17*, 4581–4587.

Gourlay, G. (2005). Advances in opioid therapy. *Supportive Care in Cancer, 13*, 153–159.

Hanks, G., & Reid, C. (2005). Contributions to the variability in response to opioids. *Supportive Care in Cancer, 13*, 145–152.

Inturrisi, C., & Lipman, A. (2010). Opioid analgesics. In *Bonica's management of pain* (pp. 1172–1181). Philadelphia, PA: Lippincott Williams & Wilkins.

Jannetto, P., & Bratanow, N. (2011). Pain management in the 21st century: Utilization of pharmacogenomics and therapeutic drug monitoring. *Expert Opinion in Drug Metabolism Toxicology, 7*(6), 745–752.

Knotkova, H., Fine, P., & Portenoy, R. (2009). Opioid rotation: The science and limitations of the equianalgesic dose table. *Journal of Pain & Symptom Management, 38*(3), 426–439.

Mercadante, S., & Bruera, E. (2006). Opioid switching: A systematic and critical review. *Cancer Treatment Reviews, 31*, 304–315.

Miaskowski, C. (2009). Understanding the genetic determinants of pain and pain management. *Seminars in Oncology Nursing, 25*(2) Suppl 1, S1–S7.

Mogil, G., & Max, M. (2006). The genetics of pain. In S. B. McMahon, M. Koltzenburg (Eds.), *Wall & Melzack's textbook of pain* (5th ed., pp. 159–174). Philadelphia, PA: Elsevier/Churchill Livingstone.

Mogil, J. S. (2009). Animal models of pain: Progress and challenges. *Nature Reviews. Neuroscience, 10*(4), 283–294.

Nagashima, M., Katoh, R., Sato, Y., Tagami, M., Kasai, S., & Ikeda, K. (2007). Is there genetic polymorphism evidence for individual sensitivity to opiates? *Current Pain and Headache Reports, 11*(2), 115–123.

Pasternak, G. (2005). Molecular biology of opioid analgesia. *Journal of Pain & Symptom Management, 29* (Suppl 5), S2–S9.

Pasternak, G. (2010). Molecular insights into mu opioid pharmacology. *Clinical Journal of Pain, 26*(1), S3–S9.

Quigley, C. (2010). Opioid switching to improve pain relief and drug tolerability. The Cochrane Collaboration. *The Cochrane Library*, Issue 11.

Reyes-Gibby, C., Shete, S., Rakvig, T., Bhat, S., Skorpen, F., Bruera, E., . . . Klepsted, P. (2007). Exploring joint effects of genes and the clinical efficacy of morphine for cancer pain: OPRMI and COMT gene. *Pain, 130*, 25–30.

Reyes-Gibby, C., Spitz, M., Yennrajalingam, S., Swartz, M., Gu, J., Wu, X., . . . Shete, S. (2009). Role of inflammation gene polymorphisms on pain severity in lung cancer patients. *Cancer Epidemiology, Biomarkers, and Prevention, 18*(10), 2636–2642.

Shaheen, P., Walsh, D., Lasheen, W., Davis, M., & Lagman, R. (2009). Opioid equianalgesic tables: Are they all equally dangerous? *Journal of Pain & Symptom Management, 38*(3), 409–417.

Shi, Q., Cleeland, C., Klepstad, P., Miaskowski, C., & Pedersen, N. (2010). Biological pathways and genetic variables involved in pain. *Quality of Life Research, 19*, 1407–1417.

Slatkin, N. (2009). Opioid switching and rotation in primary care: Implementation and clinical utility. *Current Medical Research and Opinions, 25*(9), 2133–2150.

Thapa, D., Reastogi, V., & Ahuja, V. (2011). Cancer pain management-current status. *Journal of Anesthesiology and Clinical Pharmacology, 27*(2), 162–168.

Tremblay, J., & Hamet, P. (2010). Genetics of pain, opioids and opioid responsiveness. *Metabolism Clinical and Experimental, 59*(Suppl. 1), S5–S8.

Vadalouca, A., Moka, E., Argyra, E., Sikioti, P., & Siafaka, I. (2008). Opioid rotation in patients with cancer: A review of the current literature. *Journal of Opioid Management, 4*(4), 213–250.

Wilson, J. F. (2006). The pain divide between men and women. *Annals of Internal Medicine, 144*(6), 461–464.

World Health Organization (WHO). (1996). *Cancer pain relief* (2nd ed.). Geneva, Switzerland: Author.

12

Opioid Addiction, Dependency, and Tolerance in Patients With Cancer

Yvonne D'Arcy

OVERVIEW

Since opioids are so commonly used to treat pain in cancer, the question of addiction is also a frequent concern. In the acute or diagnostic phase, patients recognize that opioids will treat their pain, but they fear addiction. It can be a tough sell to reassure patients that the risk of addiction may be low and pain relief is more of a priority. In today's world, patients can read about the risks of pain medication use and abuse in newspapers, magazines, and over the Internet.

Trying to encourage patients to report their pain and problems with medication use can be difficult. As one elderly lady told me, "I would never tell my doctor I stopped taking those pain pills. He gave them to me and I wouldn't want to offend him." Why patients have a difficult time accepting the need for medications and have trouble reporting side effects such as dizziness, nausea, or constipation to their health care providers still needs more research.

In an analysis of 106 patients who were undergoing radiation therapy for cancer, an Internet questionnaire revealed that 58% reported pain from their cancer treatment and 46% reported pain from their cancer (Simone, Vapiwala, Hampshire, & Metz, 2008). Most (80%) did not use medication to treat their pain. The reasons that the respondents gave for this lack of medication use were as follows:

- Health care provider did not recommend use (87%)
- Fear of addiction or dependence (79%)
- Inability to pay (79%) (Simone et al., 2008)

For these patients, alternative therapies provided a source for pain relief.

The fear of addiction is not just something that affects patients; it is also very prevalent in most health care providers, nurses, and caregivers of all types. The advent of REMS (Risk Evaluation and Mitigation Strategies) for extended-release opioids may create a barrier for the average health care provider who prescribes opioids at least several times per day, but REMS also provides a means of providing protection. In a survey of 400 nurse practitioners who were asked about the biggest barrier to prescribing opioids, the largest group of respondents said cost was the greatest barrier, while the number two and three responses indicated a fear of increased regulatory oversight and addiction (D'Arcy, 2009).

Very little is written about addiction, substance abuse, and medication misuse in patients with cancer. This chapter will provide information about addiction and try to determine the long-term effects of treating the acute stage cancer patient with pain as the patient progresses into the post-treatment survivor stage of the disease.

OPIOID USE IN PATIENTS WITH CANCER

Opioids have long been considered the mainstay of treating pain in patients with cancer (APS, 2005). The onset of pain is often quite severe with decreasing pain levels over the continuum of the illness (Balantyne, 2007). Pain in the acute phase can come from a variety of sources such as tumor growth, tissue impingement, organ compression, and treatment-related sources such as postradiation pain, postmastectomy and post-thoracotomy syndromes, and chemotherapy-related neuropathies. Opioids are considered a first-line option for patients with cancer pain and most practitioners feel very comfortable prescribing an opioid for a patient with cancer in the acute phase.

More than 50% of patients with cancer live at least 2 years (Starr, Rogak, & Passik, 2010). Approximately 90% of all addictions occur by the age of 35 (Starr et al., 2010). This means that the majority of older patients who are diagnosed with cancer have significantly less risk of developing a true addiction to opioid medications.

There are no definitive data for substance abuse in cancer patients. The best estimate is 7.7% for cancer pain patients of all types (Ballantyne, 2007). However, the best general estimate is that the rates are similar to aged-matched cohorts outside of tertiary care. Overall, the best estimates for addiction are that 6% to 10% of people in our society are addicted to illicit drugs, 15% to alcohol, 21% to nicotine, and many more millions are using prescription drugs nonmedically (Kircher et al., 2011). With cancer patients living much longer with painful conditions, it seems only logical that health care providers will need to become familiar with addiction, learn to screen for addiction indicators, and prescribe using universal precautions.

Addiction, Dependency, Tolerance, and Pseudoaddiction

Patients who are diagnosed with cancer may also have chronic pain conditions or develop chronic pain as a result of treatment or of cancer itself. Each patient needs to be individually assessed for addiction potential related to long-term use of opioids. Addiction is a common fear for both the patient and the health care provider. However, many of the fears arise from a misperception of what true addiction really means.

True addiction has distinctive characteristics. The *Diagnostic and Statistical Manual of Mental Disorders, fourth edition* (*DSM-IV*) criteria for diagnosing addiction, called *substance dependence*, states that patients not only have dependence and tolerance but need to have at least one behavioral element as well. This behavior is identified as compulsive drug-seeking behavior (Ballantyne, 2007). More clinically useful definitions are included in the next section for the major elements of addiction, tolerance, and dependency.

Addiction also known as *psychological dependence,* is defined as a primary chronic neurobiologic disease with genetic, psychosocial, and environmental factors influencing its development and manifestation. It is characterized by the *four Cs* (American Academy of Pain Medicine [AAPM], American Pain Society [APS], American Society of Addiction Medicine [ASAM], 2001; D'Arcy, 2011):

- Control over drug use is impaired
- Compulsive use
- Continued use despite harm
- Craving

Physiologically, addiction is governed by the neural pathways that also govern reward and pleasure. Opioids have both a direct and indirect effect on these centers within the brain. The centers that are most involved are the mesocorticolimbic dopamine systems originating in the ventral segmental section of the brain and extending into the nucleus accumbens, amygdala, and prefrontal cortex (Ballantyne, 2007). The activation of this neural area by opioids can produce euphoria and reinforce reward-seeking behaviors. The fear of withdrawal also tends to stimulate continued drug taking (Ballantyne, 2007).

Continued use of a drug such as heroin increases the body's desire for the drug since reward and pleasure follow drug use, creating reward-related learning and memory (Kircher et al., 2011). As drug use continues, there is a dopaminergic release from the ventral tegmental area (VTA) to the mesocorticolimbic system, causing a cascade of cellular and molecular changes that lead to neuroplastic changes in the neural system and reinforce the learning pattern and memory for reward-seeking behavior (Kircher et al., 2011). Addiction creates a vicious cycle of drug use, creating physiologic changes, increasing desire for more drugs, and leading to continued use.

At the same time, neuroadaptations and cellular changes are taking place that make relapse more of a reality. Patients who are in withdrawal or abstinence from drugs such as heroin have a stress response and hormonal activation that can lead to compulsive drug use (Kircher et al., 2011). The stress response can cause the release of excessive levels of norepinephrine, adrenocorticotropic hormone (ACTH), corticotrophin-releasing factor (CRF), beta-endorphin, cortisol, vasopressin, and dynorphin (Kircher et al., 2011). These physiologic changes make it difficult to control pain in these patients and opioid requirements may be higher than expected.

In the acute phase of cancer, during the diagnosis and treatment phase, opioids are often prescribed. Long-term opioid use for chronic pain presents a different situation where prescribers may be more reluctant to continue to prescribe opioids for the residual chronic pain. Many health care providers also fear readdicting a patient who has stopped using illicit drugs but who has a history of illicit drug use. It is wise to consider that in a primary care practice, the prevalence of true opioid addiction in chronic noncancer pain is 5% or less, meaning that 95% of the patients do well (Fishbain, Cole, Lewis, Rossamoff, & Rossamoff, 2008). Each patient's pain and opioid use need to be carefully monitored over the course of long-term opioid therapy.

Health care providers cannot prescribe opioids to patients to support addiction but they can prescribe opioids to treat pain. Patients who have a history of opioid addiction are at risk for relapse when opioids are used to treat cancer pain. These patients need to have pain relief, but should be made fully aware of the consequences and risks and benefits. For an addicted patient, a team approach to pain management is needed using clinicians skilled in addiction such as psychologists, counselors, addiction specialists, and pain management specialists. No matter what the patient's status is, each patient deserves adequate pain control to relieve cancer pain.

Dependency is often confused with addiction. *Physical dependence* is defined as a state of adaptation that is manifested by a class-specific withdrawal syndrome that can be produced by the following (AAPM, APS, ASAM, 2001; D'Arcy, 2011):

- Abrupt cessation of the drug
- Rapid dose reduction
- Decreasing blood levels of the drug and/or the administration of an opioid antagonist

All patients with pain who take opioids for longer than 7 to 14 days become dependent on the medication. This only means that if the opioids are suddenly stopped or the dose is decreased rapidly, a withdrawal syndrome will occur. This condition manifests as shaking, chills, pain, nausea, vomiting, or diarrhea. All addicts are psychologically and physiologically dependent on the opioid substance, but not all physiologically dependent patients are addicts. The focus on treating a patient with long-term opioids is to treat the pain not fuel addiction. Knowing the difference between the two categories will ensure that opioid-dependent patients will not be categorized as addicts.

Tolerance is a state of adaptation to the effects of the opioid such as sedation, or nausea, and thus, can be a helpful phenomenon (AAPM, APS, ASAM, 2001). However, tolerance may decrease the drug's effectiveness, especially with long-term use, and does not indicate addiction. In the cancer patient worsening pain must be evaluated for progression of disease before assuming that it is related to development of tolerance.

Opioid Misuse

Opioid misuse can occur when patients use their own opioid prescriptions for other than the intended purpose or abuse prescription medications (their own or others). An example of this is the patient who uses opioid medication with alcohol to get "a buzz."

Opioid Pseudoaddiction

Opioid pseudoaddiction is a condition that occurs when pain is being undertreated. A patient who has unrelieved pain may develop behaviors such as clock watching or being focused on obtaining pain medications, and demonstrate behaviors that are often considered drug seeking such as hoarding or use deception. Patients who are trying to achieve adequate pain relief may be seen by the professional staff as manipulative. If the patient is suspected of having opioid pseudoaddiction, the best approach is to increase medications or decrease dosing intervals, or use adjuvant medication to increase pain relief. Once pain is well controlled, the dysfunctional behaviors will resolve if pseudoaddiction is the source.

Universal Precautions

Universal precautions is a term often used in infectious disease practices to indicate the minimum level of precaution taken for all patients to avoid infection or contamination. For pain management, universal precautions refer to using standards and guidelines to minimize the risk of opioid prescribing (Gourlay, Heit, & Almahrezi, 2005). It is not possible to assess all risks when prescribing opioids, so applying the minimum level of precautions to all patients utilizing opioids is recommended. These steps from the guidelines include the following:

- Making a diagnosis with an appropriate differential
- Psychologic assessment, including the risk of addictive disorders
- Informed consent
- Treatment agreement
- Pre- and postintervention assessment of pain level and function
- Appropriate trial of opioid therapy with or without adjunctive medication
- Reassessment of pain score and level of function
- Regularly assessing the four As of pain medicine: analgesia, activities of daily living, adverse effects, and aberrant behaviors
- Periodically reviewing pain diagnosis and comorbid conditions, including addictive disorders
- Performing documentation that is complete and that addresses all elements of assessment, medications, and treatment indications such as pain (Gourlay et al., 2005)

Screening for Opioid Abuse and Identifying Aberrant Drug-Taking Behaviors

Prescribers who provide long-term opioids to patients with cancer pain have a variety of screening tools that they can use to monitor risk with opioid use, occurrence of aberrant behaviors, and compliance with opioid agreements. Behaviors that are considered to be aberrant include the following:

- Hoarding medications
- Taking someone else's medication for pain
- Raising drug doses without a prescription

■ Drinking alcohol when in pain
■ Smoking more cigarettes when in pain
■ Using opioids to treat symptoms other than pain (Fine & Portenoy, 2007)
    These dysfunctional behaviors are aimed at increasing pain relief but are less predictive of addiction.
    Behaviors that are more predictive of addiction include the following:
■ Concurrent use of illicit drugs
■ Stealing or selling prescription drugs
■ Injecting oral medications
■ Obtaining medications from nonstandard sources such as street dealers (Fine & Portenoy, 2007)

Tools for Screening

Using a tool for screening prior and during opioid use should not be considered as a lie detector. Rather, these tools should be used to identify patients who are risk of developing aberrant behaviors or have a higher potential for addiction when long-term opioids are used. Sometimes, simple questions such as the following can give an idea of the patient's potential for addictive behavior or willingness to engage in illegal activity:

■ Are you a smoker?
■ Do you have a personal or family history of alcoholism?
■ Have you ever used marijuana?
■ Have you ever purchased medications off the street?
■ Have you ever been in a substance-use treatment program? Prior addicts can be treated for pain but more structure and closer monitoring will be needed (Kircher et al., 2011).

There are several other simple screening tools that can help identify patients who will be at risk for difficulty with long-term opioids. These tools are not meant to disqualify patients with a positive screen from opioids to treat their pain; they are only meant to determine whether more care and careful monitoring will be needed.

The CAGE-AID Screen uses a set of questions centered on alcohol or drug use. The higher the number of positive responses, the greater the likelihood that the patient has a drug or alcohol abuse disorder. The CAGE questions are as follows:

■ Have you ever tried to *c*ut down on your alcohol or drug use?
■ Have people *a*nnoyed you by commenting or critiquing your drug or alcohol use?
■ Have you ever felt bad or *g*uilty about your drinking or drug use?

▪ Have you ever needed an *e*ye opener first thing in the morning to steady your nerves or get rid of a hangover?

The Trauma Screen uses personal injury as a measure of risk for using opioids. If the patient has two or more positive answers, there is a high potential for abuse. The questions of the Trauma Screen include the following:

Since your 18th birthday, have you:

▪ Had any fractures or dislocations to your bones or joints, excluding sports injuries?
▪ Been injured in a traffic accident?
▪ Injured your head, excluding sports injuries?
▪ Been in a fight or assaulted someone while intoxicated?
▪ Been injured while intoxicated?

Using a simple screen is enough information to rule out any potential opioid-related issues from some patients. For others, there is a need for more complex screening tools that can identify the magnitude of risk when opioids are used for pain relief. In a study of 48 patients who attended a pain clinic but were discontinued from opioid therapy for aberrant behavior, the patients were interviewed by a psychologist and completed three complex assessment tools: the Screener and Opioid Assessment for Patients with Pain (SOAPP-R), the Opioid Risk Tool (ORT), and the Diagnosis, Intractability, Risk, and Efficacy Inventory (DIRE). The clinical interview part of the study protocol had the highest sensitivity for predicting aberrant drug-taking behaviors (0.77). The tool with the highest sensitivity rating for predicting aberrant drug-taking behaviors was the SOAPP-R (0.72), followed by the ORT (0.45), and the DIRE (0.17) (Moore, Jones, Browder, Daffron, & Passik, 2009).

Using a more complex opioid risk screening tool can help identify those patients who will develop aberrant behaviors or who are at higher risk for misuse or abuse of opioids:

▪ The SOAPP-R uses a 14-item self-report format to assess for abuse potential. This is a reliable and valid measure, where a score of 8 or greater indicates a high risk of misuse or abuse.
▪ The ORT screens for aberrant behaviors in patients using long-term opioids. It is a simple five-item, yes/no format for self-report. Questions center on the patient's personal and family history of drug use, age, any history of preadolescent sexual abuse, and the presence of any psychologic disease such as depression, obsessive–compulsive disorder, schizophrenia, or bipolar disease. Each question has several subsections for specific substances or disease states. Scores of 0 to 3 are considered low risk, 4 to 7 are considered moderate risk, with 8 and over indicating high risk.

- The DIRE Score is a clinician-rated scale with questions in four categories: diagnosis, intractability, risk, and efficacy. The categories are then broken down into psychologic, chemical health, reliability, and social support. The higher the score, the better the risk for opioid therapy. A score of 14 and above indicates that the patient is a good risk for opioid therapy and those with lower scores are considered higher risk for opioid misuse or abuse.
- The COMM is a 17-item self-report tool used to identify aberrant drug-related behaviors for patients on long-term opioid therapy. This tool is to be used once opioid therapy has started. The COMM uses questions that can identify emotional/psychiatric issues, evidence of lying, appointment patterns, and medication misuse and noncompliance (D'Arcy, 2011; Passik, Kirsch, & Casper, 2008).

Copies of these tools are available at www.painedu.com

These tools are meant to be used as a part of a comprehensive treatment plan and not as a sole measure of suitability for opioid therapy.

Patient Agreement

Patient agreements consist of a document that outlines the rules and regulation of opioid therapy for that practice. It protects both the patient and prescribers and clearly outlines what medication will be provided, when prescriptions will be provided, information on the medication being used for pain, the risk of addiction or readdiction, and the use of random urine screening.

Although it may seem harsh to use a patient agreement for patients with cancer pain, it also can serve as an educational opportunity and a means to set goals. Once the patient agrees to opioid therapy, the patient agreement is explained to the patient. Elements of the patient agreement include the following:

- Risks and benefits of the treatment
- Goals of treatment
- Side effects of medications
- Definitions of addiction, dependence, and tolerance
- Rationale for changing or discontinuing behaviors
- Expected patient behaviors (D'Arcy, 2011)

Examples of expected patients behaviors include: taking the prescription as ordered, not using alcohol or other sedating medications concomitantly, only receiving opioid prescriptions from the prescribers on the patient agreement, having the prescription filled at one pharmacy only, and an in-clinic visit required for early prescription refill requests (D'Arcy, 2011).

Each practice is individual and how the patient agreements are enforced may vary. However, having a patient agreement allows the patient and the prescriber to interact within the parameters of the agreement and decreases conflict over what was intended with the opioid medications.

In the next chapter, more information will be provided on how to use the tools and techniques from this chapter. In addition, information on urine drug screening and safe prescribing will be included to provide an in-depth discussion of how to best use long-term opioid therapy for patients with cancer pain.

Case Study

Lydia has had colon cancer for 2½ years. She took a full course of chemotherapy after her colon surgery and still complains of significant abdominal pain. She has stopped smoking but she has a history of intermittent heroin use. She continues to see her primary health care provider for her abdominal pain. He continues to monitor Lydia's drug use with random urine screens but since she is on hydromorphone for her abdominal pain, she always has a positive report; however, no other drugs of abuse have been detected. She continues to request dosage increases because she states that her pain is severe at times. What options do you have for treating Lydia's complaints of increased pain? Does her heroin use affect her pain complaint?

Questions to Consider

1. Can you safely treat Lydia's pain with opioids?
2. Is she addicted, dependent, or tolerant to opioids?
3. Does Lydia's use of heroin affect her abdominal pain?
4. What types of screening should be used to monitor Lydia?
5. Does Lydia need a medication for breakthrough pain, dose increases, or the addition of a coanalgesic?

REFERENCES

American Academy of Pain Medicine (AAPM), American Pain Society (APS), American Society of Addiction Medicine (ASAM). (2001). *Definitions related to the use of opioids for the treatment of pain.* Retrieved from http://www.painmed.org/productpub/statements/pdfs/definition.pdf

American Pain Society (APS). (2005). *Cancer pain guidelines.* Glenview, IL: Author.

Ballantyne, J. (2007). Opioid misuse in oncology pain patients. *Current Pain and Headache Reports, 11,* 276–282.

D'Arcy, Y. (2009). Be in the know about pain management. *The Nurse Practitioner, 34*(4), 43–47.

D'Arcy, Y. (2010, August). How to manage pain in addicted patient. *Nursing 2010, 60–*64.

D'Arcy, Y. (2011). *Compact clinical guide to chronic pain management.* New York, NY: Springer Publishing.

Fine, P., & Portenoy, R. (2007). *A clinical guide to opioid analgesia.* New York, NY: Vendome Group.

Fishbain, D., Cole, B., Lewis, J., Rossamoff, H., & Rossamoff, R. (2008). What percentage of chronic nonmalignant pain patients exposed to chronic opioid analgesic therapy develop abuse/addiction and or aberrant drug related behaviors? A structured evidence based review. *Pain Medicine, 9,* 444–459.

Gourlay, D., Heit, H., & Almahrezi, A. (2005). Universal precautions in pain medicine: A rational approach to the treatment of chronic pain. *Pain Medicine, 6*(2), 107–112.

Kircher, S., Zacny, J., Apfelbaum, S., Passik, S., Kirsch, K., Burbage, M., & Lofwell, M. (2011). Understanding and treating opioid addiction in a patient with cancer pain. *The Journal of Pain, 12*(10), 1025–1031.

Moore, T. M., Jones, T., Browder, J. H., Daffron, S., & Passik, S. D. (2009). A comparison of common screening methods for predicting aberrant drug-related behavior among patients receiving opioids for chronic pain management. *Pain Medicine, 10*(8), 1426–1433.

National Institutes of Health (NIH). (2002). NIH State of the Science Statement on symptom management in cancer: Pain, depression, and fatigue. *NIH Consensus State Sciences Statement, 19,* 1–29.

Office of Cancer Survivorship. (n. d.). *About cancer survivorship research: Survivorship definitions.* Retrieved from http://cancercontrol.cancer.gov/ocs/definitions.html

Passik, S., Kirsch, K. L., & Casper, D. (2008). Addiction-related assessment tools and pain management instruments for a screening, treatment planning, and monitoring compliance. *Pain Medicine, 9*(S2), S145–S166.

Shi, Q., Smith, T. G., Michonski, J., Stein, K., Chiewkwei, K., & Cleeland, C. (2011). Symptom burden in cancer survivors 1 year after diagnosis. A report from the American Cancer Society's Cancer Studies of Cancer Survivors. *Cancer, 117,* 2779–2790.

Simone, C., Vapiwala, N., Hampshire, M., & Metz, J. (2008). Internet-based survey evaluating the use of pain medications and attitudes of radiation oncology patients toward pain interventions. *International Journal of Radiation Oncology, Biology, Physics, 72*(1), 127–133.

Slevin, K., & Ashburn, M. (2011). Primary care physician opinion survey on FDA opioid risk evaluation and mitigation strategies. *Journal of Opioid Management, 7*(2), 109–115.

Starr, T., Rogak, L., & Passik, S. (2010). Substance abuse in cancer patients. *Current Pain and Headache Report, 14,* 268–275.

13

Developing a Comprehensive Plan of Care and Prescribing Safely

Yvonne D'Arcy

OVERVIEW

Caring for patients with cancer pain requires a multimodal approach to the pain and a comprehensive plan of care in order to obtain the best outcomes. Pain management in these patients is not just a matter of providing medication for their pain. It requires a holistic, empathic, and supportive approach where the patient is an integral part of the plan. Listening to the patient is an important tool for the nurse who is caring for the patient. Learning what the patient values and expects is also a part of this process. Including the family as allies in treating pain and decreasing symptom burden can provide information that can make a difference in the success of the care plan. Helping the patients to set realistic expectations for pain management up front can avoid frustration and noncompliance.

A comprehensive plan of care for cancer pain should include both medications and nonpharmacologic interventions. Medication use should include regular reassessment for pain relief and side effects, and nonpharmacologic techniques should be evaluated regularly to see if the patient still finds them helpful or if they were stopped for some reason. Documentation of each visit is also needed to track changes or improvements in pain.

On the other side, the prescriber needs to make sure all the risks and benefits have been described to the patient and that the patient fully understands what the opioid medication is, how it should be used, and who to call if there are side effects or other problems with the medication. Using a patient agreement as described in Chapter 12 can help formalize this process. Although it sounds hard to ask patients with cancer pain to sign agreements and undergo urine screening, if opioids are being prescribed for long-term use, health care providers should ensure that they are protecting their prescriptive practice.

SETTING UP THE PAIN MANAGEMENT PLAN

When developing a plan of care for a patient with cancer pain, the first element should be a full pain-focused history and physical. Assessing the patient's pain can be done with any number of tools, as indicated in Chapter 2. However, using a tool such as the Brief Pain Inventory (BPI) as described in Chapter 2 can provide more insight into the patient's expectations and past medication use. For patients who have chronic cancer pain, a multidimensional pain scale such as the BPI or a combination of BPI with the Edmonton Functional Assessment Tool can provide a better picture of the patient's pain and current ability to function in daily life. Using the Numeric Rating Scale (NRS) at each visit can track the decrease in pain with the use of the prescribed interventions. No matter what pain rating scale is used, there should be consistent use of the same scale at subsequent patient visits.

After reviewing all previous studies and laboratory testing, further diagnostic tests can be considered if needed. The physical examination of the patient may reveal testing needs that have previously not been addressed. No matter if the patient's pain is a result of the cancer itself or is treatment related, all aspects of the pain complaint should be discussed.

The treatment plan should include not only medication management but also some nonpharmacologic options that the patient expresses interest in pursuing. Behavioral techniques such as biofeedback or relaxation can be included in the plan of care and patients can keep a diary to record their progress or lack thereof and indicate what they value or dislike about the individual therapies so that on each office visit there is a frame of reference for discussion. Patients can also record progress about increasing levels of activity through their diary.

For more complex patients especially, it is prudent to include as many additional health care practitioners as needed. Some patients need a structured physical therapy regimen, so including physical and occupational therapists and physiatrists may be necessary. Other patients may need counseling or coping strategies developed, so adding in a psychologist, social worker, or formal counselor may help develop the plan of care in this area. If interventional pain management options are needed, adding in pain specialists or anesthesiologists can help clarify what can be added for treating pain that is responsive to interventional pain management.

If opioids are used for long-term care, using a patient agreement, opioid risk screening, and setting goals and expectations can help reduce any potential for future problems. Being clear and developing a trusting relationship with the patient can go a long way toward the success of the plan of care. Using a risk–benefit analysis can help the patient understand the full scope of the plan for treating the pain. Tools for opioid risk screening can alert the health care provider to any potential issues with opioids so that extra care and monitoring can be set up.

Once the plan of care is developed and the patient is aware of the elements of the plan, opioid therapy and integrating the nonpharmacologic methods can start. Reassessment of the plan is essential so that any needed adjustments can be made. Documentation is a necessity so that the entire process can be tracked in the records. If by some chance the patient does not comply with the plan, fails to progress with the identified goals, has difficulty complying with the patient agreement, or fails repeated urine screening, then a contingency strategy should be developed. This does not mean that the patient is dismissed from the clinic, or that opioid prescribing will be stopped when there is active cancer causing pain. Rather, closer monitoring, more frequent visits, and smaller quantities of opioid prescriptions may be needed to contain inappropriate behaviors. Developing a plan and working the plan will help the patient progress toward the identified goals and provide the best pain outcomes possible for the patient.

SAFE PRESCRIBING

Since opioids are such a big part of treating cancer pain, health care providers need to be aware of the risks and benefits, and of ways to produce safe, effective pain management for the patient. Reducing the legal risks and exposure for prescribers is also an essential part of the process.

Safe prescribing is defined as using national standards and guidelines, and following recommended practices when prescribing controlled substances. These elements include the following:

- Being aware of all the requirements for a legal prescription in their licensing state
- Using national guidelines information and recommendations to guide practice
- Performing a complete and thorough history and physical examination to establish a diagnosis and treatment plan

▓ Screening patients for opioid risk and using treatment strategies that mitigate risk of misuse and assist in adherence (D'Arcy & Bruckenthal, 2011). Opioids are recognized as the mainstay for treating cancer pain, so for health care providers treating these patients, knowing how to prescribe safely is essential.

Most states have laws that govern opioid prescribing and the federal government requires a license to prescribe opioids.

Many prescribers are afraid of prescribing long-term opioids, fearing addicting the patient or increased regulatory oversight for continued prescribing of opioids. Nurse practitioners in a national survey indicated that they felt less prepared to assess and treat chronic pain such as that from cancer and cancer-related conditions. Yet it seems that these patients are being seen in primary care, with 77% of a 259-respondent cohort of primary care providers indicating that they prescribe opioids for cancer pain (Slevin & Ashburn, 2011). Knowing how to write prescriptions and following national recommendations can help to decrease legal exposure and increase confidence in prescribing practices.

Clinical Pearl	Elements of a safe prescription for opioids are as follows:
	• Date of issue
	• Patient's name and address
	• Practitioner's name, address, and DEA registration number
	• Drug name, strength, and dosage form
	• Quantity prescribed
	• Directions for use
	• Number of refills
	• Manual signature of prescriber

There are also some practices that are not considered as safe: postdating a prescription or signing a prescription and allowing another provider to fill it in (D'Arcy, 2011). Making sure that each prescription is legible and reviewed with patients so they understand how to use the medication is essential to success. To ensure proper documentation, the prescriber must document what medication was prescribed for the patient and what was explained to the patient about the medication and use.

LEGAL CONSIDERATIONS

Health care providers may fear increased regulatory oversight if the patient is going to need long-term opioids. As time passes, the prescriber may feel there could be a different way of managing the pain while the patient continues to use the opioids safely to control pain. This fear on the part of the prescriber and the desire to reduce opioid use may not be justified.

Although there may be a fear by prescribers related to regulatory oversight and DEA sanction, the true rate of sanctions is very low. In fiscal year 2003, 50 physicians (0.005% of all physicians registered) were arrested for activities that were knowingly beyond the scope of legal action (D'Arcy, 2011). Knowing what the scope of practice is when prescribing opioids can ensure that prescribing practice falls within the accepted standard of care.

Findings from a survey with 963,385 registered physicians found that when adequate documentation exists in the medical record, the risk of legal action against any physician who prescribes opioids for chronic pain is very small. The key here is that adequate documentation can go a long way to ensuring the prescriber is protected from legal actions.

In 2003, there were 47 arrests related to opioid prescribing and the DEA issued 56 DEA revocations from 2003 to 2004. Most of the physicians involved in these legal actions did not have a primary patient–physician relationship that would merit continued opioid prescribing. Some of the legal actions were based on the following:

- Prescriber substance abuse
- Fraud
- Loss of medical license
- Sex in exchange for prescriptions
- Prescribing without seeing the patient

Although these are extreme cases, it does indicate the level and types of offenses that are considered for legal action. In most cases, physicians and prescribers are aware of the standard of care and do not engage in illegal or unethical behaviors.

Health care providers are also responsible for the legal consequences of their pain management actions. In a landmark case, *Hillhaven vs. the estate of Henry James*, a patient with a pathologic femur fracture had well-controlled pain in the acute care facility using around-the-clock doses of oral morphine. When the patient was admitted to a second extended-care facility, the admitting nurse documented on the admission form that the patient was addicted to the morphine. Doses of the oral morphine were given in reduced numbers and another nonopioid medication was substituted for the oral morphine. The patient lived for 23 days and was in severe pain. After the patient's death, the estate sued and won $15 million dollars for punitive damages and pain and suffering. The settlement was reviewed and a private settlement arranged. The facility was found liable, as was the nurse. This landmark case was the first to identify patient rights to adequate pain management (Angolara, 1991).

This case points out the need to make all efforts to adequately manage the patient's pain and for each caregiver to assess his or her own knowledge and attitude toward addiction. In this case, the patient had a discernable source for pain yet the health care provider had misinformation about what constituted addiction. No patient should have to endure pain just because the health care provider does not understand the true meaning of addiction and uses the misinformation to impact care.

USING URINE SCREENING RESULTS

Most patient agreements include random urine screens as part of the plan of care. As the patient begins opioid therapy, a baseline urine drug screen should be considered, especially in patients at high risk of opioid misuse. It should never be used alone but in conjunction with the patient agreement and opioid screen. It can help determine appropriate treatment choices. The random urine drug screen is a way of testing for the presence of those opioid medications being prescribed and monitoring for the presence of any illicit substances. Two problems with the rapid "point of care" or "dipstick" urine drug screen test is that some substances will not show on the screen. Another problem is the possibility of a false-positive or false-negative result. If the patient has been prescribed opioid medications and the drug screen comes back without a positive finding for opioids, diversion is a consideration. This type of result may also be indicative of a patient who metabolizes the drug rapidly, a delay in the time of drug ingestion, a clerical error, or lack of sensitivity of the laboratory to detect the drug. Therefore, the reason for the negative result should be fully examined (D'Arcy & Bruckenthal, 2011).

Guidelines for urine drug testing include the following:
- Ensure proper collection, handling, and documentation of the specimen.
- Know the appropriate tests to order and how to interpret the results.
- Be prepared to address unanticipated results.
- Document the discussion of the urine drug test with the patient (D'Arcy & Bruckenthal, 2011).

Interpreting urine drug testing results can be confusing. The presence or absence of a drug depends on when it was last taken, the drug's half-life, the patient's overall physical condition and fluid intake, and the method and frequency of ingestion. Most drugs will show in the patient's urine test if taken within 1 to 3 days. There are some specific instances of cross reactivity and false positives and false negatives, such as the following (Bruckenthal, 2007):

- Several quinolone antibiotics can potentially produce false-positive results for opioids by immunoassay but are not misidentified by gas chromatography.
- Codeine and heroin metabolize to morphine, so both substances may be identified in the urine following codeine or heroin use, resulting in a false positive for morphine.
- Hydrocodone can be metabolized to hydromorphone.
- Marijuana is not usually detected in the urine from passive smoke inhalation.
- Marijuana can be detected in the urine after cessation of use for up to 80 days in heavy users.
- Cocaine may be present in urine for 2 to 3 days if used as a topical anesthetic in dental or other procedures, and medical records should be reviewed to confirm this.
- Coca leaf teas can produce false-positive results for cocaine.
- Poppy seed may cause a false-positive opioid result in gas chromatography test.
- Vicks nasal inhaler, selegiline, and some diet pills can cause a false-positive result for amphetamines in a rapid assay "point of care" test. Specialized gas chromatograph/mass spectrometry (GC/MS) testing may be required to ascertain the exact drug. A finding of methamphetamine always indicates aberrant behavior.
- Heroin is difficult to detect based on a half-life of 5 to 30 minutes, resulting in false-negative results.
- Some patients metabolize opioids rapidly, especially oxycodone, resulting in false negatives in a rapid "point of care" assay.

For most clinics, using the rapid assay "point of care" (dipstick) immunoassay type of test is sufficient to determine results. However, confirmatory gas chromatography/mass spectrometry should be used to confirm unexpected results and detect specific compounds and metabolites within a given class.

DOCUMENTING OUTCOMES

Staff working with patients on long-term opioid therapy should be aware of the development of aberrant behaviors. See Chapter 12 for more information on addiction and aberrant behaviors. For patients who repeatedly (more than three times) call in for early refills, have repeated prescription problems such as lost prescriptions, have spilled or stolen medications, have more than three visits where the sole focus is entirely on opioid issues, or have continued calls to administrative offices related to opioid use, the development of these aberrant behaviors must be documented.

Using a formal documentation tool such as the Pain Assessment and Documentation Tool (PADT) can help organize and record patient information. The PADT is a specialized chart note designed to aid clinicians during long-term opioid therapy. Its primary use is for non-cancer pain but it can be adapted for use in those patients who are cancer survivors with chronic pain. The elements of the tools include the use of the *four As:* analgesia, presence of aberrant behaviors, adverse effects, and activity. In a pilot study of PADT patients on long-term opioid therapy, the patients achieved relatively positive outcomes in terms of analgesia, functionality, and tolerable side effects. Although aberrant drug-taking behaviors were common in the pilot patients, they only became problematic in 10% of the patients (D'Arcy, 2011). Although the PADT is not entirely necessary for pain assessment, in every case the basic elements of the tools can be incorporated into documentation to include the following:

- Current analgesic regimen
- Level of analgesia: average to worst amount of analgesia from pain medication
- Activities of daily living: physical, family, and social relationships; mood, and sleep
- Adverse events
- Aberrant drug-related behaviors
- Clinician assessment/impression of opioid therapy
- Specific plan and progress toward goals

Copies of the PADT can be obtained from the Janssen Pharmaceuticals website: www.janssenpharmaceuticalsinc.com.

Developing a comprehensive, solid plan of care for patients with cancer pain can yield excellent outcomes. Making a plan and working the plan with the patient as a partner can provide the base for providing pain management that will improve quality of life without many of the drawbacks to opioid therapy.

CANCER PAIN GUIDELINES

- **American Pain Society (APS):** A general guideline for cancer in adults and children with recommendations for care that include non-pharmacologic recommendations; available at www.ampainsoc.org
- **National Comprehensive Cancer Network's (NCCN)** *Adult Cancer Pain*: A general guideline with practice recommendations and algorithms to guide treatment decisions; available at www.nccn.org

■ **World Health Organization's (WHO)** *Cancer Pain Relief*: An older guideline with a comprehensive overview of cancer pain including medications use; also includes a guide to opioid availability

■ **Oncology Nursing Society's** *Putting Evidence Into Practice: What Are the Pharmacologic Interventions for Nociceptive and Neuropathic Pain in Adults?* The goal of the guideline is to provide recommendations in the treatment of nociceptive and neuropathic pain in adult cancer patients. Discusses a wide variety of medications considering pain intensity, mobility, quality of life, and side effects of pharmacologic agents. Available from www.guideline.gov

■ **American College of Physicians' Evidence-Based Interventions to Improve the Palliative Care of Pain, Dyspnea, and Depression at the End of Life:** Discusses pain assessment and treatment options, which includes medications only and advance care planning. Includes information from 33 systematic reviews and 89 intervention studies. Recommends use of regular assessment and use of therapies of proven effectiveness to provide symptom management. Reinforces the need for advance planning for all patients with serious illness. Available at www.guideline.gov

Case Study

John J., aged 47, is a recovering addict who used heroin daily along with prescription opioids when he could get them. He has now been diagnosed with rectal cancer that has metastasized to his spine. He has multiple bone lesions that are painful. Radiation is reducing the pain, but since John is a former addict the pain medications being used are at very high doses and adequate pain relief is difficult to achieve. His movement is being limited and he has difficulty sleeping because of increased pain when he tries to lie in bed. He always rates his pain in the severe intensity range of 7 to 10/10. He has difficulty managing his pain at home and has been admitted to the hospital on three separate occasions recently for pain management. His oncologist has mentioned a medication, a bisphosphonate that he can get to help reduce his pain, but he will still need opioids. You have been prescribing opioids, both extended-release and short-acting medications for breakthrough pain, for John over the last 6 months. His doses continue to escalate. How will you provide better pain relief for John and protect your prescribing practices?

Questions to Consider

1. It looks like you will be prescribing opioids for a period of time for John. How you protect yourself from any legal difficulties?
2. Should you use universal precautions and opioid screening tools for aberrant behaviors? If so, which one would be the best tool to use since John is already using opioids?
3. Should John have a patient agreement and random drug screening?
4. Should you try to limit John's opioids because he has a history of addiction?

REFERENCES

Angolara, R., & Donato, B. (1991). Inappropriate pain management results in high jury award. *Journal of Pain and Symptom Management*, 6(7), 407.

Bruckenthal, P. (2007). Controlled substances: Principles of safe prescribing. *The Nurse Practitioner*, 32(5), 7–11.

D'Arcy, Y. (2011). *Compact clinical guide to chronic pain management*. New York, NY: Springer Publishing.

D'Arcy, Y., & Bruckenthal, P. (2011). *Safe prescribing for nurse practitioners*. New York, NY: Oxford University Press.

Slevin, K., & Ashburn, M. (2011). Primary care physician opinion survey on FDA opioid risk evaluation and mitigation strategies. *Journal of Opioid Management*, 7(2), 109–115.

Cancer Pain Emergencies

Pamela Stitzlein Davies

When patients present to their health care provider with new or worsening pain, a thorough assessment of the complaint is essential to determine the correct diagnosis and implement treatment. There are two cancer pain emergencies that the nurse must be aware of in order to prevent progression to an uncontrolled situation: spinal cord compression and pain crisis. Each will be described in this chapter, with approaches to management.

SPINAL CORD COMPRESSION

Metastatic epidural spinal cord compression (SCC) occurs when cancer spreads to the spine, epidural space, or the cauda equina, and results in pressure and compression of the spinal cord. When this occurs, the patient experiences signs and symptoms similar to other spinal cord injury. This is a medical emergency. If left untreated, virtually 100% of patients will become paraplegic or quadriplegic (Fitzgibbon & Loeser, 2010). If caught early, neurologic deficits can be prevented, minimized, or possibly reversed (Bucholtz, 1999).

New back pain is the first symptom of SCC in 83% to 95% of all cases, and typically appears about 2 months prior to onset of paralysis (Cole & Patchell, 2008). Complaints of new neck or back pain in the cancer patient should always be immediately investigated to prevent catastrophic neurologic damage, especially if the patient has known metastatic disease. The pain associated with advanced SCC can be very difficult to control if not aggressively managed. If the condition is promptly diagnosed and treated, the pain can be controlled, and patients may remain ambulatory if they were walking at the time of diagnosis (Bucholtz, 1999). Unfortunately, median survival for patients diagnosed with SCC is in the range of 3 to 6 months (Cole & Patchell, 2008).

SCC occurs in about 5% of all cancers. Although nearly all cancers have the potential to spread to the spine, SCC is most commonly diagnosed in breast, lung, and prostate cancer (15%–20% for each); less commonly from renal cell carcinoma, multiple myeloma, or non-Hodgkin's lymphoma (5%–10% each); and the remainder of the cases in sarcoma, colorectal, and cancer of unknown primary (Prasad & Schiff, 2005). Occasionally, pain from SCC is the presenting symptom, which ultimately leads to a new diagnosis of cancer, particularly in lung cancer. Sixty percent of SCCs occur in the thoracic spine, 25% in the lumbosacral spine, and 15% in the cervical spine (Cole & Patchell, 2008). Multiples sites of compression occur in 17% to 30% of cases (Fitzgibbon & Loeser, 2010).

Nurses are commonly the first health care provider contacted by the patient with the symptoms of SCC, and the nurse can play a primary role in recognition of the condition (Bucholtz, 1999). Neurologic "alarm" symptoms indicating possible SCC are listed in the following box. The key to diagnosis is to have a high clinical suspicion of the condition. The nurse must always keep this emergency condition in mind when the patient calls reporting troublesome new symptoms, especially new back pain or leg weakness.

ALARM SYMPTOMS FOR SPINAL CORD COMPRESSION

The following are "alarm symptoms" for spinal cord compression, which should be evaluated within 24 hours to assess for possible spinal cord compression (Prasad & Schiff, 2005):

- New onset back pain, especially in the thoracic spine
  - Usually severe and localized to one spot
  - Typically worse at night when lying down
  - Worse with Valsalva maneuver (holding breath and bearing down)
  - May present as a "band" of pain around the torso
- New radicular pain (sciatica-like pain in the legs or arms), unilateral or bilateral
- New weakness in the legs or arms
  - May be described as "heaviness" or "clumsiness" of the limbs
- Saddle anesthesia (numbness in the perineum, lower buttocks, and posterior proximal thighs)
- Other sensory changes in the legs or arms
- Loss of bowel and bladder control
  - Urinary retention with overflow incontinence
  - Loss of anal sphincter tone

Diagnosis of Spinal Cord Compression

Magnetic resonance imaging (MRI) is the "gold standard" for diagnosis of metastatic epidural spinal cord compression (Bucholtz, 1999). Computed tomography (CT) assesses the bony spine well, but does not provide clear visualization of the spinal cord and soft tissues. Positron emission tomography (PET) scans will reveal "hot spots" of metastatic disease in the spine, but are less specific at showing the soft tissues such as the spinal cord. Bone scans will reveal patients at risk of SCC due to metastatic disease in the spine, but provide a vague picture and cannot be used for diagnosis of cord compression. History and clinical examination are important, but lack sensitivity and specificity compared to MRI (Prasad & Schiff, 2005).

Treatment of Spinal Cord Compression

Patients are typically admitted to the hospital for management of SCC. However, depending on the patient's status, goals of care, and proximity to death, they can be managed at home on oral steroids alone, or admitted to an inpatient hospice center if recovery of neurologic function is not a primary goal. Aggressive pain management is always appropriate regardless of the patient status. The ability to walk after treatment is dependent on the speed of initiating therapy, the rapidity of symptom onset (slower onset of symptoms is more favorable), and the overall functional status of the patient (Cole & Patchell, 2008).

Steroids

Corticosteroids, usually dexamethasone (Decadron), are the initial treatment for both pain management and decompression of metastatic epidural spinal cord compression. There is wide variability on the loading and maintenance doses used, and no specific dose recommendations were provided in a recent Cochrane Review (George et al., 2008). Cole and Patchell (2008) suggest a "high dose" of dexamethasone if the patient is unable to walk, and a "moderate" dose if the patient retains the ability to walk. One suggested regimen is (Bobb, 2010):

- "High dose" corticosteroid for patients who are unable to walk due to SCC
  - Loading dose: dexamethasone 100 mg IV bolus
  - Maintenance dose: dexamethasone 24 mg IV QID for 3 days, then taper over 10 days
- "Moderate dose" corticosteroid for patients who are still able to walk despite SCC
  - Loading dose: dexamethasone 10 mg IV bolus
  - Maintenance dose: dexamethasone 4 mg IV QID for 3 days, then taper over 14 days

Higher dose corticosteroids are more likely to reverse neurologic-damage from compression of the spinal cord, thereby effectively reducing pain. However, high doses are also associated with serious side effects, including hyperglycemia, mood changes (depression, euphoria, psychosis), gastric bleeding, and myopathy (proximal weakness in the legs) (Bobb, 2010).

Radiation Therapy

Radiation to the affected areas of the spine improves pain, preserves neurologic function, may reverse paralysis, and improves overall quality of life. Treatment is typically given as 30 Gray (Gy, a standard radiation unit) over 10 fractions (10 daily sessions), although other schedules are also used, such as 4 Gy over 5 fractions, or 8 Gy in a single treatment (Cole & Patchell, 2008). The shorter therapies are used for patients with limited prognosis or lower functional level. Patients typically tolerate the radiation well. Common radiation side effects are fatigue and skin changes.

Surgery

New techniques allow for circumferential decompression of the spine, with overall improved outcomes for surgery alone, or surgery plus radiation, compared to radiation alone (Quraishi, Gokaslan, & Boriani, 2010 Tacioni et al., 2010). Surgery allows for immediate decompression of the spinal cord, removes tumor, and provides mechanical stabilization of unstable fractures. However, it also carries the risk of any major surgery, and patients must be fit enough to undergo the procedure. Some authors suggest that the patient should have at least a 3-month prognosis if considered for surgery. According to Cole and Patchell (2008), surgery is indicated for true displacement of the spinal cord as assessed by MRI, a single area of cord compression, unstable spine or pathologic fractures, unknown primary tumor, or relapse after or progression on radiotherapy. In addition, paraplegia cannot be present for more than 48 hours for the patient to be a surgical candidate. Surgery is commonly followed by radiotherapy.

All providers working with oncology patients must be aware of the signs and symptoms of metastatic epidural spinal cord compression. Any new complaint of back pain, especially in the thoracic region, must be assessed. Rapid identification and treatment of this oncologic emergency can make an enormous difference in the quality of life of the patient's final days: ambulation versus paraplegia.

PAIN CRISIS

Most worsening cancer pain can be treated with appropriate upward titration of opioids, adjuvant agents, antineoplastic therapies, and nonpharmacologic treatments throughout the course of the disease and at end of life. However, the oncology nurse will occasionally face a patient with an acute "pain crisis" or "pain emergency"; that is, a sustained, uncontrolled pain that is excruciating, intolerable, and distressing to the patient or family (Moryl, Coyle, & Foley, 2008). It is managed with rapid titration of opioids or other intervention (Hagen, Elwood, & Ernst, 1997).

Causes of a Cancer Pain Crisis

A pain emergency may occur for a variety of physiologic reasons, including the following (Hagen et al., 1997; Koh & Portenoy, 2010; Paice, 2010):

- Progression of disease, causing worsening somatic, visceral, or neuropathic pain from tumor compression
- Acute biliary or ureteral obstruction from tumor compression
- Perforated viscus or abscess
- New or impending pathologic fracture
- Epidural cord compression
- Unable to swallow or lack of absorption of analgesics
- Pain escalation associated with end of life
- Patient stopped taking medicine (e.g., ran out of medicines, decided to stop using opioids after family members expressed concern, or caregiver not giving analgesics regularly)
- Other less common causes of acute pain crisis include opioid-induced hyperalgesia (see Chapter 6); rapid development of an oncologic emergency such as cardiac tamponade, superior vena cava syndrome, or leptomeningeal disease.

In addition, a pain crisis may be precipitated by acute psychosocial issues, such as severe anxiety, fear, or existential distress related to advanced illness. Severe terminal agitation or anxiety may mimic a pain crisis, but responds to antipsychotics (such as haloperidol) or benzodiazepines (such as lorazepam), rather than increasing doses of opioids (see Chapter 19) (Quill et al., 2010). Close coordination with the multidisciplinary team, including medicine, social work, and chaplaincy, will assist in identification of the source of the crisis, whether related to a physiologic or psychosocial cause.

Treatment of a Cancer Pain Crisis

The key to management of a pain emergency is to act rapidly to decrease the pain. Moryl and colleagues state that we should consider an acute cancer pain episode "as much of a crisis as a code (2008, p. 1457). Protocols should be available to assist nurses in approaching a pain crisis, especially in the hospice or palliative care setting (Hagen et al., 1997).

For pain emergencies from physiologic causes, treatment choice is impacted by the site of care (inpatient hospital, inpatient hospice, skilled nursing facility, home setting, adult family home); access to parenteral route of administration (intravenous) or access to care providers who can administer medications by the subcutaneous route; and whether the patient is opioid naïve or opioid tolerant (Hanks et al., 2001; National Comprehensive Cancer Network [NCCN], 2011).

Clinical Pearl

What defines an "opioid-naïve" and "opioid-tolerant" patient? (Food and Drug Admininstration [FDA], 2011; NCCN, 2011; Stokowski, 2010):

- Opioid naive: patients who *are not* chronically receiving opioid analgesics on a daily basis
- Opioid tolerant: patients who *are* chronically receiving opioid analgesics on a daily basis, for 1 week or longer, in the following doses or more:
  - 60 mg oral morphine/day;
  - 25 mg transdermal fentanyl/hr;
  - 30 mg oral oxycodone/day;
  - 8 mg oral hydromorphone/day;
  - 25 mg oral oxymorphone/day; or
  - An equianalgesic dose of any other opioid

Treatment of acute cancer pain crisis is as follows (Moryl et al., 2008; NCCN, 2011). Note that in a pain emergency, patients will achieve pain control more rapidly with the use of intravenous [IV] medication compared to oral medication (Harris, Kumar, & Rajagopal, 2003).

■ For opioid-naïve patient, start with morphine 2 to 5 mg IV or morphine 5 to 15 mg oral (PO), sublingual (SL) or rectal (PR).

▧ For opioid-tolerant patients, give the medicine dose ordered for breakthrough pain, or calculate and give 10% to 20% of the total opioid dose received in the last 24 hours.

▧ If no or minimal pain relief, repeat the same dose in 15 minutes for IV administration, or 60 minutes for oral administration.

▧ If severe pain persists at an intensity of 7 or higher (on a 0-10 scale), increase the dose by 50% and administer in 15 minutes for IV or 60 minutes for PO/SL/PR.

▧ Continue to administer the prior dose every 15 minutes IV or every 60 minutes PO/SL/PR until the patient experiences at least 50% reduction in pain, becomes drowsy, or significant opioid-related side effects occur.

▧ Consider adjuvant or coanalgesic agents IV or PO/SL/PR (corticosteroids, NSAIDs, acetaminophen, benzodiazepines).

▧ After pain is controlled, calculate the new 24-hour opioid requirement based on the total doses received, and increase the new baseline opioid dose, with 10% to 20% of the baseline dose for breakthrough pain.

▧ If significant opioid side effects occur with dose escalation, rotate to another opioid (see Chapter 4).

▧ While treating the pain, assess for the cause of the pain emergency; if opioids are not being swallowed or absorbed, change the route of administration.

▧ Provide emotional support to the patient and family. Assess for psychosocial issues, such as existential distress, that may have triggered or contributed to the pain crisis.

Nurses must be aware of how to approach and manage a pain emergency. Having protocols available in the inpatient nursing unit or the home hospice service will allow nurses to bring pain relief to the patient more quickly.

SUMMARY

Nurses are strategically positioned to assess and manage cancer pain emergencies. The key to spinal cord compression is early diagnosis. Having a high index of suspicion and knowledge of the tumors that are likely to cause this condition will aid in rapid evaluation, medical management, and possibly retention of neurologic integrity. Pain crises occur in all settings, including the home and hospital. By being aware of a treatment algorithm for acute pain crisis, such as suggested in this chapter, the nurse can promote the highest level of comfort for the person experiencing severe cancer pain.

Case Study

Marcia, a 34-year-old woman, has a 6-year history of breast cancer. She presents for follow-up after recently being diagnosed with recurrent disease with metastasis to the bone. She has new left thigh pain from metastatic disease in the femur, mild right upper quadrant pain from liver metastases, and left arm discomfort from lymphedema. As you check her vital signs, she also incidentally complains of new thoracic pain, which she blames on lifting boxes over the weekend. She discounts this as "just aches and pains from doing too much."

She describes the new back pain as sharp and tender in the mid-back; she also recalls a new ache that has been developing today "like a band around my chest." It was 5/10 today, but was 8/10 last night, interfering with her sleep. That new pain is worse when lying down.

Questions to Consider

1. What additional information would be useful?
2. What is your greatest concern regarding Marcia's pain report?

REFERENCES

Bobb, B. (2010). Urgent symptoms at the end of life. In B. Ferrell & N. Coyle (Eds.). *Oxford textbook of palliative nursing*. New York, NY: Oxford University Press.

Bucholtz, J. (1999). Metastatic epidural spinal cord compression. *Seminars in Oncology Nursing, 15*(3), 150–159.

Cole, J., & Patchell, R. (2008). Metastatic epidural spinal cord compression. *Lancet Neurology, 7*, 459–466.

Fitzgibbon, D. R., & Loeser, J. D. (2010). *Cancer pain: Assessment, diagnosis, and management*. Philadelphia, PA: Wolters Kluwer/Lippincott, Williams & Wilkins.

Food and Drug Administration (FDA). (2011, October 2). *FDA for Health Professionals*. Retrieved from http://www.fda.gov

George, R., Jeba, R., Ramkumar, G., Chacko, A., Leng, M., & Tharyan, P. (2008). Interventions for the treatment of metastatic extradural spinal cord compression in adults. *Cochrane Database of Systematic Reviews*, (4), Art. No.: CD006716.

Hagen, N., Elwood, T., & Ernst, S. (1997). Cancer pain emergencies: A protocol for management. *Journal of Pain and Symptom Management, 14*(1), 45–50.

Hanks, G., De Conno, F., Cherny, N., Hanna, M., Kalso, E., McQuay, H., . . . Ventafridda, V. (2001). Morphine and alternative opioids in cancer pain: The EAPC recommendations. *British Journal of Cancer, 84*, 587–593.

Harris, J., Kumar, K., & Rajagopal, M. (2003). Intravenous morphine for rapid control of severe cancer pain. *Palliative Medicine, 17*, 248–256.

Koh, M., & Portenoy, R. (2010). Cancer pain syndromes. In E. Bruera & R. Portenoy (Eds.), *Cancer pain: Assessment and management* (2nd ed., pp. 53–85). New York, NY: Cambridge University Press.

Moryl, N., Coyle, N., & Foley, K. (2008). Managing an acute pain crisis in a patient with advanced cancer. "This is as much of a crisis as a code." *Journal of the American Medical Association, 299*(12), 1457–1467.

National Comprehensive Cancer Network (NCCN). (2011). *National Comprehensive Cancer Network guidelines: Adult cancer pain.* Retrieved from http://www.nccn.org/professionals/physician_gls/f_guidelines.asp

Paice, J. (2010). Pain at the end of life. In B. Ferrell & N. Coyle (Eds.), *Oxford textbook of palliative nursing* (3rd ed., pp. 161–185). New York, NY: Oxford University Press.

Prasad, D., & Schiff, D. (2005). Malignant spinal-cord compression. *Lancet Oncology, 6*, 15–24.

Quill, T. E., Holloway, R. G., Shah, M. S., Caprio, T. V., Olden, A. M., & Storey, J. C. (2010). *Primer of palliative care* (5th ed.). Glenview, IL: American Academy of Hospice and Palliative Medicine.

Quraishi, N., Gokaslan, Z., & Boriani, S. (2010). The surgical management of metastatic epidural compression of the spinal cord. *Journal of Bone and Joint Surgery, 92*, 1054–1060.

Stokowski, L. (2010). *Opioid-naive and opioid-tolerant patients.* Retrieved from http://www.medscape.com/viewarticle/733067_2

Tancioni, F., Navarria, P., Lorenzetti, M., Pedrazzoli, P., Masci, G., Mancosu, P., . . . Scorsetti, M. (2010). Multimodal approach to the management of metastatic epidural spinal cord compression (MESCC) due to solid tumors. *International Journal of Radiation Oncology, Biology, Physics, 78*(5), 1467–1473.

15

Neuropathic Pain

Pamela Stitzlein Davies

Recognizing the presence of neuropathic pain (NP) in the cancer patient is an essential skill for the nurse, as the management is different from the pain of a nociceptive source. NP tends to be less responsive to opioid therapy, usually requires multiple medication regimens for control, and is generally more difficult to treat (Gordon & Love, 2004). Untreated NP may cause intense discomfort, debility, poor quality of life, and increased suffering. In the long-term cancer survivor, NP may last for years, even decades. The estimated cost of chemotherapy-induced NP is estimated at $2.3 billion in the United States (Lema, Foley, & Hausheer, 2010).

DEFINITION OF NP

NP is defined by the International Association for the Study of Pain (IASP) Task-force on Taxonomy as "pain caused by a lesion or disease of the somatosensory nervous system" (IASP Taskforce on Taxonomy, 2011; http://www.iasp-pain.org/AM/Template.cfm?Section=Pain_Definitions). Other authors define it as "abnormal persistent pain that results from a direct injury to the nervous system" (Cruciani, Strada, & Knotkova, 2010, p. 479). The IASP emphasizes that NP is a *clinical description*, and not a diagnosis. Unlike nociceptive pain, NP is a maladaptive and pathologic pain, caused by dysfunction in the peripheral nerves, or in the central processing of signals (Fitzgibbon & Loeser, 2010). This causes pain to be perceived even when there is no input from the periphery to the CNS. Clifford Woolf has described NP as "pain with no braking mechanisms" (D'Arcy, 2011, p. 293). While pain from nociceptive input provides a useful warning system of injury (e.g., pain from a sprained ankle), NP serves no useful purpose (Pasero, 2004; Suzuki, Sikandar, & Dickenson, 2010).

> | *Clinical* | Neuropathic pain is a *maladaptive* and *pathologic* phenome- |
> | *Pearl* | non, caused by dysfunction either in the peripheral nerves, or |
> | | in the central processing of pain signals. |

A Brief Review of Normal Pain Processing

To understand NP, a brief review of *normal* nociceptive pain perception is needed. There are four key stages to pain perception: (1) transduction, (2) transmission, (3) perception, and (4) modulation (Vanderah, 2007). In the periphery, noxious external stimuli activate free nerve endings called *nociceptors*. This stimulation is called *transduction*. The nociceptive fibers respond only to potentially damaging stimuli, such as mechanical (e.g., tumor, surgery), thermal (e.g., burn), chemical (e.g., chemotherapy), or infectious (e.g., herpes zoster) sources (Marchand, 2008). Nociceptive stimulation results in the release of numerous chemical transmitters in the periphery, such as prostaglandins, bradykinin, substance P, hydrogen ions, serotonin, and histamine, which activates a complex cascade leading to inflammation (Costigan, Scholz, & Woolf, 2009; Marchand, 2008). Pain signals are relayed via *transmission*, from the periphery to the spinal cord, by small unmyelinated C-fibers or thinly myelinated A-delta fibers. The signal then synapses to a second-order neuron, crosses the spinal cord, and travels up the spinothalamic (or other) tract to the thalamus. It synapses again to a third-order neuron, and is passed on to the sensory cortex. *Perception* is the awareness and interpretation of the pain signal. The final, and key, element in this process is *modulation*, in which pain signals are selectively *inhibited*, limiting the perception of pain. Inhibition of the pain signal occurs by a number of methods at a variety of levels in the CNS (Vanderah, 2007). Examples include inhibiting interneurons, endogenous chemicals (such as opioids), and the descending modulatory system. Modulation is the way in which pain therapies such as analgesics—as well as complementary treatments like hypnosis, meditation, and imagery—do their work to reduce pain intensity.

PATHOPHYSIOLOGY OF NEUROPATHIC PAIN

The pathophysiology of NP is complex, and is the result of multiple mechanisms (Cruciani et al., 2010). After a nerve is injured, *plasticity* of the nervous system plays an important role in the development of NP. Plasticity refers to structural and functional changes of the peripheral nervous system (PNS) and central nervous system (CNS) in response to injury (Costigan et al., 2009). Maladaptive plasticity promotes abnormal functioning of the nerves, which leads to NP.

NP is subdivided into peripheral and central mechanisms. Peripheral mechanisms include the development of *peripheral sensitization*. Damage to nerve and other cells causes the release of an "inflammatory soup" of chemical mediators (Gordon & Love, 2004). Exaggerated responses to pain stimuli occur from hyperexcitable nerve endings, lowered nerve depolarization threshold, and "cross-talk" between the normally isolated nerve cells (Pasero, 2004). Spontaneous discharge of signals from the periphery results, even in the absence of external stimuli. Voltage-gated sodium channels play a significant role in peripheral mechanisms of NP, and are the target of many anticonvulsants and tricyclic antidepressants (TCAs; Beydoun & Backonja, 2003).

Central sensitization occurs in the CNS, leading to hyperexcitability of the central neurons. The ongoing barrage of signals from the injured peripheral nerves is theorized to trigger development of central sensitization (Costigan et al., 2009). By means of neuroplasticity mechanisms, the CNS reorganizes synaptic connectivity, with lower activation thresholds and increased response to stimuli (Costigan et al., 2009). Plasticity leads to anatomic changes, with sprouting of collateral neurons, which leads to abnormal "cross-talk" between the nerves of the CNS (Fitzgibbon & Loeser, 2010). This pathologic "cross-excitation" results in recruitment of additional neurons, leading to a larger receptor field being affected. This process, along with lower activation thresholds and increased response to stimuli, creates a phenomenon known as *"wind up"* (Pasero, 2004). In addition, descending inhibitory mechanisms, which help to reduce pain, become suppressed. The overall result of the multitude of complex mechanisms is the development of NP.

Prevalence of Neuropathic Pain

Estimates of the pevalence of NP depend on the criteria for defining NP, the method of assessment (self-report, interview, or the "gold-standard" clinician examination) (Haanpää et al., 2009). In 2008, the IASP Neuropathic Pain Special Interest Group (NeuPSIG) created diagnostic criteria for NP research, which will help define prevalence more clearly in future studies.

In a 2012 systematic review of 22 studies involving 13,683 patients with cancer pain, the prevalence of NP is estimated at 20% for those with definite or probable "pure" NP, and up to 40% if possible or "mixed" NP is included in the analysis (Bennett et al., 2012). In a subanalysis of six studies that met the new NeuPSIG diagnostic criteria for NP, the estimated prevalence of NP ranged from 13% to 36%.

Most cancer patients report two to three different types of pain. This systematic review also analyzed seven papers that reported on the mechanism of each pain complaint. There were 8,174 different pains in 4,049 patients, for a mean of 2 pains per patient. Seventy four percent were determined to be nociceptive in origin, 19% neuropathic, 3% were mixed origin, and 5% were unknown/other. Furthermore, in four studies the etiology of NP was determined. Of the 1,674 NP recorded, 64% were caused directly by the cancer, 20% by cancer treatment, 4% associated with having cancer, 10% unrelated to cancer, and 2% unknown etiology (Bennett et al., 2012).

PREVALENCE AND ETIOLOGY OF NEUROPATHIC PAIN

In a systematic review of seven papers, 4,049 cancer patients reported 8,174 different pains. Of those:

- 20% had "pure" NP, and 40% had "mixed" NP
- The source of NP was:
  - 64% directly from the cancer
  - 20% from cancer treatment
  - 4% associated with having cancer (e.g., herpes zoster or postherpetic neuralgia)
  - 10% unrelated to cancer; 2% unknown etiology

(Bennett et al., 2012)

Other authors have reported similar or higher incidence of cancer-related NP (Lema, et al. 2010). Early studies reported ranges of prevalence from 34%, 40%, to more than 50% of those with cancer pain (Miguel, 2006; Reyes-Gibby, Morrow, Bennett, Jensen, & Shete, 2010). In a 2010 study of breast cancer *survivors* with pain, the incidence of NP was 19% to 39%, depending on the assessment tool utilized (Reyes-Gibby et al., 2010). Similarly, a study of neuropathy and NP measures in patients receiving taxanes and platinum compounds found the NP incidence of 30% (Smith, Cohen, Pett, & Beck, 2011).

Rates of chemotherapy-induced peripheral neuropathy (CIPN) are very high, from 57% to 92%, depending on the agent used. However, these rates combine *nonpainful* peripheral neuropathies (e.g., numbness) with painful neuropathies (e.g., painful tingling, burning). Additional information about long-term effects from chemotherapy can be found in Chapter 17.

SOURCES OF CANCER-RELATED NEUROPATHIC PAIN

NP in the cancer patient is caused by three primary conditions: direct tumor involvement, cancer treatment, and indirect etiologies or unrelated comorbidities (Fitzgibbon & Loeser, 2010).

Tumor Sources of Neuropathic Pain in Cancer

Cancer as a direct cause of NP is estimated at 64% incidence (Bennett et al., 2012). Tumor invasion of nerves or nerve plexus, or tumor bulk pressure on surrounding tissues that increase the pressure on nerves, are the most common causes of cancer-related NP. Examples include the following:

- 38-year-old woman with metastatic lung cancer who develops a 3-cm tumor in the axilla with direct compression of the nerves of the brachial plexus, causing severe uncontrolled arm pain
- 30-year-old man with a 10-cm sarcoma in the pelvis that invades the gluteal muscle; the tumor causes compression of the sciatic nerve, leading to severe radicular pain in the leg

Involvement of the CNS is another source of tumor-related pain. Primary or secondary (metastatic) brain tumors frequently cause headache, as well as nausea, motor impairment, incoordination, and seizures. Leptomeningeal metastasis, also known as *carcinomatous meningitis*, is the result of tumor spread to the meniges and cerebral spinal fluid, which can cause headaches and nausea. It occurs most commonly in lung cancer, breast cancer, melanoma, and lymphoma (Fitzgibbon & Loeser, 2010).

Treatment Sources of Neuropathic Pain in Cancer

Treatment sources as a cause of NP in the cancer setting are estimated at 20% for those in active cancer treatment (Bennett et al., 2012). The incidence of treatment as the source of NP may be higher once the patient is free of disease and left with residual chronic pain. Chemotherapy, surgery, radiation, and other therapies are the causes of treatment-related NP. These sources will be briefly reviewed in the next section, but more detailed information is available in Chapter 17 and Appendices 17.2 and 17.3.

Chemotherapy Agents Causing Neuropathic Pain

Certain chemotherapy agents have a very high incidence of chemotherapy-induced peripheral neuropathy (CIPN), from 57% to 92%. However, as noted earlier, these numbers reflect both *nonpainful* peripheral neuropathies (such as numbness), as well as *painful* neuropathies (such as burning.). In addition to CIPN, other forms of painful or nonpainful chemotherapy-induced neuropathy may develop; for example, autonomic neuropathy from vincristine (e.g., constipation, cardiovascular dysfunction), and cranial nerve neuropathy leading to ototoxicity from cisplatin (Driver, Cata, & Phan, 2006).

Painful neuropathies from chemotherapy occur most commonly from the following classes of agents (Wickham, 2007; Wilkes, 2007):
- **Platinum** compounds (e.g., cisplatin, carboplatin, oxaliplatin)
- **Taxanes** (e.g., paclitaxel, docetaxel, nab-paclitaxel)
- **Vinca alkaloids** (e.g., vincristine, vinblastine, vinorelbine)
- Other classes (e.g., bortezomib, thalidomide)

CIPN may develop within the first few cycles of therapy. However, an interesting phenomenon occurs with several chemotherapy agents called "coasting," in which a painful neuropathy may develop *weeks* or even *months* after completion of chemotherapy (Wickham, 2007; Wilkes, 2007). Patient education regarding this possibility will aid decreasing anxiety if it does occur. Many cases of CIPN resolve within months of cessation of chemotherapy, but other cases may last for years (Wickham, 2007).

Chemotherapy most commonly causes a *distal symmetrical sensory polyneuropathy*, also referred to as a *"stocking-glove"* distribution. The injury is *polyneuronal*, meaning it affects multiple nerves (Wilkes, 2007). This causes sensory changes and/or pain in the longest nerves: those of the hands and feet. CIPN may extend proximal to include the wrists and forearms or the ankles and calves. It is common to have a predominance of involvement in either the hands or the feet. CIPN may cause sensory, motor, or autonomic neuropathy.
- Sensory neuropathy: Changes in sensation including numbness, pain, dysesthesias, hyperalgesias (common)
- Motor neuropathy: Changes in motor function including loss of deep tendon reflexes, foot drop, limb weakness, ataxia (less common)

■ Autonomic neuropathy: Changes in sympathetic or parasympathetic function, such as changes in heart rate, blood pressure, bladder emptying, or changes in bowel motility such as delayed gastric emptying or constipation (less common)

Patients at higher risk of developing chemotherapy-induced peripheral neuropathy include those with the following (Wickham, 2007; Wilkes, 2007):

■ Higher doses of neurotoxic chermotherapy agents
■ "Dose-dense" schedules of neurotoxic chemotherapy (more frequent administration)
■ Higher overall cumulative doses of neurotoxic agents
■ Administration of multiple neurotoxic agents
■ Presence of pre-existing neuropathy conditions, such as diabetes or HIV peripheral neuropathy
■ Older age

Surgery as a Source of Neuropathic Pain

Postsurgical pain syndromes are well-known phenomena after cancer surgery. Common postoperative cancer pain syndromes include the following (Burton, Fanciullo, Beasley, & Fisch, 2007; Cohen, Gambel, Raja, & Galvagno, 2011; Polomano, Ashburn, & Farrar, 2010):

■ Postamputation pain
■ Postthoracotomy pain
■ Postmastectomy pain
■ Post–radical neck dissection pain

With improvements in perioperative pain management, the incidence of surgical NP appears to be declining (Polomano et al., 2010). Increased utilization of "multimodal" pain therapy in the perioperative period is showing promise at preventing development of postsurgical pain syndromes (Fassoulaki, Triga, Melemeni, & Sarantopoulos, 2005; Gebhardt, 2006). Examples of multimodal therapy include perioperative intravenous infusions of lidocaine, neuroaxial blocks (intrathecal, epidural), regional blocks (brachial plexus), or injections of local anesthetic into the incision.

Radiation Therapy as a Source of Neuropathic Pain

NP syndromes from radiation primarily involve plexopathies, as follows (Driver et al., 2006; Levy, Chwistek, & Rohtesh, 2008; Polomano & Farrar, 2006; Polomano et al., 2010):

- Brachial plexopathy: NP in dermatomal patterns of the arm after radiation to the axilla; for example, in breast and lung cancers, Hodgkin's disease
- Lumbosacral plexopathy: NP in dermatomal patterns of the leg after radiation to the pelvis; for example, in gastrointestinal or gynecologic cancers or Hodgkin's disease
- Myelopathy: A rare syndrome causing burning back pain due to damage to the spinal cord; may be accompanied by loss of sensation, motor weakness, and paralysis

More precise radiotherapy techniques have resulted in fewer chronic NP syndromes attributed to radiation. In addition, newer treatment regimens, which combine radiation with chemotherapy or surgery, have allowed for overall lower doses of radiation. Radiation-related NP syndromes typically arise weeks or months after completion of radiation, but occasionally may present years, even decades, after therapy (Levy et al., 2008).

Indirect Etiologies and Unrelated Comorbidities Causing Neuropathic Pain in the Cancer Patient

About 4% of NP cases are an "indirect" result of having cancer (Bennett et al., 2012). The primary indirect etiology of NP in cancer is the development of herpes zoster (HZ) infection from cancer-related immunosuppression, with the resulting complication of postherpetic neuralgia (PHN) (Alvarez, Galer, & Gammaitoni, 2006).

Herpes Zoster

Also known as a "shingles" outbreak, HZ results from reactivation of the varicella zoster virus (VZV, or chickenpox virus), which spreads from a single dorsal root ganglion or cranial nerve ganglion, with an eruption of painful vesicles on the skin of the innervated dermatome. The thoracic dermatomes are the most commonly affected sites, at 50% to 70% of all cases, followed by the trigeminal nerve (primarily the ophthalmic division), cervical, and lumbar dermatomes (Dworkin & Schmader, 2001). Severely immunocompromised patients are at risk of developing *disseminated herpes zoster*, which may be life threatening. The pain of HZ may be quite severe. It has been described as "the belt of roses from hell" in ancient literature (Watson & Gershon, 2001). The HZ outbreak is considered an acute NP, and typically lasts for a few days to several weeks. The herpetic lesions then crust and the pain gradually diminishes.

The two primary risk factors for developing HZ is age over 50 and immunosuppression. Both of these risk factors describe the typical oncology patient. The hematologic malignancies have greater incidence of HZ outbreaks, with Hodgkin's disease the highest (Alvarez et al., 2006). Anecdotal experience finds an association between the site of previous surgery (mastectomy, thoracotomy, craniotomy) and the site of HZ outbreak, although the literature is equivocal on this topic.

Postherpetic Neuralgia

Postherpetic neuralgia (PHN) is a separate persistent pain syndrome from HZ, which develops in only some cases. It is defined as persistent pain lasting longer than 1 to 4 months after crusting and healing of the HZ rash. PHN is a NP occurring in the affected unilateral HZ dermatome, and often "recruiting" nearby dermatomes to a wider swath of pain by means of central sensitization. Patients usually describe the chronic postherpetic pain as having a different sensation compared to the pain of acute zoster outbreak. The pain intensity may range from severe and life altering, to mild and not requiring any treatment.

In the general population, the primary risk factor for developing and maintaining PHN is older age. Patients over the age of 70 who develop HZ have a 50% chance of developing PHN that never resolves. Younger persons (40 or younger) rarely develop chronic PHN lasting more than 1 year (Watson & Gershon, 2001). Although the majority of cancer patients are at risk for HZ and PHN due to increased age and immunosuppression, it is not clear if having cancer independently adds an *additional* risk for the development of HZ or PHN (Alvarez et al., 2006).

Unrelated Causes of Neuropathic Pain

Approximately 10% of cancer pain patients have a NP problem unrelated to cancer, cancer treatment, or "indirect" causes from cancer (Bennett et al., 2012). The two most common sources of pre-existing NP are painful diabetic peripheral neuropathy and painful sciatica (lumbar radiculopathy). Other pre-existing NP sources may include central pain conditions (such as poststroke pain, or pain from multiple sclerosis or spinal cord injury), or peripheral sources (complex regional pain syndrome, trigeminal neuralgia, or HIV/AIDS-related neuropathy). Patients with painful peripheral neuropathies are at higher risk of developing chemotherapy-induced peripheral neuropathy, and may require modification of their regimen dose or schedule (Wickham, 2007).

ASSESSMENT OF NEUROPATHIC PAIN

Assessment of NP is the key to management. For recalcitrant pain problems, the nurse should always consider NP as a possible source, especially if the patient uses certain verbal descriptors, or has received therapies that place them at higher risk, as mentioned earlier.

Verbal Descriptors of Neuropathic Pain

Classically, NP has been described by the following three hallmark characteristics, although not every patient suffers from all three components (Dworkin et al., 2003; Rowbotham & Fields, 1989):

- **Continuous** pain: Burning, "hot," aching pain
- **Lancinating** pain: Shooting, sharp, stabbing, "electrical shocks"
- **Abormal sensations** or cutaneous sensitivity: Numbness, pins and needles

Other descriptors may include: painful numbness, tingling, itching, abnormal temperature perception (e.g., "When I touch something cold it feels burning hot"), or unusual hypersensitivity to touch (e.g., "I can't stand to have the sheet touch my feet when I'm in bed"). Athough such descriptions are not diagnostic of NP, their use should flag the clinician to assess for NP as a possible contributor to the pain complaint (Haanpää et al., 2009). The nurse should assess for neurologic manifestations of pain by asking about these descriptors (Wickham, 2007).

Researchers have long been interested in correlating the mechanism of NP and the specific pain descriptors to the choice of drug class for initial treatment (Beydoun & Backonja, 2003; Dworkin et al., 2003; Rowbotham, 2005). For example, complaints of lancinating pain may be more amenable to treatment with anticonvulsants. However, results in this area have been mixed.

A recent study sought to further clarify prescribing based on the proposed mechanism of NP. Using NP scales, patient reports of pain were divided into two factors (Mackey et al., 2012).

- **Factor 1: Stabbing pain** (described as stabbing, sharp, shooting)
- **Factor 2: Heavy pain** (described as heavy, gnawing, aching)

They proposed that the mechanism of action of "stabbing pain" is carried by thinly myelinated A-delta fibers ("first pain"); while the mechanism of "heavy pain" is carried by slower unmyelinated C-fibers ("second pain"). The researchers found that patients with high levels of "heavy pain" had improved response to intravenous lidocaine over placebo compared to those in the other group (Mackey et al., 2012).

Neuropathic Pain Terminology

Sensory abberations from neuropathy are divided into *positive* and *negative* phenomena (Haanpää et al., 2011). Positive sensory changes include the sensation of pain from innoculous touch (*allodynia*) and an increased sense of pain from a pin prick (*hyperalgesia*). Negative sensory changes include numbness (*hypoesthesia*) or minimal painful sensation from a pinprick (*hypoalgesia*). The IASP Taskforce on Taxonomy has defined pain terminology. The following box lists several terms related to NP.

NEUROPATHIC PAIN TERMS
The following selected terms are useful to know when caring for the patient with NP (IASP Taskforce on Taxonomy, 2011):

- **Allodynia**: A painful sensation produced by a stimulus that does not normally cause pain (e.g., the touch from clothes or bedsheets causes pain, similar to what is experienced after a bad sunburn)
- **Paresthesia**: An abnormal sensation, not unpleasant, evoked or nonevoked (e.g., numbness, tingling)
  - *Evoked* refers to an outside stimulus, such as a pin prick or a brush stroke; *nonevoked* means the sensation is spontaneous
- **Dysesthesia**: An unpleasant sensation, whether evoked or non-evoked (e.g., uncomfortable pins and needles, painful itching, formication [sensation of bugs crawling under skin])
- **Hyperesthesia**: Increased sensation to a stimulus (nonpainful; e.g., cold metal feels more intensely cold)
- **Hyperalgesia**: Increased pain from a stimulus that is normally painful (e.g., a pin prick feels sharper and more painful)
- **Hyperpathia**: Abnormally painful reaction to a stimulus, especially a repetitive stimulus; occasionally pain is explosive in character
- **Hypoesthesia:** Decreased sensitivity to stimulation
- **Hypoalgesia:** Diminished pain in response to a normally painful stimulus

Focused Physical Examination for Neuropathic Pain

The nurse can perform a focused physical examination for neuropathy with a cotton tip applicator, safety pin, alcohol swab, tuning fork, and reflex hammer (Haanpää et al., 2011). Abnormalities and deficits from neuropathy may or may not be evident on clinical examination; the presence of abnormalities does not diagnose NP, nor does the absence eliminate the possibility of NP. However, clinical examination provides supporting data toward a clinical diagnosis. Testing includes the following (Bickley, Szilagyi, & Bates, 2008; Fuller, 1999; Haanpää et al., 2009; Wickham, 2007):

- **Sensory examination** (testing small fibers: A-delta and C)
  (Test the affected area [e.g., fingertips, thigh, chest wall], then compare it to a normal area.)
  - **Light touch perception**
    - Using a cotton tip applicator, stroke the affected area lightly.
    - Is touch perceived? Is it a normal or abnormal sensation (*paresthesia, dysesthesia, numbness*)? Is it painful or unpleasant with light touch (*allodynia*)?
  - **Pinprick perception**
    - Lightly tap the painful area with a clean safety pin.
    - Is there a normal sensation of pinprick? Or is there an "exaggerated" response sensation of pain (*hyperalgesia*) or a diminished response (*hypoalgesia*)?
    - Tap repeatedly (e.g., 5 to 10 times) in one spot. Does the patient feel single pin pricks or does it summate with an "explosion" of pain (*hyperpathia*)?
    - Two-point discrimination: using two pins, touch the fingertip simultaneously, alternating with a single-point touch. Find the minimal distance that two points are discriminated. A normal finding is 2–3 mm on the fingertip.
  - **Cold temperature perception**
    - Use the flat side of a tuning fork, or an alcohol swab. Is cool temperature appreciated? Is the cool sensation quite pronounced (*hyperesthesia*) or minimal (*hypoesthesia*)? Is it painful or uncomfortable (*dysesthesia*)?.
- **Motor, proprioception, and vibratory sense** (testing large fibers)
  - **Motor function**
    - Check motor strength in the major muscle groups: deltoid, biceps, triceps, wrist extensor/flexor, interrosseous (fingers), hip flexor/extensor/abbductor/adductor, quadraceps, hamstring; test dorsiflexion, plantarflexion, great toe flexion.
      - Grade on a scale of 0 to 5 (0 is flaccid, 5 is normal strength)
  - **Stretch reflexes**
    - Use the reflex handle to check for brachial, brachioradialis, patellar, and ankle reflexes.
      - Grade on a scale of 0 to 4 (0 is no response, +2 is normal, +4 is very brisk (abnormal))
    - Plantar reflex (Babinski sign)
      - Present or absent

- **Proprioception**
  - Grasp the sides of the great toe and hold it away from the other toes. Demonstrate the test by moving the toe upward (flexion) or downward (extension), while explaining the position to the patient. To perform the test, have the patient close his or her eyes and tell you which direction you are moving the toe joint. This can also be performed on the thumb.
- **Tandem walk**
  - Have the patient walk heel to toe in a straight line (e.g., the "drunk driving test"). Can the patient maintain balance? (You are checking for ataxia.)
- **Vibratory sense**
  - Briskly tap the tuning fork against your hand to make it vibrate.
  - Place the base of the tuning fork on the bony prominence at the great toe interphalangeal joint (other testing sites include the ankle lateral malleolus, or thumb interphalangeal joint).
  - Have the patient tell you if he or she can sense vibration, and when he or she can no longer feels vibration.
  - Can you still feel significant vibration between your fingers when the patient no longer feels it? If yes, how many seconds until your fingers no longer sense vibration?

Neuropathic Pain Assessment Tools

A number of tools have been developed specifically for NP. These tools can be divided into two categories: screening versus assessment tools for NP (D'Arcy, 2011), which are described in the following list:

- *Screening* tools are brief, verbal or written, and intended for use in the clinic or at the bedside to detect for the presence or absence of NP.
- *Assessment* tools are more detailed, typically take longer to complete, and are more appropriate to a specialized pain or neurology clinic, or a research setting.

Two screening tools that have been tested in the cancer population include the *ID Pain* and the *S-LANSS* (Bennett, Smith, Torrance, & Potter, 2005; Portenoy, 2006; Reyes-Gibby et al., 2010). More detailed assessment tools include the Neuropathic Pain Scale (see the next section), Neuropathic Pain Symptom Inventory, Neuropathic Pain Diagnostic Questionnaire, and the Neuropathic Pain Questionnaire (long and short forms) (Jensen, 2006; Mercadante et al., 2009):

- **ID Pain**
  - This is a brief screening tool with a body diagram, and six simple yes or no questions about sensations of pain in the last week.

- Five of the questions include items related to NP (e.g., pins and needles, hot/burning, numb, electric shocks, allodynia). Each "yes" response receives 1 point. The sixth question is related to nociceptive pain (pain limited to joints); a positive response receives a negative point.
- Scores range from −1 to 5. A score of 3 or higher is indicative of NP.
- **S-LANSS** (Self-report Leeds Assessment of Neuropathic Symptoms and Signs)
  - This is a brief screening tool to identify patients with NP.
  - It includes a body diagram, a 0 to 10 numerical rating scale, and a 7-item binary (yes or no) questionnaire.
  - Five questions ask about symptoms (pins and needles, electric shocks, burning), and two ask the patient to self-test for signs of NP (gently rub and press the painful area).
  - Scores can range from 0 to 24, and anything greater than 12 is highly suggestive of NP.
- **Neuropathic Pain Scale** (Galer & Jensen, 1997)
  - This is a 10-item, pen, and paper, NP assessment tool.
  - Each descriptor (hot, sharp, sensitive, itchy, dull) is rated on a 0 to 10 Likert box scale, with 0 being no symptom and 10 being the most intense symptom imaginable.
  - This tool has been shown useful in the intial assessment of NP and to evaluate treatment effects.

TREATMENT OF NEUROPATHIC PAIN

Management of NP has proved challenging to patient and clinician alike, primarily because NP is more resistant to therapy. The approach to NP management usually requires multiple pharmacologic agents and higher doses, as well as other therapies (Dworkin et al., 2003). Because patients commonly have a partial response to individual drugs, the concept of *"rational polypharmacy"* or *"multimodal therapy"* has been advanced for management of NP (Allen, 2008; Argoff et al., 2006). This refers to the use of two or more drugs to treat the same condition (Kingsbury, Yi, & Simpson, 2001). The concern with use of polypharmacy is increased risk for drug interactions and side effects, especially in the elderly (Brant, 2010). But the desired benefit is for improved pain control by targeting different sources of NP with drugs of different mechanisms (Ziegler, 2011).

There are no FDA-approved oral drugs in the United States specifically for cancer-related NP. This is because the vast majority of world research on NP is performed on two noncancer pain conditions: diabetic peripheral neuropathy (DPN) and postherpetic neuralgia (PHN) (Beydoun & Backonja, 2003). These two conditions are favored for research due to a relatively good understanding of the disease mechanism and, in the case of HZ and PHN, a distinct onset of the painful condition. Drugs with an FDA approval for management of NP, such as duloxetine (Cymbalta), gabapentin (Neurontin), or lidocaine 5% (Lidoderm) patch are usually approved for DPN and/or PHN.

For patients on chemotherapy, drug interactions are important considerations. It is prudent to check with the oncology pharmacist prior to initiating any therapy for management of NP. In addition, patients in Phase 1 chemotherapy studies typically have restrictions on the addition of other drugs, such as adjuvant agents.

Treatment of NP is provided with the following classes of drugs, as well as other agents:

- Anticonvulsants
- Antidepressants
- Topicals
- Opioids

Anticonvulsants to Manage Neuropathic Pain

Anticonvulsants, also known as *antiepileptic drugs*, are a primary treatment for NP. The two first-line agents in cancer settings are gabapentin (Neurontin) and pregabalin (Lyrica) (Argoff et al., 2006). These drugs have the best evidence for efficacy, FDA approval for DPN (pregabalin) or PHN (gabapentin), and fewer drug interactions (Moulin et al., 2007). Other anticonvulsants used in NP, but without an FDA indication, include topiramate (Topamax), lamotrigine (Lamictal), or oxcarbazepine (Trileptal) (Forde, 2007).

Older agents include carbamazepine (Tegretol), which is FDA approved for trigeminal neuralgia. Valproic acid (Valproate) and phenytoin (Dilantin) have only limited evidence for efficacy in NP (Argoff et al., 2006). These older drugs cost less, but they have more drug interactions and require laboratory monitoring for possible impact on the hematologic or hepatic system. For more information on these drugs, see Chapter 5.

Gabapentin is tolerated better when it is started at a lower dose (100 to 300 mg), and titrated over a period of days to weeks. It takes a minimum of 2 weeks for gabapentin to start having an analgesic effect, whereas the analgesic effect of pregabalin starts as early as 1 to 2 days, and a more rapid titration schedule is tolerated. Both drugs cause sedation (in approximately 20% of patients), dizziness (in approximately 30%), and peripheral edema (in approximately 8%) (Forde, 2007). Dose adjustments must be done in kidney disease. Example orders follow:

- **Gabapentin** 100 to 300 mg PO at bedtime × 3 to 7 days, then 100 to 300 mg at dinnertime and bedtime for 3 to 7 days, then 100 to 300 mg TID. May be titrated to 900 to 3,600 mg per day, administered in 2 to 3 doses per day.
  - For those with decreased creatinine clearance, the maximum dose is 100 to 600 mg per day given in 1 to 3 doses.
- **Pregabalin** 75 to 150 mg PO at bedtime for 3 to 4 days, may titrate to 150 to 600 mg daily given in 2 to 3 doses per day.
  - For elders and decreased creatinine clearance, start at 25 to 50 mg daily, and titrate to 25 to 150 mg in 1 to 2 doses.

Antidepressants to Manage Neuropathic Pain

Two classes of antidepressants (ADs) have been proven effective at reducing the severity of NP: the serotonin-norepinephrine reuptake inhibitor (SNRI) drugs (duloxetine [Cymbalta] and venlafaxine [Effexor]), and the older TCAs (e.g., nortriptyline, desipramine, amitriptyline). The other major class of antidepressants, selective serotonin reuptake inhibitors (SSRIs, e.g., citalopram [Celexa], paroxetine [Paxil], fluoxetine [Prozac]) are not effective in management of NP. The monoamine oxidase inhibitor (MAOI) drugs are not used for management of NP.

Like anticonvulsants, there are no antidepressants specifically FDA approved for use in NP caused by cancer or cancer treatment. The efficacy of ADs in treating painful neuropathies has been shown to be separate from their ability to treat depression. In a seminal study, two TCA drugs, desipramine and amitriptyline, were compared to the effect of fluoxetine or placebo in painful diabetic peripheral neuropathy (DPN). The two TCA drugs improved the pain of DPN, whereas fluoxetine was no better than placebo. Study participants were evaluated by a psychiatrist for the presence or absence of depression. In an interesting cross-over design, the authors concluded that the antidepressants worked for pain whether or not the subjects were depressed (Max et al., 1992). A similar result was found by Rowbotham in 2005 (Rowbotham, Reisner, Davies, & Fields, 2005). The theorized mechanism of action for pain relief is the noradrenergic effect of TCAs and SNRIs that are not present in the SSRI drugs (Max et al., 1992).

The antidepressant dose for analgesia is lower than what is required for depression management (Rowbotham et al., 2005). In a recent Cochrane Review, TCAs and venlafaxine were shown effective for management of NP, with a number needed to treat of 3 (Saarto & Wiffen, 2010). However, the role of TCAs in *preventing* NP may be limited. In a study of 114 patients without neuropathy who were starting chemotherapy that would put them at risk for chemotherapy-induced neuropathy (CIN), the use of amitriptyline failed to prevent development of this problem (Kautio et al., 2009).

SNRI and TCA drugs have significant side effects, which impact tolerability. These include sedation, dizziness, lightheadedness, orthostatic hypotension, constipation, and urinary retention (Argoff et al., 2006). These side effects tend to be dose related, meaning the higher the dose, the more significant the side effects. SNRIs can cause hypertension; therefore, blood pressure should be monitored after therapy is initated (Gordon & Love, 2004). TCAs can lead to prolonged QTc intervals, seen on ECGs. Such prolongation predisposes a patient to a higher risk of *torsade de pointes*, a dangerous cardiac arrhythmia that can lead to sudden cardiac death (Straus et al., 2006). This is especially concerning for patients taking concomitant TCAs and methadone, as both of these drugs prolong the QTc. TCAs tend to have more drug interactions than SNRIs, and their use may be limited when patients are receiving chemotherapy or enrolled in cancer clinical trials. These drugs need to be titrated slowly to improve tolerance to the side effects.

Sample doses of antidepressants to manage NP follow (Forde, 2007; Moulin et al., 2007):

- SNRIs:
  - Duloxetine: Start at 20 to 30 mg once daily, and increase over several weeks to 30 mg BID or 60 mg once daily.
  - Venlafaxine: Start at 37.5 to 75 mg once daily, and titrate over several weeks to 150 to 225 mg per day in two or three divided doses.
- TCAs:
  - Amitriptyline or desipramine, nortriptyline: Start with 10 to 25 mg at bedtime for 1 to 2 weeks, then increase by 25 mg every 1 to 2 weeks. Maximum dose is 150 to 200 mg at hs for amtriptyline or desipramine. Maximum dose for nortriptyline is 150 mg.

Topical Agents to Manage Neuropathic Pain

Two primary topical agents are used to manage NP: lidocaine 5% (Lidoderm) patches, and capsaicin. Other topical analgesics, such as diclofenac (Flector) patch or diclofenac (Voltaren) gel will not be discussed, as they are not useful in NP.

Lidocaine Patch

The lidocaine 5% patch is FDA approved for use in postherpetic neuralgia, with a NNT of 4.4 (Davies & Galer, 2004). Its efficacy has been examined off-label in multiple other NP conditions, including painful peripheral neuropathy, postthoractomy pain, postmastectomy pain, intercostal neuralgia, HIV pain, low back pain, and amputation stump pain (Gordon & Love, 2004; Wallace, Galer, & Gammaitoni, 2006). Lidocaine is a sodium channel blocker that can decrease both spontaneous and evoked NP. The patches are made of soft felt backing with an aqueous gel adhesive. It must be placed at the site of pain, up to three patches may be applied for 12 hours of each 24-hour period. The systemic blood levels of lidocaine are minimal and not clinically relevant (Campbell, Rowbotham, Davies, Jacob, & Benowitz, 2002).

Capsaicin

The active component of chili peppers, capsaicin is made from the oil of this plant. Capsaicin is believed to exert its effects by depleting substance P in sensory nerve endings (McCleane, 2007). The cream or gel is applied to the painful area four times a day for a minimum of 2 weeks. It causes intense burning, which may be intolerable to patients. Capsaicin is available over the counter in the United States. Patients should be instructed to start with low-dose capsaicin (Zostrix) 0.025%. Once this is tolerated, they may increase to the more potent capsaicin (Zostrix-HP) 0.075%. Some authors recommend premedication with a eutectic mixture of local anesthetic (EMLA) cream 30 minutes prior to application of capsaicin during initial usage.

Patients must be warned to wear gloves during application (or apply with a commercially available applicator stick) to avoid getting the drug on the hands. Hands should be thoroughly washed after application, and efforts should be made to avoid touching or scratching the treated area and transferring the drug to the eyes or mucous membranes. Such accidental exposure may cause severe pain and burning. Although it is not dangerous, it can be quite uncomfortable, similar to eating a hot chili pepper.

Lidocaine patches or capsaicin may be helpful for management of NP syndromes such as postthoractomy pain, postmastectomy pain, or chemotherapy-induced painful peripheral neuropathy (Gordon & Love, 2004; McCleane, 2007).

Opioids to Manage Neuropathic Pain

Opioids have not traditionally been considered useful in the treatment of NP (Cruciani et al., 2010). However, several studies have shown efficacy in NP, although higher doses may be required (Gordon & Love, 2004; Watson, Moulin, Watt-Watson, Gordon, & Eisenhoffer, 2003).

In a study of 81 patients with NP from peripheral origin (postherpetic neuralgia, painful peripheral neuropathy) or central origin (poststroke pain, incomplete spinal cord injury pain, multiple sclerosis pain), a dose-response design revealed a 33% improvement in pain from high-dose opioid therapy (Rowbotham et al., 2003). However, even with modified dosing schedules, 27% of patients dropped out of the study due to side effects. The drug used in this study was levorphanol, a long-acting mu agonist, which patients could self-titrate within strict guidelines. Pain of peripheral origin appears to be more responsive to opioids than pain of central origin (Mercadante et al., 2009; Rowbotham et al., 2003).

Other Agents to Manage Neuropathic Pain

First- and second-line therapies for NP management include anticonvulsants, antidepressants, opioids, and topical agents. When those agents fail to manage refractory NP, the addition of less commonly used drugs is considered (Cruciani et al., 2010). These include lidocaine or ketamine infusions, or cannabis.

Lidocaine

There have been a variety of small studies on the use of lidocaine infusions or subcutaneous injections for NP syndromes, including painful diabetic neuropathy, postherpetic neuralgia, as well as some cancer pain syndromes (Galer, Harle, & Rowbotham, 1996). Although local anesthetics are commonly used for nerve blocks, infusions of these agents is not common in the clinical setting (Cruciani et al., 2010). In a cancer pain crisis, a lidocaine infusion may be helpful to "break" the uncontrolled pain. ECG and vital sign monitoring is required during infusion. Doses start at 1 to 2 mg/kg over 30 to 45 minutes. For those requiring frequent IV infusions, another option is a continuous subcutaneous infusion at 1 to 2 mg/kg/hr to a plasma concentration of 2 to 5 mcg/mL (Cruciani et al., 2010). Side effects include paresthesias, lightheadedness, nausea, tremor, bradycardia, hypotension, and arrhythmias. Parenteral lidocaine should be used for management of NP only by a provider familiar with the necessary precautions and protocols.

Ketamine

Ketamine is a dissociative anesthetic with analgesic and psychedelic properties. It has analgesic properties through NMDA receptor antagonism. Ketamine is used in cancer pain management for refractory NP, postoperative pain in patients with significant opioid tolerance, and opioid hyperalgesia syndrome. It has an opioid-sparing effect, allowing for tapering of very high doses of opioids by half (Fitzgibbon & Loeser, 2010). The loading dose is 0.25 to 0.5 mg/kg over 10 minutes, then a continuous infusion is started at 0.1 mg/kg/hr and titrated as tolerated. Like lidocaine, this drug should only be given in a setting where continuous monitoring can be performed, with knowledgeable staff and protocols for use. A sample infusion protocol is available in Pasero and McCaffery (2011).

Cannabinoids

Cannabis (marijuana) binds with the endogenous cannabinoid system to provide analgesia as well as a wide variety of other effects, including appetite stimulation, sedation, and psychologic effects. Nabiximols (Sativex) is a cannabis-derived oromucosal spray approved in Canada and the United Kingdom for management of NP, pain related to multiple sclerosis, and spasticity (Fitzgibbon & Loeser, 2010). Medical marijuana is prescribed in some settings for cancer-related pain, chronic pain, nausea and vomiting, anorexia, as well as other chronic conditions (Cruciani et al., 2010). However, the efficacy of medical marijuana for analgesia continues to be debated (Fitzgibbon & Loeser, 2010). The primary side effects are sedation, dizziness, and dry mouth. In addition, some may experience significant psychologic effects, such as hallucinations or paranoia, which can be quite frightening. Anectodal experience has revealed that patients who are best suited to use cannabinoids are those who have enjoyed using marijuana recreationally in the past without problematic psychomimetic effects.

SUMMARY

Management of NP is challenging, as it tends to be more resistant to standard therapies than nociceptive pain. Consideration should be given to NP as a possible source of symptoms, especially if the cancer pain is not responding to analgesics as expected. Due to the difficulty of treating NP, multiple drugs from a variety of classes are typically needed, referred to as *rational polypharmacy* or *multimodal therapy*. Drug classes typically used include anticonvulsants, antidepressants, opioids, and topical agents.

Other drugs, such as ketamine or lidocaine infusions, are used rarely for refractory cases of NP. NP is amenable to interventional blocks, such as brachial plexus block. These are performed by an anesthesiologist, under CT or fluoroscopy guidance. See Chapters 8 and 9 for additional information.

The nurse's role is to carefully assess the patient for NP, discuss management with the team, and educate the patient on the variety of medications that may be prescribed. Patient education on prevention of falls is essential, as several of these drugs (e.g., opioids, TCAs) can cause lightheadedness or orthostatic hypotension. Vigilance will help prevent complications and help the patient maintain the therapeutic regimen to improve comfort in the setting of NP.

Case Study

Jean is a 69-year-old female with advanced multiple myeloma. She has diffuse bone pain, as well as plasmacytoma deposits. She is currently on a fentanyl patch 50 mcg/hr every 72 hours for pain, with hydromorphone 4 mg tablets, taking 6 tablets per day. Jean reports her pain intensity is 6 out of 10 most of the time. She does not feel her pain is well controlled on these medicines, but does not want to increase the dose due to side effects of constipation, sedation, and occasional instability. She reports feeling "down" and "hopeless" with the worsening pain.

As the nurse, you take a careful history, and discover that Jean has new, worsening pain in the left gluteus muscle with radiation down the left leg in the L5–S1 dermatome. Jean describes the pain as burning, deep, aching, occasional "electric shocks," and says she cannot get comfortable at night. You review the current medication list in detail, and discover that Jean is not on any medicines for NP. You report your findings to Jean's oncologist. Together, you review the recent CT scan results, which show extensive growth of a large plasmacytoma deposit in the left gluteus, near the sciatic nerve. The oncologist orders an MRI scan of the pelvis for follow-up.

Questions to Consider

1. What class of medication should you recommend to the oncologist? What starting dose would be optimal for Jean?
2. What psychologic screening is essential to perform before Jean leaves the visit today? Are there other providers that should talk to Jean today?
3. Given the current medication side effects Jean is coping with, what additional nursing education pointers are needed?

REFERENCES

Allen, S. (2008). Neuropathic pain—The case for opioid therapy. *Oncology, 74*(Suppl. 1), 76–82.

Alvarez, N., Galer, B., & Gammaitoni, A. (2006). Postherpetic neuralgia in the cancer patient. In O. de Leon-Casasola (Ed.), *Cancer pain: Pharmacologic, interventional and palliative care approaches* (pp. 123–137). Philadelphia, PA: Saunders.

Argoff, C., Backonja, M., Belgrade, M., Bennett, G., Clark, M., Cole, B., . . . McLean, M. J. (2006). Consensus guidelines: Treatment planning and options. Diabetic peripheral neuropathic pain. *Mayo Clinic Proceedings, 81*(4, Suppl.), S12–S25.

Bennett, M., Rayment, C., Hjermstad, M., Aass, N., Caraceni, A., & Kaasa, S. (2012). Prevalence and aetiology of neuropathic pain in cancer patients: A systematic review. *Pain, 153,* 359–365.

Bennett, M., Smith, B., Torrance, N., & Potter, J. (2005). The S-LANSS score for identifying pain of predominantly neuropathic origin: Validation for use in clinical and postal research. *Journal of Pain, 6*(3), 149–158.

Beydoun, A., & Backonja, M. (2003). Mechanistic stratification of antineuralgic agents. *Journal of Pain Symptom Management, 25*(5S), S18–S30.

Bickley, L., Szilagyi, P., & Bates, B. (2008). *Bates' guide to physical examination and history taking.* Philadelphia, PA: Wolters Kluwer/Lippincott Williams & Wilkins.

Brant, J. (2010). Practical approaches to pharmacologic management of pain in older adults with cancer. *Oncology Nursing Forum, 37*(5, Suppl.), S17–S26.

Burton, A., Fanciullo, G., Beasley, R., & Fisch, M. (2007). Chronic pain in the cancer survivor: A new frontier. *Pain Medicine, 8*(2), 189–198.

Campbell, B., Rowbotham, M., Davies, P., Jacob, P., & Benowitz, N. (2002). Systemic absorption of topical lidocaine in normal volunteers, patients with post-herpetic neuralgia, and patients with acute herpes zoster. *Journal of Pharmaceutical Sciences, 91*(5), 1343–1350.

Cohen, S., Gambel, J., Raja, S., & Galvagno, S. (2011). The contribution of sympathetic mechanisms to postamputation phantom and residual limb pain: A pilot study. *Journal of Pain, 12*(8), 859–867.

Costigan, M., Scholz, J., & Woolf, C. (2009). Neuropathic pain: A maladaptive response of the nervous system to damage. *Annual Review of Neuroscience, 32*, 1–32.

Cruciani, R., Strada, E., & Knotkova, H. (2010). Neuropathic pain. In E. Bruera & R. Portenoy (Eds.), *Cancer pain: Assessment and management* (pp. 478–505). New York, NY: Cambridge University Press.

D'Arcy, Y. (2011). *Compact clinical guide to chronic pain management: An evidence-based approach.* New York, NY: Springer Publishing.

Davies, P., & Galer, B. (2004). Review of lidocaine patch 5%: Studies in the treatment of postherpetic neuralgia. *Drugs, 64*(9), 937–947.

Driver, L., Cata, J., & Phan, P. (2006). Peripheral neuropathy due to chemotherapy and radiation therapy. In O. de Leon-Casasola (Ed.), *Cancer pain: Pharmacological, interventional and palliative care approaches* (pp. 107–121). Philadelphia, PA: Saunders.

Dworkin, R., & Schmader, K. (2001). The epidemiology and natural history of herpes zoster and postherpetic neuralgia. In C. Watson & A. Gershon (Eds.), *Herpes zoster and postherpetic neuralgia* (2nd ed., pp. 39–64). New York, NY: Elsevier.

Dworkin, R., Backonja, M., Rowbotham, M., Allen, R., Argoff, C., Bennett, G., . . . Weinstein, S. M. (2003). Advances in neuropathic pain: Diagnosis, mechanisms and treatment recommendations. *Archives of Neurology, 60*, 1524–1534.

Eidelman, A., & Carr, D. (2006). Taxonomy of cancer pain. In O. de Leon-Casasola (Ed.), *Cancer pain: Pharmacological, interventional and palliative care approaches* (pp. 3–12). Philadelphia, PA: Saunders.

Fassoulaki, A., Triga, A., Melemeni, A., & Sarantopoulos, C. (2005). Multimodal analgesia with gabapentin and local anesthetics prevents acute and chronic pain after breast surgery for cancer. *Anesthesia & Analgesia, 101*, 1427–1432.

Fitzgibbon, D. R., & Loeser, J. D. (2010). *Cancer pain: Assessment, diagnosis, and management.* Philadelphia, PA: Wolters Kluwer/Lippincott, Williams & Wilkins.

Forde, G. (2007). Adjuvant analgesics for the treatment of neuropathic pain: Evaluating efficacy and safety profiles. *Journal of Family Practice*, (Suppl.), 3–12.

Fuller, G. (1999). *Neurological exam made easy* (3rd ed.). New York, NY: Churchill Livingstone.

Galer, B., & Jensen, M. (1997). Development and preliminary validation of a pain measure specific to neuropathic pain: The neuropathic pain scale. *Neurology, 48*, 332–338.

Galer, B., Harle, J., & Rowbotham, M. (1996). Response to intravenous lidocaine infusion predicts subsequent response to oral mexiletine: A prospective study. *Journal of Pain Symptom Management, 12*(3), 161–167.

Gallagher, R. (2005). Rational integration of pharmacologic, behavioral, and rehabilitation strategies in the treatment of chronic pain. *American Journal of Physical and Medical Rehabilitation, 84*(Suppl. 3), S64–S76.

Gebhardt, R. (2006). Pain following extremity amputation. In O. de Leon-Casasola (Ed.), *Cancer pain: Pharmacological, interventional and palliative care approaches* (pp. 103–105). Philadelphia, PA: Saunders.

Gordon, D., & Love, G. (2004). Pharmacologic management of neuropathic pain. *Pain Management Nursing, 5*(4, Suppl.), 19–33.

Haanpää, M., Attal, N., Backonja, M., Baron, R., Bennett, M., Bouhassira, D., . . . Treed, R. D. (2011). NeuPSIG guidelines on neuropathic pain assessment. *Pain, 152*, 14–27.

Haanpää, M., Backonja, M., Bennett, M., Bouhassira, D., Cruccu, G., Hansson, P., . . . Baron, R. (2009). Assessment of neuropathic pain in primary care. *American Journal of Medicine, 122*, S13–S21.

International Association for the Study of Pain (IASP) Taskforce on Taxonomy. (2011, July 14). *IASP Taxonomy.* Retrieved from http://www.iasp-pain.org/AM/Template. cfm?Section=Pain_Defi...isplay.cfm&ContentID=1728

Irving, G. (2005). Contemporary assessment and management of neuropathic pain. *Neurology, 64*(Suppl. 3), S21–S27.

Jensen, M. (2006). Review of measures of neuropathic pain. *Current Pain and Headache Reports, 10*, 159–166.

Kautio, A., Haanpaa, M., Leminen, A., Kalso, E., Kautiainen, H., & Saarto, T. (2009). Amitriptyline in the prevention of chemotherapy-induced neuropathic symptoms. *Anticancer Research, 29*, 2601–2606.

Kingsbury, S., Yi, D., & SImpson, G. (2001). Rational and irrational polypharmacy. *Psychopharmacology, 52*(8), 1034–1035.

Lema, M., Foley, K., & Hausheer, F. (2010). Types and epidemiology of cancer-related neuropathic pain: The intersection of cancer pain and neuropathic pain. *Oncologist, 15*(Suppl. 2), 3–8.

Levy, M., Chwistek, M., & Rohtesh, R. (2008). Management of chronic pain in cancer survivors. *Cancer Journal, 14*(6), 401–409.

Mackey, S., Carroll, I., Emir, B., Murphy, K., Whalen, E., & Dumenci, L. (2012). Sensory pain qualities in neuropathic pain. *Journal of Pain, 13*(1), 58–63.

Marchand, S. (2008). The physiology of pain mechanisms: From the periphery to the brain. *Rheumatic Disease Clinics of North America, 34*(2), 285–309.

Max, M., Lynch, S., Muir, J., Shoaf, S., Smoller, B., & Dubner, R. (1992). Effects of desipramine, amitriptyline, and fluoxetine on pain in diabetic neuropathy. *New England Journal of Medicine, 326*, 1250–1256.

McCleane, G. (2007). Topical analgesics. *Medical Clinics of North America, 91*, 125–139.

McWhinney, S., Goldberg, R., & McLeod, H. (2009). Platinum neurotoxicity pharmacogenetics. *Molecular Cancer Therapeutics, 8*(1), 10–16.

Mercadante, S., Gebbia, V., David, F., Aielli, F., Verna, L., Casuccio, A., . . . Ferrera, P. (2009). Tools for identifying cancer pain of predominantly neuropathic origin and opioid responsiveness in cancer patients. *Journal of Pain, 10*(6), 594–600.

Miguel, R. (2006). Initial approach to the paitent with cancer pain. In O. de Leon-Casasola (Ed.), *Cancer pain: Pharmacological, interventional and palliative care approaches* (pp. 25–32). Philadelphia, PA: Saunders.

Moulin, D., Clark, A., Gilron, I., Ware, M., Watson, C., Sessle, B., . . . Velly, A. (2007). Pharmacological management of chronic neuropathic pain – Consensus statement and guidelines from the Canadian Pain Society. *Pain Research & Management, 12*(1), 13–21.

Pasero, C. (2004). Pathophysiology of neuropathic pain. *Pain Management in Nursing, 5*(4 (Suppl 1)), 3–8.

Pasero, C., & McCaffery, M. (2011). *Pain assessment and pharmacologic management.* St. Louis, MO: Mosby Elsevier.

Polomano, R., & Farrar, J. (2006). Pain and neuropathy in cancer survivors. *American Journal of Nursing, 106*(Suppl. 3), 39–46.

Polomano, R., Ashburn, M., & Farrar, J. (2010). Pain syndromes in cancer survivors. In E. Bruera & R. Portenoy (Eds.), *Cancer pain: Assessment and management* (2nd ed., pp. 145–163). New York, NY: Cambridge University Press.

Portenoy, R. (2006). Development and testing of a neuropathic pain screening questionnaire: ID Pain. *Current Medical Research & Opinion, 22*(8), 1555–1565.

Reyes-Gibby, C., Morrow, P., Bennett, M., Jensen, M., & Shete, S. (2010). Neuropathic pain in breast cancer survivors:Using the ID pain as a screening tool. *Journal of Pain Symptom Management, 39*(5), 882–889.

Rowbotham, M. (2005). Mechanisms of neuropathic pain and their implications for the design of clinical trials. *Neurology, 65*(Suppl. 4), S66–S73.

Rowbotham, M., & Fields, H. (1989). Post-herpetic neuralgia: The relation of pain complaint, sensory disturbance, and skin temperature. *Pain, 39*(2), 129–144.

Rowbotham, M., Reisner, L., Davies, P., & Fields, H. (2005). Treatment response in antidepressant-naïve postherpetic neuralgia patients: Double-blind, randomized trial. *Journal of Pain, 6*(11), 741–746.

Rowbotham, M., Twilling, L., Davies, P., Reisner, L., Taylor, K., & Mohr, D. (2003). Oral opioid therapy for chronic peripheral and central neuropathic pain. *New England Journal of Medicine, 348*(13), 1223–1232.

Saarto, T., & Wiffen, P. (2010). Antidepressants for neuropathic pain: A Cochrane review. *Journal of Neurological & Neurosurgical Psychiatry, 81*, 1372–1373.

Smith, E., Cohen, J., Pett, M., & Beck, S. (2011). The validity of neuropathy and neuropathic pain measures in patients with cancer receiving taxanes and platinums. *Oncology Nursing Forum, 38*(2), 133–142.

Straus, S., Kors, J., DeBruin, M., van der Hooft, C., Hofman, A., Heeringa, J., . . . Witterman, J. C. (2006). Prolonged QTc interval and risk of sudden cardiac death in a population of older adults. *Journal of the American College of Cardiologists, 47*(2), 362–367.

Suzuki, R., Sikandar, S., & Dickenson, A. (2010). Nociception: Basic principles. In E. Bruera & R. Portenoy (Eds.), *Cancer pain: Assessment and management* (2nd ed., pp. 3–22). New York, NY: Cambridge University Press.

Treede, R., Jensen, T., Campbell, J., Cruccu, G., Dostrovsky, J., Griffin, J., . . . Serra, J. (2008). Neuropathic pain: Redefinition and a grading system for clinical and research purposes. *Neurology, 70*(18), 1630–1635.

Vanderah, T. (2007). Pathophysiology of pain. *Medical Clinics of North America, 91*, 1–12.

Wallace, M., Galer, B., & Gammaitoni, A. (2006). Topical and oral anesthetics. In O. de Leon-Casasola (Ed.), *Cancer pain: Pharmacological, interventional and palliative care approaches* (pp. 327–335). Philadelphia, PA: Saunders.

Watson, C., & Gershon, A. (Eds.). (2001). *Herpes zoster and postherpetic neuralgia* (2nd ed.). New York, NY: Elsevier.

Watson, C., Moulin, D., Watt-Watson, J., Gordon, A., & Eisenhoffer, J. (2003). Controlled-release oxycodone relieves neuropathic pain: A randomized controlled trial in painful diagetic neuropathy. *Pain, 105*, 71–78.

Wickham, R. (2007). Chemotherapy-induced peripheral neuropathy: A review and implications for oncology nursing. *Clinical Journal of Oncology Nursing, 11*(3), 361–376.

Wilkes, G. (2007). Peripheral neuropathy related to chemotherapy. *Seminars in Oncology Nursing, 23*(3), 162–173.

Yawn, B., Wollan, P., Weingarten, T., Watson, J., Hooten, W., & Melton, L. (2009). The prevalence of neuropathic pain: Clinical evaluation compared with screening tools in a community population. *Pain Medicine, 10*(3), 586–593.

Ziegler, D. (2011). Current concepts in the management of diabetic polyneuropathy. *Current Diabetes Review, 7*(3), 208–220.

16

Myofascial Pain

Pamela Stitzlein Davies

Successful cancer pain management is dependent on a establishing a clear understanding of the *source* of the pain. As noted in previous chapters, neuropathic pain (NP) is best managed with adjuvant agents, such as anticonvulsants or antidepressants. Nociceptive pain from somatic or visceral sources are typically managed with opioids, whereas nociceptive pain from metastasis to the bone is managed not only with opioids, but with addition of nonsteroidal anti-inflammatory drugs (NSAIDs), or corticosteroids (e.g., dexamethasone), as well as radiation therapy.

Likewise, the management of nociceptive pain that arises from muscles or tissues, also known as *myofascial pain*, is managed differently than other nociceptive pain. It is essential to establish myofascial pain as the pain generator, as it will usually respond to touch therapies such as massage, trigger point release, or stretching and strengthening exercises. Pharmacologic therapy, such as tizanidine, may help somewhat, but myofascial pain typically is less responsive to opioid therapy than other nociceptive pain (Marcus, 2005). This chapter discusses the sources of myofascial pain in the cancer setting, with therapeutic options for management.

MYOFASCIAL PAIN

Myofascial pain refers to discomfort that arises from the muscles, causing sustained muscle contractions, or from the surrounding fascia and connective tissue causing fibrosis and restriction in mobility, which leads to pain. These pain syndromes are common in the general population, and may be present prior to diagnosis and treatment of malignancy, or may be caused, or exacerbated, by cancer treatment (Stubblefield, 2011). Muscle pain is described as aching, diffuse, and difficult to localize, and is more common in the elderly (Dommerholt & Shah, 2010). Myofascial pain is a frequent cause of severe pain and disability in society. It commonly affects the neck, shoulder girdle, low back, and gluteal area; it less commonly affects the chest and ribs (Sola & Bonica, 2001). Multiple authors point out that myofascial pain is frequently misdiagnosed as bursitis, arthritis, or even visceral disease (Dommerholt & Shah, 2010; Lavelle, Lavelle, & Smith, 2007; Sola & Bonica, 2001).

Clinical *Pearl*	Myofascial pain is extremely common in the general population, but is frequently misdiagnosed as arthritis, bursitis, or visceral pain. The neck, shoulder girdle, low back, and gluteal muscles are most commonly affected. Physical therapy and regular aerobic activity are the primary treatments.

Despite the prevalence in the general population, the diagnostic criteria for myofascial pain are variable, and the existence of the syndrome itself is questioned by some (Marcus, 2005). In a survey sent to members of the American Pain Society (APS) members in 1997, 88.5% of the 403 respondents indicated that myofascial pain syndrome is a "legitimate and distinct" diagnosis that is separate from fibromyalgia syndrome (Harden, Bruehl, Gass, Niemiec, & Barbick, 2000). The majority of respondents agreed that the diagnosis of myofascial pain syndrome includes the three essential elements identified by Travel and Simons in their seminal work on myofascial pain: regional pain, the presence of trigger points, and a normal neurologic examination (Simons & Travel, 1998). Eighty percent of study participants included these additional elements of myofascial pain syndrome: pain described as dull, deep, or aching; muscular tender points, taut bands in the muscles; muscle ropiness; muscle nodules; decreased range of motion; pain worsened by stress; and pain improved by trigger point injection or specialized "spray and stretch" techniques (Harden et al., 2000). A tender point is a nonspecific area of focal tenderness that may be associated with myofascial trigger points or with other conditions such as fibromyalgia syndrome.

Clinical Pearl

Following are signs and symptoms of myofascial pain syndrome (Harden, Bruehl, Gass, Niemiec, & Barbick, 2000; Lavelle, Lavelle, & Smith, 2007; Simons & Travel, 1998):

- Regional (vs. diffuse) pain complaint
- Pain described as dull, deep, or aching
- The presence of muscular trigger points (TPs) and tender points
- A palpable taut band in the muscle correlating to the trigger point
- A "local twitch response" (the examiner feels a snapping sensation in the muscle when the trigger point is palpated)
- Reproducible referred pain when the trigger point is palpated (see Figures 16.1 through 16.3)
- Muscle "ropiness" and muscle nodules
- Decreased range of motion with sensitivity to stretching
- Pain worsened by stress
- Pain improved by trigger point injection or "spray and stretch" techniques
- Weak muscles with or without atrophy
- Normal neurologic examination

Myofascial pain occurs less frequently in workers whose jobs involve intense muscle activity on a daily basis when compared to the sedentary worker or the person with intermittent activity (Sola & Bonica, 2001). An acute injury (such as whiplash) may produce myofascial pain, as well as microtrauma from repetitive stress injury (Cummings & Baldry, 2007). *Peripheral sensitization* of muscle nociceptors and *central sensitization* are mechanisms that are theorized to perpetuate the myofascial pain syndrome (see Chapter 15 for details) (Dommerholt & Shah, 2010). For this reason, some authors hypothesize that myofascial pain is a form of neuropathic pain. Indeed, some authors advocate use of membrane-stabilizing drugs typically used in neuropathic pain, such as gabapentin and tricyclic antidepressants, for the management of myofascial pain (Fitzgibbon & Loeser, 2010).

Physical examination includes palpation of the muscles for trigger points, tender points, taut or ropy muscles, nodules within the muscles, and a localized twitch response (see the next section). In addition, muscles and joints in the area surrounding the pain should be tested for strength and range of motion, and a basic neurologic examination should be performed (Marcus, 2005).

Although half of human body weight is attributed to skeletal muscle, the cause of muscle pain remains debated. Some theorize that muscle pain is a type of neuropathic pain; others believe it is primarily a somatoform disorder (i.e., a medically unexplained [psychogenic] physical complaint); and others believe that it occurs only secondary to inflammation, muscle strain, or tendonitis (McCarron, Xiong, & Henderson, 2009; Harden et al., 2000). However, many now hold to the "integrated trigger point" hypothesis. In this model, virtually all acute and chronic musculoskeletal pain—such as headaches, back pain, and osteoarthritis—can be traced to myofascial trigger points (Dommerholt &Shah, 2010).

Myofascial Trigger Points

A trigger point (TP or TrP) is a "hyperirritable spot in skeletal muscle that is associated with a hypersensitive palpable nodule in a taut band" (Dommerholt & Shah, 2010). Pressure on the trigger point causes pain, and creates a characteristic and reproducible referred pain pattern, often to distant sites. This referral pattern is a different and distinct pattern from those of neurologic dermatome distributions or dermatologic skin patterns (Lavelle et al., 2007). For example, pressure on a trigger point in the upper trapezius muscle will refer pain to the ipsilateral temple, jaw, occipital area, and anterolateral neck (see Figure 16.1). Pressure on a trigger point in the lower trapezius will refer pain to the posterior neck and ipsilateral shoulder (see Figure 16.2). Trigger point activation in the piriformis will radiate pain to the posterior gluteal area and midthigh (see Figure 16.3).

Trigger points are identified by simple physical examination. The patient is asked to point to the area of pain with a single finger. The examiner then palpates the muscle with moderate to deep pressure. At the site of the trigger point, the patient will often involuntarily jerk from discomfort; this is known as the "jump sign," and is one of the most reliable indicators of the presence of a trigger point (Cummings & Baldry, 2007). Trigger points may be active or latent. Active trigger points cause spontaneous pain at rest, usually at both the trigger point site and the referred area. Latent trigger points do not cause spontaneous pain, but can be identified upon examination by the "jump sign" and taut muscle bands (Cummings & Baldry, 2007). Taut muscle bands are commonly found on exam, and "strumming" the band perpendicular to the fiber direction may result in a local twitch response, in which the

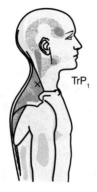

Figure 16.1 ■ Trapezius trigger point 1 (TrP$_1$) causing pain in the head and neck.
X: Indicates location of the myofascial trigger point on the trapezius muscle
Stippled gray area: Site of referred pain
Solid gray area: Typical site of most intense referred pain
[http://www.triggerpoints.net/triggerpoints/trapezius.htm] *Source:* © The Trigger Point and Referred Pain Guide, www.Triggerpoints.net and www .MyoRehab.net. Used with permission.

examiner palpates a "snapping" sensation in the muscle as it is stroked (Dommerholt & Shah, 2010).

MYOFASCIAL PAIN IN THE CANCER SETTING

Myofascial pain may be related or unrelated to the cancer. Pre-existing problems are typically worsened, and latent trigger points may become active in the oncology setting. The primary cause of myofascial pain in the cancer patient is inactivity, deconditioning, and fatigue. Muscle disuse from excessive time spent in a chair or bed leads to increased incidence of muscle pain, trigger points, and muscle injury (Marcus, 2005). Fatigued patients may be hesitant to be active, concerned that it will make them even more tired. Generalized debility makes patients appropriately fearful of falls. This leads to more deconditioning, leading to worsening myofascial pain. Thus, a vicious cycle develops and may require significant persuasion on the part of the medical team to help break the pathologic cycle (Biondolillo, 2006).

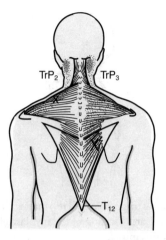

Figure 16.2 ▦ Trapezius trigger points 2 and 3 causing pain in the neck
and shoulder. Trigger Point 2 (TrP$_2$) and 3 (TrP$_3$):
X: indicates location of myofascial trigger point on trape-
zius muscle
Stippled gray area: site of referred pain
Solid gray area: Typical site of most intense referred pain
[http://www.triggerpoints.net/triggerpoints/trap23.htm] *Source:* © The
Trigger Point and Referred Pain Guide, www.Triggerpoints.net and www
.MyoRehab.net. Used with permission.

However, the cancer patient may experience pain in the muscle or
fascia from direct tumor involvement, such as a soft-tissue sarcoma, or
referred pain from a nearby diseased area (Marcus, 2005). An example of
tumor-related muscle pain is *malignant psoas syndrome*, a rarely described,
but occasionally observed condition associated with bulky metastatic
disease from ovarian, colorectal, or other cancers (Agar, Broadbent, &
Chye, 2004). Tumor pressure causes psoas muscle spasm and lumbosacral
plexopathy leading to severe pain with flexion of the hip. Patients undergoing treatment for cancer face several unique myofascial pain issues. This
has been well documented in head and neck cancers, breast cancer, and
as sequelae to mantle radiation for Hodgkin's lymphoma. Details are provided in the following sections.

In the physical examination of the cancer patient, care should be taken
to avoid deep tissue palpation if the platelets are less than 100,000, or the

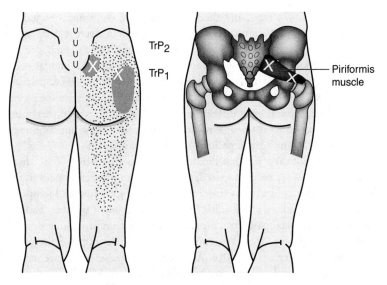

Figure 16.3 ■ Piriformis trigger point causing pain in the gluteus
and posterior thigh. Trigger Points 1 (TrP₁) and 2 (TrP₂):
X: indicates location of myofascial trigger point on pirifor-
mis muscle
Stippled gray area: site of referred pain
Solid gray area: Typical site of most intense referred pain
[http://www.triggerpoints.net/triggerpoints/piriformis.htm] *Source:* © The
Trigger Point and Referred Pain Guide, www.Triggerpoints.net and www
.MyoRehab.net. Used with permission.

patient is on anticoagulation therapy, as significant bruising could result.
In addition, it is this author's experience that new nodules related to soft-
tissue sarcomas may initially mimic trigger points in both the pain report
and physical examination. Should there be any doubt about the source of a
palpable nodule, the oncologist should be contacted immediately.

Shoulder Problems in Head and Neck Cancer

First described in 1952, postsurgical shoulder morbidity has been a known
complication of radical neck dissection (RND) for head and neck cancer
(Bradley et al., 2010). Shoulder problems include pain; limitations in range

of motion (ROM), especially shoulder abduction; deformities including shoulder droop; and scapular flaring. These problems were attributed to loss of the spinal accessory nerve from the radical surgery (which also included resection of the sternocleidomastoid muscle, internal jugular vein, and complete removal of lymph nodes), affecting 60% to 80% of patients after RND. However, as surgical techniques were refined, with transition to a modified radical neck dissection (MRND), which spared the recurrent laryngeal nerve, the problems decreased in frequency, but continued to persist in 18% to 72% of patients (Bradley et al., 2010).

The current theory is that shoulder problems after MRND, in which the spinal accessory nerve is spared, are likely from myofascial pain in the shoulder girdle, contractures (from fibrosis of the glenohumeral joint due to immobility), adhesive capsulitis (painful restriction of shoulder ROM), neuropathic cervical pain, or trauma to the nerve from stretching or traction during surgery. The latter can take 12 to 18 months for the nerve to recover (Bradley et al., 2010). An even less invasive procedure, called *selective neck dissection*, has fewer complications than MRND. Radiation therapy to the neck, with or without neck surgery, is another source of posttreatment shoulder dysfunction, although it is less common if radiation therapy alone is done. In addition to these shoulder issues, pain and limited neck ROM are common after head/neck cancer surgery. This dysfunction is felt to be from adhesion of neck muscles to the overlying platysma muscle after removal of fascia, subcutaneous tissue, and lymph nodes during surgery.

Prevention of postoperative myofascial pain and adhesive capsulitis involves early shoulder mobilization and stretching, with physical therapy referral for supervision and management of complications. Physical therapy has been shown to improve quality of life (QOL) after RND or MRND. Shoulder problems are prevalent in the general population, and heal slowly. Therefore, aggressive management is needed when a trigger therapy, such as head/neck surgery or radiation is performed, to prevent a viscous cycle of impaired mobility, causing pain, leading to further decrease in ROM, and development of painful fibrosis.

Diagnosis of shoulder girdle ROM issues involves patient history and a simple physical examination. First, observe the patient at rest with the shirt removed. Look for asymmetry aside from the obvious surgical defect. This may include shoulder droop on the ipsilateral side, atrophy of the trapezius muscle, or lack of scapula movement with shoulder ROM. Finally, have the patient stretch the arm straight up, over the head, and bend the elbow to reach down and touch the ipsilateral scapula (external rotation of the shoulder); then reach straight down and behind, bending the elbow to reach up and touch the scapula (internal rotation) (Marcus, 2005). Compare the nonsurgical side to the surgical side. Additionally, a mental health assessment is appropriate, as depression has been shown to worsen shoulder pain and dysfunction after RND (Bradley et al., 2010).

Shoulder Dysfunction After Mastectomy

Patients treated for early or locally advanced breast cancer typical undergo a modified radical mastectomy (MRM) or lumpectomy as the foundational therapy. However, the prevalence of shoulder dysfunction can be as high as 51% postoperatively (Chan, Lui, & So, 2010). This includes limitations in ROM, and pain and weakness. In a review of six studies, Chan and colleagues found early initiation of exercises (within the first few days postoperatively) improved shoulder function, especially flexion and abduction (2010).

Neck, Shoulder, and Chest Wall Dysfunction With Hodgkin's Lymphoma

Pain, muscle spasms, and limitations of range of motion are common long-term sequelae after extended-field radiation for Hodgkin's lymphoma. Although not commonly used now, extended-field radiation, such as "mantle field" or "inverted-Y field" radiated a large area. This included the affected lymph nodes, adjacent areas, and clinically uninvolved sites in the radiation field (Freedman & Friedberg, 2012). Mantle field radiation included the neck, medial shoulders, midchest, and axillae in the radiation field in order to treat the cervical, supraclavicular, mediastinal, and axillary lymph nodes. The inverted-Y radiation field included the periaortic, iliac, inguinal, and femoral lymph nodes (Stubblefield, 2011).

Although mantle-field radiation is not used often today, the late effects on muscles and tissues may occur many years, even decades, after treatment. Radiation fibrosis in the treated area may cause muscle spasms, pain, weakness, myopathy, plexopathy, and neuropathy among other problems (Stubblefield, 2011).

Myalgias and Arthralgias From Aromatase Inhibitors in Breast Cancer

Aromatase inhibitors (AIs) are well-known causes of arthralgias and my-algias. AIs are adjuvant agents for prevention of breast cancer recurrence and have been shown to extend survival. AIs are the preferred drug in post-menopausal women, as they prevent disease recurrence better than tamoxifen. Drugs include anastrozole (Arimidex), exemestane (Aromasin), and letrozole (Femara). Since 75% of breast cancer patients are postmenopausal, the majority will be on an AI at some point in their treatment. However, the incidence of musculoskeletal pain from AIs is 30%, compared to 24% incidence with tamoxifen (Winters, Habin, & Gallagher, 2007). Problems include myalgias (muscle pain), arthralgias (joint pain), or arthritis (joint pain with inflammation, swelling, or erythema). Very low levels of estro-gen are theorized to cause such pain. However, it is important to note that myalgias, arthralgias, and arthritis are common complaints in women. In a study of 251 premenopausal, perimenopausal, and postmenopausal women in primary care, there was a 57% incidence of muscle and joint pain, but the reports were not correlated to menopausal status (Xu, Bartoces, Neale, Dailey, Northrup, & Schwartz, 2005).

Other drugs used in breast cancer treatment that cause myalgias and arthralgias include taxanes (75% incidence), pegfilgrastim (Neulasta) for treatment-related neutropenia, or drugs for osteoporosis, such as alendro-nate (Fosamax) or risedronate (Actonel). The discomfort from these treat-ments may severely impact QOL.

Management includes over-the-counter analgesics, such as acetamin-ophen or NSAIDs. Regular exercise is one of the primary effective treat-ments for AI-induced myalgias.

TREATMENT OF MYOFASCIAL PAIN IN THE CANCER SETTING

Clinicians typically respond to the cancer patient's complaints of pain with an increased dose of opioids. However, most myofascial pain does not re-spond well to opioid therapy (Fitzgibbon & Loeser, 2010). When increased doses of opioids only cause worsening side effects without appreciable im-provement in pain, other sources, such as myofascial pain, should be con-sidered as the pain source. Nurses are in an excellent position to assess for myofascial pain and educate patients about the importance of regular aerobic activity and a home exercise program.

Nonpharmacologic Therapies for Myofascial Pain

Nonpharmacologic therapies are the primary treatments for myofascial pain, with physical therapy and regular aerobic exercise being the key strategies for management (Biondolillo, 2006; Marcus, 2005; Stubblefield, 2011). As noted earlier, deconditioning and debility are primary sources of myofascial pain in the oncology patient. It is essential that the nurse provide ongoing education on the importance of regular physical exercise, and compliance with physical therapy programs.

Physical Therapy

Physical therapy usually includes education about a home exercise program designed to strengthen the core (abdominal and back) muscles and those of the upper and lower extremities, as well as improve ROM, balance, and coordination (Biondolillo, 2006). Supervised gait training is provided, with instruction on proper use of a cane or walker. Management of trigger points by physical therapy or a massage therapist may include manual "pin and stretch" techniques to help release the trigger points, and passive and active ROM exercises.

Trigger Point Injection (TPIs) or "Dry Needling"

Initially developed as injections of local anesthetic or corticosteroids into the trigger points, clinicians later discovered that the effect inexplicably lasted for hours to days longer than the pharmacologic effect of the injected substance. Studies revealed that the "dry needling" technique produced similar results to trigger point injection, and many centers now use this instead of trigger point injection. The technique involves a solid filament needle (without a lumen) inserted 5 to 10 mm into the trigger point for 30 seconds (Dommerholt & Shah, 2010). No medication is injected, and each painful trigger point must be individually needled for effect. A key component of this therapy is postprocedure stretching to loosen and release the trigger point. Elicitation of the twitch response is hypothesized to release of endogenous endorphins, or possibly oxytocin, leading to prolonged pain relief from the procedure (Dommerholt & Shah, 2010). As noted earlier, platelets should be greater than 100,000 for use of this technique, and it is usually contraindicated for cancer patients on anticoagulation therapy.

Spray and Stretch

Simons and Travel developed use of the "spray and stretch" technique, which was used for many years (1998). This technique involves use of a vapocoolant spray to anesthetize the skin. The target trigger point is firmly anchored with one hand, and the other hand is used to passively stretch the muscle several times (Lavelle et al., 2007). Active stretching exercises by the patient were then done after treatment. Unfortunately, the various vapo-coolants (such as fluoromethane) are agents that worsen greenhouse gasses, and their use is either banned or discouraged (Dommerholt & Shah, 2010).

Thermal Modalities
Hot and cold packs can be extremely helpful to reduce myofascial pain, especially before or after physical therapy and stretching. Nurses can encourage regular use of thermal packs by writing a "prescription" to apply a hot or cold pack for 10 minutes every 6 hours. Their use should be avoided on radiated skin until a year after completion of treatment. Care should be used in patients with sensory abnormalities, such as peripheral neuropathy, and avoided in those with vascular disorders or open wounds. To prevent burns, patients must be instructed to insulate cold packs and avoid placing ice directly on the skin. In addition, patients should be taught to avoid falling asleep with a heating pad (Biondolillo, 2006).

Other Nonpharmacologic Therapies
Other nonpharmacologic therapies that may improve myofascial pain include the following (Biondolillo, 2006; Dommerholt & Shah, 2010; Lavelle et al., 2007):
- Massage
- Acupuncture or acupressure
- Transcutaneous electrical nerve stimulation (TENS)
- Ultrasound
- Laser therapy to trigger points
- Extracorporeal shockwave therapy (ECST)

Pharmacologic Therapies for Myofascial Pain
Pharmacologic therapy has a minor role in management of myofascial pain, including that from trigger points. Few drugs are FDA approved for myofascial pain, and most of the studies of oral drugs have been done on acute low back pain (LBP). Several treatments that are mentioned in the literature are listed in the next section.

Trigger Point Injection
Trigger point injection with local anesthetics such as lidocaine or procaine, corticosteroids, sterile saline, or sterile water may be effective, but is proba-bly no more effective than dry needling (Staal, de Bie, de Vet, & Nelemans,

2008). Botulinum toxin (Botox) is useful for spasticity caused by upper motor neuron lesions. Its use in trigger point management is controversial (Dommerholt & Shah, 2010; Swarm, Karanikolas, & Cousins, 2005).

Skeletal Muscle Relaxants

It is essential for the nurse, as well as the patient, to understand that the so-called *skeletal muscle relaxants* do not actually relax the muscles. This group of drugs includes a number of different agents with different mechanisms of action, most of which were approved in the mid-20th century. Few of these drugs have been subjected to rigorous studies, and their efficacy for myofascial pain management is controversial, especially in the setting of chronic pain (Jackson & Argoff, 2010). However, a 2003 Cochrane Review showed evidence of improvement of acute LBP with skeletal muscle relaxants compared to placebo, but due to the side effects, the authors indicated that other therapies may be effective without the sedating properties of this class of drug (van Tulder, Touray, Furlan, Solway, & Bouter, 2003). Their use has not been studied in cancer pain.

Tizanidine (Zanaflex) is a centrally acting alpha-2 agonist, and has FDA approval for management of spasticity from multiple sclerosis or spinal cord injury. Of all the drugs listed in this section, tizanidine has the best evidence of management of low back pain, especially when combined with ibuprofen. Baclofen (Lioresal) and diazepam (Valium) are classified as GABA-agonist muscle relaxants. Baclofen has FDA approval for spasticity from CNS disorders, and may be given intrathecally. Diazepam has long been used for acute muscle spasms with back injury, but there is little evidence to support its use (Jackson & Argoff, 2010).

Methocarbamol (Robaxin), metaxalone (Skelaxin), and carisoprodol (Soma) are classified as *sedative–hypnotic* muscle relaxants. They have been used for decades to manage muscle spasm from acute and chronic low back pain as well as other conditions. However, the evidence for efficacy is sparse at best. Carisoprodol use should be avoided, as there are significant dependency and abuse issues associated with its use. The metabolite of carisoprodol is meprobamate, a Schedule IV anxiolytic. The European Medicines Agency has removed carisoprodol from production. In the United States, several states have reclassified it as a Schedule IV drug (European Medicines Agency, 2007).

Antidepressants

Duloxetine (Cymbalta) is FDA approved for use in chronic musculoskeletal pain and fibromyalgia syndrome and may be a useful adjuvant to nonpharmacologic therapy in myofascial pain. Tricyclic antidepressants

(TCAs) are mentioned in the literature as muscle relaxants, but have little data to support their use. However, because myofascial pain is theorized to have a possible neuropathic component, a trial of a TCA may be attempted as an adjuvant therapy, especially to see if the sedation effects lead to improvement in sleep and overall quality of life. Cyclobenzaprine (Flexeril), although classified as a skeletal muscle relaxant, is more similar to TCAs in structure and function. Like TCAs, it may have a small role in decreasing pain from myofascial sources. Due to the structural similarity to TCAs, it should not be given concurrently. A 2009 Cochrane Review found insufficient evidence to support the use of cyclobenzaprine in myofascial pain (Leite et al., 2009).

Anticonvulsants

Although the literature mentions use of anticonvulsants, such as gabapentin or pregabalin, for low back pain or muscle spasms, there is little evidence to support the use specifically in myofascial pain (Fitzgibbon & Loeser, 2010).

Topical Agents

Topical NSAIDs include the diclofenac epolamine (Flector) patch, which is FDA approved for acute pain from minor strains and sprains. It is applied twice a day for a few days until the acute injury pain subsides. Diclofenac sodium (Voltaren) gel is FDA approved for pain from osteoarthritis, and is applied to painful joints four times a day. The lidocaine 5% (Lidoderm) patch is FDA approved for postherpetic neuralgia. Up to three patches are applied to the painful area for 12 out of 24 hours. Counterirritant balms, such as capsaicin, menthol, or camphor, may provide some relief of myofascial pain. These are applied several times a day. None of these agents is specifically FDA approved for myofascial pain (Jackson & Argoff, 2010).

SUMMARY

Myofascial pain problems are common in the general population as well as those with cancer. Deconditioning, debility, surgery, and radiation therapy contribute to a high incidence in the oncology patient. However, myofascial contributors are usually overlooked as a source of pain, leading to further decline and debility.

Shoulder and neck problems are common after head, neck, or breast surgery for cancer. Including physical therapy into the postoperative rehabilitation program is essential for prevention and management of musculoskeletal problems. Postoperative or postradiation lymphedema may contribute to myofascial pain problems. In addition, breast cancer patients on aromatase inhibitors struggle with the side effects of myalgias and arthralgias.

The two major treatment regimens for myofascial pain are physical therapy and aerobic exercise. Pharmacologic therapies play a minor role in treatment. The nurse is in a key position to assess for myofascial contributors to the pain complaint, and advocate for the patient by speaking with the oncologist or physical therapist about management strategies. Patient education should focus on the importance of compliance with ROM exercises to prevent shoulder dysfunction after surgery, encouraging ongoing participation in a physical therapy home exercise regimen, and maintenance of a daily aerobic program to optimize conditioning during cancer treatment (Chan et al., 2010).

Case Study

Jean is a 68-year-old woman with "smoldering" multiple myeloma. She underwent a stem cell transplant several months ago, but with suboptimal results. She has residual disease present, but is on a variety of therapies to keep it under control. Her anticipated prognosis is at least a year or more. She became quite debilitated during the transplant process, and has not been following the physical therapy reconditioning program regularly. Recently she knelt down, and was unable to stand up without assistance due to weakness in the legs.

Jean developed a new pain in the left buttocks radiating down the left leg. It has been progressively worsening over the last 2 to 3 months. She is very worried that there is a new myeloma or plasmacytoma deposit in this area causing the pain, despite reassurances from her oncologist that the CT scan, bone scan, osseous survey, and a pelvic MRI revealed no disease present in the affected area. The oncologist is uncertain of the cause of the pain. The dose of opioid has been titrated from oxycodone CR 10 mg BID to 20 mg TID with no improvement in pain.

The nurse practitioner (NP) performs a detailed physical examination, including a thorough myofascial examination of the gluteus muscles and neurologic exam of the lower extremities. He discovers a discrete area of exquisite tenderness deep in the gluteus maximus at the location of the piriformis muscle. Pressure at this site produces

(Continued)

radiation of pain in a sciatic-like pattern, which reproduces her pain. Neurologically, her reflexes are intact and sensory check is normal. However, her lower extremity strength testing reveals generalized weakness, with +4 on a 0 to 5 scale throughout (able to resist gravity and some pressure, but not at a normal level of strength). The NP diagnoses myofascial pain syndrome, and order a comprehensive physical therapy evaluation, for stretching, strengthening, and a trial of a transcutaneous electrical nerve stimulator (TENS) unit. He recommends tapering of the opioid down to previous levels.

Questions to Consider

1. What signs and symptoms make myofascial pain a likely source of Jean's pain?
2. Why is physical therapy the primary treatment offered?
3. Why does the NP recommend an opioid taper?
4. What other drugs (if any) may be helpful for this pain?

REFERENCES

Agar, M., Broadbent, A., & Chye, R. (2004). The management of malignant psoas syndrome: Case reports and literature review. *Journal of Pain Symptom Management, 28*(3), 282–293.

Biondolillo, A. (2006). Physical therapy. In O. de Leon-Casasola (Ed.), *Cancer pain: Pharmacological, interventional and palliative care approaches* (pp. 369–378). Philadelphia, PA: Saunders.

Bradley, P., Ferlito, A., Silver, C., Takes, R., Woolgar, J. A., Strojan, P., . . . Rinaldo, A. (2010). Neck treatment and shoulder mobility: Still a challenge. *Head & Neck, 33,* 1060–1067.

Chan, D., Lui, L., & So, W. (2010). Effectiveness of exercise programmes on shoulder mobility and lymphoedema after axillary lymph node dissecxtion for breast cancer: Systematic review. *Journal of Advanced Nurssing, 66*(9), 1902–1914.

Cummings, M., & Baldry, P. (2007). Regional myofascial pain: Diagnosis and management. *Best Practice & Research Clinical Rheumatology, 21*(2), 367–387.

Dommerholt, J., & Shah, J. (2010). Myofascial pain syndrome. In S. Fishman, J. Ballantyne, & J. Rathmell (Eds.), *Bonica's management of pain* (4th ed., pp. 450–471). Philadelphia, PA: Wolters Kluwer, Lippincott Williams & Wilkins.

European Medicines Agency. (2007, November 14). *Final decisions: Carisoprodol.* Retrieved from http://www.ema.europa.eu/ema/index.jsp?curl=pages/medicines/human/referrals/Carisoprodol/human_referral_000119.jsp&mid=WC0b01ac0580024e9a

Fitzgibbon, D. R., & Loeser, J. D. (2010). *Cancer pain: Assessment, diagnosis, and management.* Philadelphia, PA: Wolters Kluwer/Lippincott, Williams & Wilkins.

Freedman, A., & Friedberg, J. (2012, January). *Initial treatment of limited stage diffuse large B cell lymphoma.* Retrieved from http://www.uptodate.com

Harden, R., Bruehl, S., Gass, S., Niemiec, C., & Barbick, B. (2000). Signs and symptoms of the myofascial pain syndrome: A national survey of pain management providers. *Clinical Journal of Pain, 16*(1), 64–72.

Jackson, K., & Argoff, C. (2010). Skeletal muscle relaxants and analgesic balms. In S. Fishman, J. Ballantyne, & J. Rathmell (Eds.), *Bonica's management of pain* (4th ed., pp. 1187–1193). Philadelphia, PA: Wolters Kluwer, Lippincott Williams & Wilkins.

Lavelle, E., Lavelle, W., & Smith, H. (2007). Myofascial trigger points. *Medical Clinics of North America, 91,* 229–239.

Leite, F., Atallah, Á., El Dib, R., Grossmann, E., Januzzi, E., Andriolo, R., & da Silva, E. M. (2009). Cyclobenzaprine for the treatment of myofascial pain in adults. *Cochrane Database of Systematic Reviews* (Issue 3. Art. No.: CD006830).

Marcus, N. (2005). Pain in cancer patients unrelated to the cancer or treatment. *Cancer Investigation, 1,* 84–93.

McCarron, R., Xiong, G., & Henderson, M. (2009). Unexplained physical symptoms-somatoform disorders. In R. McCarron, G. Xiong, & J. Bourgeois (Eds.), *Lippincott's primary care psychiatry* (pp. 135–146). Philadelphia, PA: Wolters Kluwer, Lippincott Williams & Wilkins.

Simons, D., & Travel, J. (1998). *Myofascial pain and dysfunction: The trigger point manual; Volume 1. The upper half of body* (2nd ed.). Philadelphia, PA: Lippincott Williams & Wilkins.

Sola, A., & Bonica, J. (2001). Myofascial pain syndromes. In J. Loeser, S. Butler, C. Chapman, & D. Turk (Eds.), *Bonica's management of pain* (3rd ed., pp. 530–542). Philadelphia, PA: Lippincott, WIlliams & Wilkins.

Staal, J., de Bie, R., de Vet, H., & Nelemans, P. (2008). Injection therapy for subacute and chronic low back pain. *Cochrane Database of Systematic Reviews, 3* (Art. No.: CD001824).

Stubblefield, M. (2011). Cancer rehabilitation. *Seminars in Oncology, 38*(3), 386–393.

Swarm, R., Karanikolas, M., & Cousins, M. (2005). Anaesthetic techniques for pain control. In D. Doyle, G. Hanks, N. Cherny, & K. Calman (Eds.), *Oxford textbook of palliative medicine* (3rd ed., pp. 378–396). New York, NY: Oxford University Press.

van Tulder, M., Touray, T., Furlan, A., Solway, S., & Bouter, L. (2003). Muscle relaxants for non-specific low-back pain. *Cochrane Database of Systematic Reviews* (Issue 4. Art. No.: CD004252.).

Winters, L., Habin, K., & Gallagher, J. (2007). Aromatase inhibitors and musculoskeletal pain in patients with breast cancer. *Clinical Journal of Oncology Nursing, 11*(3), 433–439.

Xu, J., Bartoces, M., Neale, A. V., Dailey, R., Northrup, J., & Schwartz, K. (2005). Natural history of menopause symptoms in primary care patients: A MetroNet study. *Journal of the American Board of Family Practice, 18,* 374–382.

17

Chronic Pain in the Cancer Survivor

Pamela Stitzlein Davies

OVERVIEW

As treatments improve and cancer-related deaths decline, the unique issues and problems related to cancer survivorship are becoming more apparent. A high proportion of cancer survivors report treatment-related long-term health concerns that negatively affect quality of life (Stein, Syrjala, & Andrykowski, 2008). The National Cancer Institute (NCI) reports there are an estimated 12 million cancer survivors—approximately 4% of the population—and 65% of these are 65 years of age and older. The most common cancer sites in survivors are breast (22%), prostate (20%), colorectal (9%), and gynecologic (8%). A large majority of adults (67%) diagnosed with cancer today will be alive after 5 years, and 75% of children will be alive after 10 years (NCI, 2011). Figures 17.1 and 17.2 from the NCI show these data graphically.

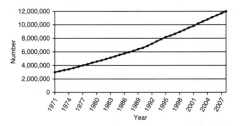

Figure 17.1 ■ Estimated number of cancer survivors in the United States from 1971 to 2008. *Source:* National Cancer Institute. Data source: Altekruse, S. F., Kosary, C. L., Krapcho, M., Neyman, N., Aminou, R., Waldron, W., . . . Edwards, B. K. (Eds.). (2011). *SEER cancer statistics review, 1975–2008.* Bethesda, MD: National Cancer Institute. Retrieved from http://cancercontrol.cancer.gov/ocs/prevalence/prevalence.html

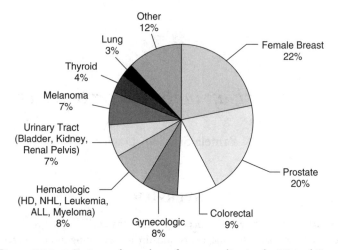

Figure 17.2 ■ Estimated number of persons alive in the United States diagnosed with cancer on January 1, 2008, by site (N = 119). *Source:* National Cancer Institute. Data source: Altekruse, S. F., Kosary, C. L., Krapcho, M., Neyman, N., Aminou, R., Waldron, W., . . . Edwards, B. K. (Eds.). (2011). *SEER cancer statistics review, 1975–2008.* Bethesda, MD: National Cancer Institute. Retrieved from http://cancercontrol .cancer.gov/ocs/prevalence/prevalence.html

Research on cancer survivorship is limited, but common long-term complaints include the following (Deimling et al., 2005; Harrington, Hansen, Moskowitz, Todd, & Feuerstein, 2010; Nail, 2001):

■ Fatigue
■ Pain
■ Cognitive problems
■ Depression
■ Anxiety
■ Functional limitations
■ Lymphedema

Complaints of pain in cancer survivors are common (Lyne, Coyne, & Watson, 2002). An analysis of the *2002 National Health Interview Survey* of over 30,000 persons found the incidence of pain in cancer survivors was much higher (34%) than controls without a history of cancer (18%) (Mao et al., 2007). In some groups, the incidence of chronic cancer-related pain can be upward of 80% (Polomano, Ashburn, & Farrar, 2010).

WHO IS THE CANCER SURVIVOR?

In this chapter, chronic pain issues in the cancer survivor will be explored. The term *cancer survivor* has different interpretations. The NCI definition is: "An individual is considered a cancer survivor from the time of cancer diagnosis, through the balance of his or her life" (NCI, 2006). However, from the perspective of long-term sequelae of cancer and cancer treatment, this definition is less useful, as it includes those both *with* and *without* evidence of disease and with or without acute treatment effects. This chapter will focus on survivors who are not in active treatment but under cancer surveillance, with cancer pain syndromes not attributed to disease progression (Mullen, 1985; Polomano et al., 2010).

Pain syndromes are typically divided into three broad categories: acute, chronic, and cancer (or malignant) pain. Classically, *"cancer pain"* referred to the patient with active disease undergoing treatment, palliation, or end-of-life care. The focus is on aggressive opioid dose escalation as the disease progressed, with minimal use of adjuvant agents. However, with the current success at treating—and sometimes curing—cancer, the numbers of long-term survivors have increased. The concept of *"cancer pain"* is now changing, and includes *chronic pain* from cancer or cancer treatment (Burton, Fanciullo, Beasley, & Fisch, 2007). The emerging approach toward the patient with *chronic cancer-related pain* is modeled on a *chronic pain* paradigm, in which the focus is on "rational polypharmacy" with anticonvulsants and antidepressants, while avoiding unlimited escalation of opioids. However, there is minimal research evidence to support this newer approach (Levy, Chwistek, & Rohtesh, 2008).

Cancer Treatment Summary

Depending on the cancer type, patients may be referred back to their primary care provider (PCP) for routine screening and surveillance 2 to 10 years after being declared free of disease (Smith, Alexander, & Singh-Carlson, 2011). Unfortunately, most PCPs do not feel equipped for this role, as training for physicians, nurse practitioners, physician assistants, and nurses rarely includes information on the unique problems and issues that may arise years, even decades, after cancer treatment (Hewitt, Greenfield, & Stovall, 2006).

To aid the PCP and oncologists in caring for the cancer survivor, the NCI, the American Cancer Society (ACS), and the Institute of Medicine (IOM) encourage oncologists to provide a comprehensive Cancer Treatment Summary and Survivorship Care Plan at the end of treatment (NCI, 2010). This should include a list of chemotherapy agents and dosages; radiation site, number of fractions, and total dose received; type of surgery; and any other therapies given, such as transcatheter arterial chemoembolization (TACE). Ideally, this should also list common side effects or late effects from the treatment received, such as chemotherapy-induced peripheral neuropathy (CIPN); cardiovascular, diabetes, or osteoporosis risks; as well as a cancer surveillance health maintenance schedule. For an example of a Cancer Treatment Summary and Survivorship Care Plan, see Table 17.1.

Table 17.1 ■ *Example of Breast Cancer Treatment Summary*

Breast Cancer Treatment Summary Date of preparation: January 13, 2012	
Patient Name: Jane Doe *Medical Record Number: 123456*	*Date of Birth: 1960*
Cancer diagnosis: Right breast cancer Infiltrating ductal carcinoma, multifocal tumor of the right breast, associated DCIS, low to intermediate grade	**Date of diagnosis:** 1/12/2010 **Age at diagnosis:** 50
Tumor stage: Stage II B **Tumor size (T):** T2 **Nodes (N):** N1 (total 2 of 22 positive) **Metastases (M):** 0	**Tumor grade: Grade 2**
Hormone receptors: Estrogen receptor (ER) positive 70% Progesterone receptor (PR) positive 80%	**HER-2:** IHC: Negative for overexpression FISH: N/A
	Genetic Counseling: 11/3/2011 at University Genetic Clinic
Family history of cancer: Sister: Breast cancer at age 40 Father: Died at age 71 of lung cancer Maternal uncle: Metastatic lung cancer Paternal uncle: Esophageal cancer Paternal cousin: Prostate cancer Paternal cousin: Lung cancer	***BRCA1* testing:** Myriad Genetics *BRCA1* mutation, 185 insertion A **BART testing:** No mutation detected ***BRCA2* testing:** No mutation detected Sister also has mutation in *BRCA1*.

(continued)

Breast Cancer Treatment Summary
Date of preparation: January 13, 2012

Patient Name: Jane Doe
Medical Record Number: 123456   *Date of Birth: 1960*

Significant past medical history: Right arm lymphedema. Generalized myalgias and arthralgias. Painful CIPN. Hypertension. Hypothyroidism. Osteopenia. Hypercholesterolemia. Depression. Past smoker, 20-pack/year history of tobacco use, quit in 2004.

Past surgical history: 12/28/2011—Prophylactic laparoscopic assisted vaginal hysterectomy and bilateral salpingo-oophorectomy for risk reduction, no evidence of malignancy.

Medications: anastrozole 1 mg daily, gabapentin 100 mg BID at dinner and HS, levothyroxine 100 mcg daily, calcium carbonate 1,000 mg daily. Vitamin D 2,000 IU daily, vitamin B_{12} daily, multivitamin daily. Hydrocodone/acetaminophen 5/500 1 QID prn pain.

Cancer Treatment

Surgery

Breast surgery:	**Lymph node surgery:**
1/12/2010: Needle localization excisional biopsy	1/29/2010: Right axillary lymph node dissection
1/29/2010: Right total mastectomy	
3/1/2010: Port-a-cath placement	
5/19/2011: Port-a-cath removal	

Reconstruction: Right DIEP flap reconstruction—05/19/2011

Systemic Therapy

Chemotherapy: 3/12/2010– 7/17/2010	Route	Dose	Reduction Y/N	Schedule	Number of Cycles
doxorubicin (Adriamycin)	IV	60 mg/m² = 126 mg 48 mg/m² = 99 mg	Yes	Every 14 days	3 1
cyclophospha-mide (Cytoxan)	IV	600 mg/m² = 1260 mg 480 mg/m² = 990 mg	Yes		3 1
docetaxel (Taxotere)	IV	100 mg/m²= 170 mg	Dose decreased to 130 mg after 2 doses	Every 14 days	4

(continued)

Table 17.1 ■ *Example of Breast Cancer Treatment Summary (continued)*

Systemic Therapy					
Chemotherapy: 3/12/2010– 7/17/2010	Route	Dose	Reduction Y/N	Schedule	Number of Cycles

Cumulative anthracycline dose administered:
Doxorubicin: 60 mg/m² × 3 doses; 48 mg/m² × 1 dose = 228 mg/m²

Growth factors used: pegfilgrastim (Neulasta) 6 mg x 8 doses

HER-2 targeted therapy: Not indicated

Endocrine (hormonal therapy): anastrozole (Arimidex) 1 mg daily starting 9/2010 for planned 5 years

Bisphosphonate therapy for breast cancer indication: zoledronic acid (Zometa) 4 mg IV every 6 months for planned 3 years—first dose 12/7/2011

Enrolled in clinical trials ? No

Radiation Therapy		
Date Start: 8/1/2010	Date Stop: 9/14/2010	Total Dose 6,200 (cGy)

Fields included: Right chest wall 5,000 cGy over 25 fractions
Superior breast tissue and right supraclavicular lymphatics 4,600 cGy over 23 fractions
Right mastectomy scar boost 1,200 cGy

Complications of therapy:
- 25% dose reduction of docetaxel (Taxotere) due to hand/foot syndrome
- Peripheral neuropathy; 20% dose reduction in doxorubicin/cyclophosphamide for hematologic toxicity
- Radiation resulted in brisk hyperpigmentation and erythema, but no moist desquamation
- Right arm lymphedema
- Postoperative wound infection following DIEP reconstruction requiring IV antibiotics

Providers	
Primary care provider: Dr. General	Surgeon: Dr. Scalpel Plastic surgeon: Dr. Implant
Radiation oncologist: Dr. Rads	Medical oncologist: Dr. Chemo

(continued)

Providers

Survivorship plan: Long-term effects and follow-up care recommendations:
• Post-treatment breast imaging:
    • Mammogram once a year, due 9/2012
    • Breast MRI once a year due 3/2012
• **Note:** The survivorship plan (not included) reviews general information on the management of common long-term effects, such as lymphedema, neuropathy, myalgias/arthralgias, and bone health. Recommendations for follow-up care, wellness checks (such as colonoscopy), and emotional and sexual health are also listed.

The author is grateful to: Theresa Wittenberg, MS, PA-C, Fred Hutchinson Cancer Research Center, Seattle Cancer Care Alliance Survivorship Clinic; and Heidi Trott, MN, ARNP, Seattle Cancer Care Alliance Breast Cancer Survivorship Clinic, for their assistance in the development of this fictional treatment summary.

IMPORTANCE OF ATTENDING TO PAIN IN THE CANCER SURVIVOR

Complaints of a new or worsening pain in a cancer survivor may herald disease recurrence, and cannot be ignored. Prompt work-up is essential to establish the source of the pain, and assess for possible new sites of disease. The approach to a new pain complaint is different for the cancer survivor than the non-cancer patient. For example, guidelines for new-onset acute back pain in the *non-cancer* patient encourage watchful waiting before initiating evaluations such as x-ray, CT scan, MRI scan, or electromyography (EMG), as most back pain conditions are self-limiting (Chou et al., 2007). However, for the patient with a history of cancer, or with certain additional worrisome signs and symptoms, the guidelines recommend prompt imaging to assess for serious conditions such as cancer recurrence, spinal cord compression, or vertebral infection; or less serious but painful conditions such vertebral compression fractures. Worrisome symptoms associated with new-onset acute back pain include progressive neurologic deficits, such as lower extremity weakness, urinary retention, fecal incontinence; unexplained weight loss; or fevers and night sweats.

Clinical Pearl	Complaints of a new or worsening pain in a cancer survivor may herald disease recurrence and cannot be ignored.

The Experience of Cancer Survivorship

Fear of cancer recurrence is ever-present in the cancer survivor. It has been referred to as a "Damocles syndrome" (Hewitt et al., 2006). Damocles, from Greek mythology, was delighted to be invited to the king's banquet, but found himself seated directly under a sword suspended by a single horsehair. Any movement could dislodge the sword and kill him instantly, making it impossible to relax and enjoy the banquet. Likewise, the persistent anxiety related to fear of cancer recurrence can be overwhelming to the point of interfering with everyday function and quality of life (Vachon, 2001).

Julia Rowland, MD, Director of the National Cancer Institute Office of Cancer Survivorship, lists several key points about cancer survivorship in her article, "What are cancer survivors telling us?" (Rowland, 2008). Her research shows that cancer affects every aspect of the survivor's life: physical, psychological, cognitive and emotional; that being disease-free does not mean being free from the effects of cancer; that transition from active treatment to recovery is stressful. Yet, the research also shows that cancer survivors are resilient, and the experience can result in inner growth and improved self-esteem. Additionally, cancer may provide a "teachable moment," and encourage smoking cessation, regular exercise, healthy diet, and moderation of alcohol intake. Factors that appear to lead to successful transition to survivorship include skilled health care providers, a strong social network, and having a sense of purpose or meaning in life (Miller, 2010a; Rowland, 2008).

PAIN IN THE CANCER SURVIVOR

For most survivors, pain is more than a physical symptom. It is a constant reminder of past cancer and represents the possible return of disease. Writers refer to chronic pain from cancer treatment as the *"price of survival"* (Hewitt et al., 2006, p. 68), but the anxiety that accompanies chronic pain can be very difficult to cope with or endure. After cancer recurrence concerns have been ruled out, the cancer survivor is left with an ongoing problem of chronic pain, among other issues. The source of the pain is most commonly caused by the cancer *treatment*, not from the cancer itself (Burton et al., 2007).

Clinical Pearl	Pain in the cancer survivor is usually caused by the cancer *treatment*, not from the cancer.

Chronic cancer treatment-related pain sources are from the following (Sun, et al. 2008):

- Chemotherapy
- Radiation therapy
- Surgery
- Other therapies

The incidence of chronic pain in survivors is high. Of patients who have completed cancer treatment, chronic pain estimates are as follows (Basen-Engquist & Bodurka, 2007; Burton et al., 2007; Harrington et al., 2010; Fossa, Travis, & Dahl, 2007; Kerns, 2010):

- Prostate: 53%
- Breast: 50%
- Ovarian: 50%
- Postthoracotomy: 50%
- Head and neck: 40%
- Colorectal: 27%
- Testicular: 20%
- Hematopoietic cell transplantation: 10%

The sources of these pain issues include surgery (such as post-thoracotomy pain), chemotherapy (e.g., painful peripheral neuropathy), radiation (e.g., brachial plexopathy pain), or other treatments (e.g., steroids causing avascular necrosis). Table 17.2 lists common chronic pain syndromes in the cancer survivor by system.

CHEMOTHERAPY-INDUCED PERIPHERAL NEUROPATHY

Chemotherapy-induced peripheral neuropathy (CIPN) is a common side effect of several classes of chemotherapy agents (see Table 17.3). These include the following (Wickham, 2007):

- Platinum compounds (cisplatin)—up to 92% incidence
- Taxanes (paclitaxel, docetaxel)—up to 78% incidence
- Vinca alkaloids (vincristine, vinblastine)—up to 57% incidence
- Other classes (bortezomib, thalidomide)—up to 81% incidence

CIPN includes both painful and nonpainful conditions. A large percentage of patients suffer from painful paresthesias (painful tingling) or other discomfort (burning, shooting), while others develop only sensory abnormalities, such as numbness, without pain. Paresthesias are distressing to patients, and negatively impact quality of life (Erb, 2011). Insensate digits or feet make it difficult to perform instrumental activities of daily

Table 17.2 ■ Chronic Cancer Pain Syndromes

System Affected	Pain Syndrome	Common Cancer Type or Patients at Risk	Common Causes in the Cancer Survivor	Treatments
Neurologic				
	Painful distal symmetrical peripheral neuropathy	Breast Ovarian	Chemotherapy	Anticonvulsants, antidepressants, opioids
	Postherpetic neuralgia (chronic pain after a herpes zoster [shingles] attack)	All, especially Hodgkin's disease, non-Hodgkin's lymphoma, and other hematologic malignancies	Immunosuppression from chemotherapy, Sites of radiation treatment	Anticonvulsants, antidepressants, opioids Lidocaine 5% patch
	Complex regional pain syndrome (CRPS)	Breast	Axillary node dissection	Anticonvulsants, antidepressants, opioids Physical therapy
	Brachial plexopathy	Lymphoma Lung Breast	Radiation, surgery	Anticonvulsants, antidepressants, opioids Physical therapy
	Lumbosacral plexopathy	Cervical Uterine Bladder Prostate Rectal Sarcoma Lymphoma	Radiation, surgery	Same as above
	Postoperative pain syndromes: post-thoracotomy, postmastectomy, postamputation (phantom limb pain, stump pain), post–radical neck dissection	Lung Breast Head/neck Sarcoma	Surgery	Same as above Interventional blocks in some cases

Rheumatic	Migratory noninflammatory myalgias and arthralgias	Breast, Hematopoietic cell transplantation	Tamoxifen, Aromatase inhibitors, Radiation, High-dose cyclophosphamide	NSAIDs, Acetaminophen, Opioids, Exercise, Physical therapy, Vitamin D
Lymphatic	Pain or discomfort from lymphedema	Breast, Pelvic tumors	Breast surgery, axillary or inguinal node dissection or radiation	Compression garments, manual lymphatic drainage
Skeletal	Osteoporosis	Postmenopausal women, Prostate cancer treated with androgen-deprivation therapy	Increased risk of fracture causing pain	Bisphosphonates, Vitamin D + calcium supplementation, Estrogen supplementation in some patients
	Osteonecrosis of the jaw	Breast, multiple myeloma, skeletal metastasis (breast, lung, prostate), history of radiation to the head and neck	Bisphosphonate therapy, More common with intravenous use of pamidronate and zoledronic acid, More common after 36 months or longer exposure to bisophosphonate therapy	Early diagnosis is important, as there is no specific treatment, Oral rinses, Antibiotics, Conservative surgical debridement of necrotic bone, although surgery, may worsen the condition.
	Avascular necrosis of femoral head, humeral head, knee	Hematopoietic cell transplantation	Long-term or high-dose steroid administration	Opioids, May require joint replacement (hip, knee, shoulder)

Sources: Baehring & Wollmann, 2010; Miller, 2010b; Hewitt, Greenfield, & Stovall, 2006; Sehbai, Mirza, Ericson, Marano, Hurst, & Abraham, 2007; Syrjala, Martin, Deeg, & Boeckh, 2007; Fitzgibbon & Loeser, 2010.

Table 17.3 ■ *Drugs Commonly Causing Chemotherapy-Induced Peripheral Neuropathy (CIPN) or Other Effects*

Class	Example Drugs	Comments
Vinca alkaloids	Vincristine Vinblastine Vinorelbine	57% incidence from vincristine, lower incidence from vinblastine Typically sensory "stocking-glove" distribution CIPN May be sensorimotor or autonomic (constipation)
Platinum compounds	Cisplatin Carboplatin Oxaliplatin	Cisplatin causes 57%–92% incidence of sensory or sensorimotor neuropathy Increased risk with higher cumulative dose "Coasting" is common Carboplatin has lower incidence (13%–42%) and less severity Increased risk with higher cumulative dose Oxaliplatin causes a self-limited acute neuropathy upon exposure to cold within 30–60 minutes of infusion in up to 92% of patients Also may develop a chronic CIPN that may persist for months after completing chemotherapy Calcium and magnesium infusions may prevent
Taxanes	Paclitaxel (Taxol) paclitaxel protein-bound (Abraxane) Docetaxel (Taxotere)	Up to 83% incidence of persistent sensory CIPN with paclitaxel; 73% with paclitaxel protein-bound; and up to 64% with docetaxel Paclitaxel up to 58% develop acute myalgias and arthralgias within 1–3 days of drug administration, usually resolves within 7 days Cumulative dose dependent Symptoms may wax and wane Coasting is common
Other	Bortezomib (Velcade)	Sensory neuropathy incidence 35% May also cause motor and autonomic neuropathy

(continued)

Table 17.3 ▨ *Drugs Commonly Causing Chemotherapy-Induced Peripheral Neuropathy (CIPN) or Other Effects (continued)*

Thalidomide	Sensory neuropathy Incidence is 25%–81%, dose related
Methotrexate, cytosine arabinoside (Cytarabine, or "Ara-C") 5-fluorouracil ("5-FU") Ifosfamide Etoposide Procarbazine	Rare incidence Cause both sensory, motor, and autonomic neuropathy
Anthracyclines (doxorubicin [Adriamycin]	Rare incidence
Alkylating agents (cisplatin, cyclophosphamide)	

Sources: Baehring & Wollmann, 2010; Miller, 2010b; Hewitt, Greenfield, & Stovall, 2006; Paice, 2011; Polomano, Ashburn, & Farrar, 2010; Wilkes, 2007; Wickham, 2007.

living such as buttoning a shirt, typing on a keyboard, walking, or driving. Patients must use great care to protect numb fingers, especially when handling hot or frozen foods or washing dishes.

CIPN may resolve within months of cessation of chemotherapy, or may last for years (Wickham, 2007). *"Coasting"* is an interesting phenomenon that occurs with certain chemotherapy agents. In this situation, a painful neuropathy may develop *weeks* or even *months* after completion of chemotherapy (Wickham, 2007; Wilkes, 2007). Patient education regarding this possibility will aid in decreasing anxiety if it does occur.

CIPN is caused by inability to effectively repair DNA damage, leading to apoptosis (cell death). It is hypothesized that certain genes protect from the development of neuropathy. Researchers are attempting to define genetic phenotype and genotype associations that may predict for chemotherapy neurotoxicity in order to individualize the dose of therapy. However, currently there appears to be a lack of correlation between the incidence of neurotoxicity and tumor response rate in platinum therapy (McWhinney, Goldberg, & McLeod, 2009).

Chemotherapy most commonly causes a *distal symmetrical sensory polyneuropathy*. More commonly referred to as a *"stocking-glove"* distribution, this causes sensory changes or pain in the hands and feet. CIPN may occasionally expand to include the wrists/forearms and ankles/calves. It is common to have a predominance of involvement in either the hands or the feet. Neuropathy may also include the loss of proprioception (perception of joint movement and position), vibratory sense, stretch reflexes (e.g., patella reflex), or loss of motor or autonomic function (McWhinney, Goldberg, & McLeod, 2009). The forms of neuropathy include the following (Wickham, 2007):

▪ Sensory neuropathy: Changes in sensation including numbness, pain, dysesthesias, hyperalgesias (common)
▪ Motor neuropathy: Changes in motor function including loss of deep tendon reflexes, foot drop, limb weakness, ataxia (less common)
▪ Autonomic neuropathy: Changes in sympathetic or parasympathetic function, such as changes in heart rate, blood pressure, bladder emptying, or changes in bowel motility such as delayed gastric emptying or constipation (less common)

Patients at higher risk of developing CIPN include those with the following (Wickham, 2007):

▪ Pre-existing painful neuropathy from diabetes or other cause
▪ Higher cumulative doses of neurotoxic agents
▪ Multiple neurotoxic agents
▪ Older age

Neuroprotectants for CIPN

Patients frequently inquire about the use of supplements or drugs during chemotherapy as a means to protect the nerves from CIPN. Multiple agents have been examined, but the majority of the studies are small, underpowered, and nonrandomized. Larger randomized controlled studies are needed, but the following agents appear promising: acetyl-L-carnitine, alpha lipoic acid, calcium and magnesium IV infusions, glutathione, and vitamin E (McWhinney et al., 2009; Visovsky, Collins, Abbott, Aschenbrenner, & Hart, 2007; Wickham, 2007).

Oncology patients should always check with their oncologist or pharmacist before taking supplements of any kind. There is a great deal of controversy on the role of supplements in cancer care due to limited data on the topic. Many scientists have theoretical concerns that antioxidants could actually "protect" cancer cells during chemotherapy or radiation therapy, rather than enhancing the antitumor effect of treatment (D'Andrea, 2005).

PAINFUL SYNDROMES FROM RADIATION THERAPY

With the advent of more precise radiotherapy techniques, chronic pain syndromes attributed to radiation are now less common than in the mid-20th century. In addition, newer treatment regimens, which combine radiation with chemotherapy or surgery, have allowed for overall lower doses of radiation. When chronic pain syndromes do arise, it is typically weeks or months after completion of radiation, but occasionally may present years, even decades, after therapy (Levy et al., 2008).

Syndromes include the following (Driver, Cata, & Phan, 2006; Levy et al., 2008; Polomano & Farrar, 2006; Polomano et al., 2010):

- Brachial or lumbosacral plexopathy; neuropathic pain in dermatomal patterns of the arm or leg after radiation to the axilla or pelvis (breast, lung, GI or GYN cancers, Hodgkin's disease)
- Lymphedema of the head and neck, arm, breast, leg, or pelvis after radiation to these regions
- Proctitis or cystitis, causing burning pain in the bladder or rectum, after pelvic radiation for prostate, rectal, cervical, or endometrial cancer
- Radiation enteritis, after pelvic radiation, causing chronic diarrhea and painful defecation from rectal excoriation, mucosal ulceration, and GI adhesions
- Chronic headache after whole brain radiation:
  - A rare headache syndrome known as *SMART: stroke-like migraine attacks after radiation therapy*, may occur years after cranial radiation, especially in pediatric populations
- Myelopathy, a rare syndrome causing burning back pain due to damage to the spinal cord; may be accompanied by loss of sensation, motor weakness, and paralysis
- Osteoradionecrosis, a rare radiation injury involving demineralization and vascularization of the bone, leading to severe pain and the need for joint replacement

POSTSURGICAL PAIN SYNDROMES IN THE CANCER SURVIVOR

Postsurgical pain syndromes are well-known phenomena, and are not unique to cancer surgery. With improvements in pain management, the incidence appears to be declining (Polomano et al., 2010). Increased utilization of "multimodal" pain therapy in the perioperative period is showing promise at preventing development of postsurgical pain syndromes (Elvir-Lazo & White, 2010; Fassoulaki, Triga, Melemeni, & Sarantopoulos, 2005; Gebhardt, 2006). Examples include perioperative intravenous infusions of lidocaine, neuroaxial blocks (intrathecal, epidural), regional blocks (brachial plexus), or injections of local anesthetic into the incision.

Common postoperative cancer pain syndromes include the following (Burton et al., 2007; Cohen, Gambel, Raja, & Galvagno, 2011; Polomano et al., 2010):

- Postamputation pain
- Postthoracotomy pain
- Postmastectomy pain
- Postradical neck dissection pain
- Lymphedema

Postamputation Pain Syndrome

Postamputation pain occurs in as many as 80% of cases. There are three distinct entities after amputation, as follows (Gebhardt, 2006):

- Phantom limb: A sensation of the amputated limb still being present
- Phantom limb pain: Pain originating from the amputated limb
- Stump pain: Pain at the site of amputation

Up to 98% of amputees experience vivid phantom limb immediately following the amputation, especially after a traumatic loss of the limb. Phantom sensations decline somewhat over time, but a significant number of amputees still experience sensations decades later. Phantom sensations are most common in a limb, but may occur after a mastectomy, hysterectomy, or colectomy (Gebhardt, 2006). Phantom limb pain is more likely to occur if the limb was painful before surgery (as in sarcoma), or if amputated from trauma. It may be severely painful, such as a sensation of the amputated foot being crushed, or simply irritating and bothersome, such as an annoying itch that will not resolve. Stump pain may be caused by a nonhealing wound, poorly fitting prosthesis, or a neuroma. Neuromas form at the site of injury and spontaneously trigger painful nerve impulses. Surgical stump revision may help this condition. Postamputation pain typically subsides over a year. However, if pain persists longer than 1 year, it is unlikely to ever improve (Cohen et al., 2011; Polomano et al., 2010).

Postthoracotomy Pain Syndrome

The incidence of pain after open thoracotomy is 80% in the first few months after surgery. This declines over time to 60% at 1 year, and 30% at 5 years (Burton et al., 2007; Polomano et al., 2010). Pain is typically moderate to severe in intensity, and is located along the site of the scar. The cause is theorized to be from damage to the intercostal nerves, although several authors have pointed out that there can be a significant myofascial component to the pain (Reddy, 2006; Sarna, Grannis, & Coscarelli, 2007). Postsurgical frozen shoulder is common and can lead to significant discomfort, as well as impact everyday activities. It is therefore important to clearly assess the various components of the complaint to sort out whether the pain will respond to treatments for neuropathic pain or physical rehabilitation strategies. Video-assisted thoracotomy surgery (VATS) is a new technique that is minimally invasive. Early reports indicate a much lower incidence of chronic pain associated with VATS compared to open thoracotomy (Burton et al., 2007; Fitzgibbon & Loeser, 2010).

Postmastectomy Pain Syndrome

Postmastectomy pain (PMP) syndrome also carries a very high incidence rate, at approximately 50%. Pain intensity may range from mild to severe, and is located on the anterior chest wall, axilla, or the medial and posterior upper arm. Some women experience *phantom breast syndrome* also, which may or may not be painful. PMP is a neuropathic pain characterized by burning or lancinating pain, hyperalgesia, and, often allodynia (painful skin sensitivity) (Reddy, 2006). This can make it difficult to wear a bra, prosthesis, and clothing, causing an impact on quality of life related to socialization. There may also be a significant component of myofascial pain in the neck, arm, shoulder, and pectoralis muscle after mastectomy, which may or may not be related to neuropathy. This is best treated with physical therapy.

Newer surgical techniques such as sentinel node biopsy rather than axillary node dissection, and partial mastectomy ("lumpectomy") instead of complete mastectomy appear to be associated with lower rates of chronic pain (Polomano et al., 2010).

Post-Neck Dissection Pain Syndrome

Post-neck dissection pain occurs in 40% to 52% of patients. The pain is both neuropathic as well as somatic (myofascial and soft tissue) in origin. Like postthoracotomy and postmastectomy pain syndromes, there is a high incidence of pain related to frozen shoulder. Not surprisingly, radical neck dissection appears to cause more chronic pain issues than a modified radical neck dissection (Polomano et al., 2010).

OTHER PAIN SYNDROMES IN THE CANCER SURVIVOR

Other pain syndromes that may affect the cancer survivor include lymphedema, osteoporosis, osteonecrosis of the jaw, avascular necrosis, postherpetic neuralgia, and myalgias and arthralgias from hormonal therapies.

Lymphedema

Lymphedema occurs when the lymph flow is disrupted as a consequence of surgery or radiation. It causes swelling, discomfort, pain, tightness, and limited range of motion. If not controlled, lymphedema can lead to skin breakdown, poor vascular circulation, and nerve entrapment in extreme cases. Even if well controlled, patients are at higher risk of cellulitis from minor traumas.

In the upper extremity, lymphedema is most commonly associated with a mastectomy and axillary node dissection for breast cancer, with an incidence of 20% to 56%. Of those patients, 30% to 60% report pain associated with the lymphedema. Lower extremity lymphedema is associated with gynecologic or other pelvic surgeries, especially if the pelvic lymph nodes and vessels are removed. The incidence is less well documented, but appears to be in the range of 10% to 15% (Polomano et al., 2010). Head and neck lymphedema is common after surgery or radiation to these areas.

Management of lymphedema, and the associated discomfort, is nonpharmacologic, with manual lymphatic drainage by a specialized physical therapist or massage therapist. This is followed by extremity wraps until the lymphedema is maximally reduced. The patient is then fitted with compression garments (arm sleeve or leg sleeve) that are worn part or full time. Occasionally, mechanized compression pumps with multichamber sleeves are utilized for more complicated cases. Unlike edema, lymphedema does not respond to diuretics. New techniques for management involve microsurgical anastomosis of the lymph vessels, or liposuction of excess subcutaneous adipose formed from absent lymph flow (Fu & Smith, 2010).

Osteoporosis

Osteoporosis leads to loss of bone density and increases the risk of painful events, such as vertebral body compression fractures. Many cancer survivors are affected by osteoporosis due to chemotherapy-induced ovarian failure, surgical menopause, aromatase inhibitors (such as letrozole [Femara], used as adjuvant therapy for estrogen receptor–positive breast cancer), androgen-deprivation therapy in prostate cancer, or steroid use. The populations at highest risk are survivors of hemopoietic cell transplantation, breast cancer, advanced prostate cancer, and lymphoma (Polomano et al., 2010). Bisphosphonates, such as pamidronate (Aredia), zoledronic acid (Zometa), or alendronate (Fosamax) prevent bone loss and reduce fracture risk significantly (Pavlakis, Schmidt, & Stockler, 2005). Although there is a small risk of osteonecrosis of the jaw (see the next section) or atypical fractures, the benefit of bisphosphonates is felt to outweigh the hazards in higher-risk patients such as breast or prostate cancer survivors (Watts & Diab, 2010).

Osteonecrosis of the Jaw

Osteonecrosis of the jaw (ONJ) is a rare but serious complication of bisphosphonate therapy. Signs and symptoms include oral or jaw pain, loose teeth, nonhealing gums, spontaneous oral ulceration, and slow healing or bone necrosis after dental surgery. Increased risk for ONJ includes a history of bisphosphonates given by the intravenous route, therapy for more than 36 months, older age, multiple myeloma, and a history of recent dental extraction (Sehbai et al., 2007). Early diagnosis is important, as there are no specific treatments for ONJ. Oral rinses and antibiotics may be used for related infections. Conservative surgical debridement of necrotic bone may be attempted, although surgery may worsen the condition.

Herpes Zoster and Postherpetic Neuralgia

Herpes zoster (HZ or "shingles") is the reactivation of the varicella zoster virus in those who had chickenpox in younger years. It spreads from a single dorsal root or cranial nerve ganglion to the innervated dermatome. Patients may experience a *prodrome* (early signal of disease) of pain before the classic herpetic vesicles appear in a dermatomal distribution on one side of the body. The thoracic dermatomes are the most commonly affected sites, at 50% to 70% of all cases, followed by the trigeminal nerve (primarily the ophthalmic division), cervical, and lumbar dermatomes (Dworkin & Schmader, 2001). Severely immunocompromised patients are at risk of developing *disseminated herpes zoster*, which may be life threatening.

The pain of HZ may be quite severe. It has been described as "the belt of roses from hell" in ancient literature (Watson & Gershon, 2001). The HZ outbreak typically lasts for a few days to several weeks, then the herpetic lesions crust over and the pain gradually diminishes.

The two primary risk factors for developing HZ is age over 50 and immunosuppression. Both of these risk factors describe the typical oncology patient. The hematologic malignancies have greater incidence of HZ outbreaks, with Hodgkin's disease the highest (Alvarez, Galer, & Gammaitoni, 2006). Anecdotal experience finds an association between the site of previous surgery (mastectomy, thoracotomy, craniotomy) and the site of HZ outbreak, although the literature is inconsistent on this topic.

Postherpetic neuralgia (PHN) is a separate chronic pain syndrome from HZ, which develops in only some cases. It is defined as persistent pain lasting longer than 1 to 4 months after healing of the HZ rash. PHN is a neuropathic pain occurring in the affected unilateral HZ dermatome, and often "recruiting" nearby dermatomes to a wider swath of pain. There are three primary types of pain: constant (burning, aching), lancinating (sharp, shooting), and abnormal cutaneous sensitivity (allodynia) (Watson & Gershon, 2001). Patients usually describe the chronic postherpetic pain as having a different sensation compared to the pain of acute zoster outbreak. The pain intensity may range from severe and life altering to mild, and not requiring any treatment.

In the general population, the primary risk factor for developing and maintaining PHN is older age. Patients over the age of 70 who develop HZ have a 50% chance of developing PHN that never resolves. Younger persons (40 or younger) rarely develop chronic PHN lasting more than 1 year (Watson & Gershon, 2001).

Musculoskeletal Symptoms in the Survivor

Musculoskeletal symptoms, such as myalgias, arthralgias, muscle cramps, generalized muscle weakness, and limitations in physical capacity are common and persistent complaints in the cancer survivor (Sreih & Obedid, 2010). The highest prevalence is seen in hematologic malignancies, especially after high-dose chemotherapies; hematopoietic cell transplantation (HCT); and in adult survivors of childhood cancer (Syrjala, Yi, Artherholt, Stover, & Abrams, 2010).

Steroids, as well as a steroid taper, may also cause significant myalgias. These drugs are used in many settings, but especially in the management of chronic graft-versus-host-disease (GVHD) after a HCT. An occasional complication of steroid treatment is proximal muscle weakness.

Myalgias and Arthralgias From Adjuvant Therapy in the Breast Cancer Survivor

Use of adjuvant therapy in breast cancer has resulted in significant improvement in disease-free survival. These agents are typically given for years after initial breast cancer therapy. Tamoxifen is used in premenopausal women; it is typically taken for 2 to 5 years then switched to an aromatase inhibitor to prevent the development of resistance. Postmenopausal women are started on an aromatase inhibitor such as letrozole (Femara), exemestane (Aromasin), or anastrozole (Arimidex), and continued for up to 5 years. Aromatase inhibitors are also used in the setting of metastatic breast cancer to slow disease progression. Aromatase inhibitors appear to have an advantage over tamoxifen for improved disease-free survival, lower rates of thromboembolic events, and secondary endometrial malignancy (Din, Dodwell, Wakefield, & Coleman, 2010).

Common side effects of hormonal therapy for breast cancer include arthralgias, myalgias, and arthritis. Although initial studies reported rates of 35%, more recent studies indicate that 50% of women suffer from aromatase inhibitor–induced musculoskeletal syndrome (AIMSS) (Goss et al., 2003; Lintermans & Nevena, 2011). The joints most commonly affected include the hands, wrists, knees, neck, shoulder, feet, and back (Lintermans & Nevena, 2011). Carpal tunnel syndrome, de Quervain's tenosynovitis, and bilateral trigger thumb have been reported (Din et al., 2010). Morning stiffness is frequently a problem. Approximately 60% of affected persons report moderate to severe symptom intensity, although some note a decrease in severity after 6 months of therapy.

Arthralgias rarely spontaneously improve while on therapy, but the vast majority of women report resolution of symptoms upon discontinuation of treatment. However, due to the length of therapy (2 to 5 years), and profound impact on overall quality of life, the musculoskeletal symptoms may lead to early discontinuation of the hormonal therapy in 5% to 20% of patients, with a resulting loss of protection from recurrent disease (Dent, Gaspo, Kissner, & Pritchard, 2011).

Treatment for painful myalgias, arthralgias, and arthritis related to hormone therapy includes standard symptomatic approaches to musculoskeletal pain management: NSAIDs or COX-2 inhibitors (celecoxib), acetaminophen, tramadol, or opioids. One report suggests use of gabapentin or pregabalin (Dent et al., 2011). Vitamin D supplementation may be helpful, as low levels are associated with the development of AIMSS, and postmenopausal women tend to have low vitamin D levels (Kaplan, 2011; Rastelli et al., 2011). Other oral supplements such as omega fish oils, glucosamine, and chondroitin have been suggested, although the studies are small. Nonpharmacologic therapies commonly used in arthritis are encouraged, such as weight-bearing exercise, physical therapy, massage, acupuncture, and transcutaneous electrical nerve stimulation (TENS). In addition, switching to another aromatase inhibitor may be helpful, especially from exemestane, which has highest incidence of AIMSS (Din et al., 2010).

Sexual Dysfunction and Dyspareunia

Sexual dysfunction, such as anorgasmia, low libido, dyspareunia, and erectile dysfunction, are well-known complaints among survivors, and have a major impact on quality of life (Vistad et al., 2011). The incidence is high, with survivors reporting 90% incidence after breast cancer (Dizon, 2009), 90% after ovarian cancer (Stavraka et al., 2011), and 25% to 80% after prostate cancer treatment (Harrington et al., 2010). Women are more impacted with sexual dysfunction after HCT (80%) than men (29%) (Lee, 2011). Dyspareunia, or painful intercourse, is quite common after breast and gynecologic cancers. Menopause, whether surgically or chemically induced, causes vaginal atrophy and dryness. Pelvic radiation leads to decreased blood flow to the vaginal wall or pelvic fibrosis (Park et al., 2007). Eighty-one percent of ovarian cancer survivors report vaginal dryness, which is a significant problem for 25% (Stavraka et al., 2011). These conditions cause discomfort or pain during coitus.

Nurses have a significant role in assessing sexual dysfunction, and providing instruction on the liberal use of vaginal lubricants for improved comfort during intercourse (Lee, 2011). Topical estrogen therapy improves vaginal atrophy, and may be permissible even in selected patients with estrogen receptor-positive breast cancer (Melisko, Goldman, & Rugo, 2010). Graduated vaginal dilators are useful in cases of vaginal constriction after pelvic surgery or pelvic radiation to decrease treatment-associated dyspareunia.

Avascular Necrosis

Avascular necrosis (AVN), also known as *aseptic necrosis*, is seen in survivors of hemopoietic cell transplantation (HCT), especially after unrelated-donor allogeneic transplant and childhood acute lymphoblastic leukemia (Campbell et al., 2009). Femoral and humeral heads are the joints most commonly affected. The cause is not well understood, but is related to disruption of the blood supply to the bone, especially at the distal circulation, and impaired bone repair mechanisms. Long-term exposure to high-dose steroids have been hypothesized to cause fat emboli in the microvasculature of the bone. The diagnosis is made with plain radiographs, bone scans, and magnetic resonance imaging (MRI); however, MRI is the most sensitive.

Avascular necrosis causes significant pain with movement, which impacts overall quality of life (Syrjala, Martin, Deeg, & Boeckh, 2007). It is a chronic degenerative condition that slowly worsens. Few treatments are helpful except joint replacement, but this option is usually deferred until the joint is at high risk of collapse, especially in younger patients. Cortical bone drilling is occasionally utilized in hopes of promoting bone circulation and delaying joint replacement surgery, although the efficacy is uncertain (Sen, 2009).

Chronic pain is a significant issue in avascular necrosis, and is managed with chronic opioid therapy, with a focus on maintaining a stable nonescalating dose. Canes and crutches help off-weight the affected joint, and physical therapy can be helpful for teaching safe mobility and fall prevention. Swimming is an excellent exercise to keep joints moving while minimizing pain.

MANAGEMENT OF CHRONIC PAIN IN THE CANCER SURVIVOR

Managing chronic pain in the cancer survivor is an emerging field, described as "a new frontier" (Burton et al., 2007); however, the literature is lacking on this important field. For example, in an informal review of four excellent textbooks on cancer pain, none has a chapter dedicated specifically to managing pain in the cancer survivor (Bruera & Portenoy, 2010; Davis, Glare, & Hardy, 2005; Fitzgibbon & Loeser, 2010; de Leon-Casasola, 2006).

Much of classic *cancer pain management* is focused primarily on the use of escalating doses of opioids, with adjuvant agents as secondary therapies. This is especially true in the advanced disease and end-of-life settings. However, for the survivor with chronic cancer-related pain, lasting for years or decades, the approach to pain management must shift toward a classic *chronic pain* model (Burton et al., 2007; Levy et al., 2008). This model emphasizes maintenance of function with a focus on rehabilitation, non-pharmacologic management (such as physical therapy, regular exercise), coping skills, and occasional use of interventional blocks. Pharmacologic management focuses on adjuvant agents (anticonvulsants, antidepressants, topicals). Opioid therapy is utilized, but is de-emphasized, with a focus on stable and non-escalating doses (Ballantyne, 2007).

This is a paradigm shift. The focus becomes one of chronic pain management strategies, rather than acute pain strategies. This may be quite unsettling to patients, who were accustomed to an opioid dose escalation anytime they complained of worsening pain during the active treatment phase. Clinicians should openly address this change in strategy and new goals of therapy once the patient graduates from active treatment to long-term surveillance. The survivor may view this as a dramatic and negative change, even punitive, and will require continual reassurance that the shift in strategy is in the patient's best long-term interest. It is important to reassure patients that any new pain complaints will always be promptly evaluated.

Rational Polypharmacy in the Management of Chronic Pain in the Cancer Survivor

Rational polypharmacy describes combining drugs with different mechanisms of action that may complement each other to treat chronic pain. These include anticonvulsants, antidepressants, NSAIDs, topical agents, and opioids (Alvarez et al., 2006). The drugs selected depend on the hypothesized source of the chronic pain, whether primarily neuropathic pain, primarily nociceptive pain (somatic or visceral), or mixed pathophysiology, as follows (Levy et al., 2008; Quill et al., 2010):

- Neuropathic source:
  - Antidepressants: Serotonin–norepinephrine reuptake inhibitor (SNRI), tricyclic antidepressant (TCA)
  - Anticonvulsants: Gabapentin, pregabalin, carbamazepine
  - Topical agents: Lidocaine patch, capsaicin
  - Opioids
  - Alpha$_2$ agonists: Clonidine
- Nociceptive source/somatic:
  - Nonsteroidal antiinflammatory drugs (NSAIDs)
  - Acetaminophen
  - Opioids

- Nociceptive source/visceral:
  - Treatment of chronic visceral pain is dependent upon the cause, such as adhesions causing small bowel obstruction, hepatosplenomegaly

Specific information on these drug classes can be found in Section II, Chapters 3, 4, and 5.

SUMMARY

As the treatment of cancer improves, more patients will survive, and some will achieve a permanent cure (Ganz, 2007). Of these survivors, a majority will suffer from chronic pain problems related to their cancer treatment. As the field of pain management in the cancer survivor emerges, it is likely that the designation of "cancer pain" will be divided into three groups, as follows (Burton et al., 2007):

- Acute cancer pain management: For the patient in active treatment
- Chronic cancer pain management: Chronic pain in the survivor after completion of treatment
- Palliative cancer pain management: In advanced disease, hospice and end-of-life settings

The classic approach to cancer-related pain, from a model of advancing disease, is focused on ever-escalating doses of opioids. However, for the person with chronic cancer-related pain lasting for years, possibly even decades, the approach to pain management must shift toward a classic *chronic* pain model (Ballantyne, 2007). This model emphasizes coping skills, nonpharmacologic management (such as physical therapy, massage, regular exercise), as well as selected pharmacologic agents. Although opioids are utilized, their use is de-emphasized as the focal point of therapy, and the goal is to keep the opioid dose stable in the setting of chronic pain in the cancer survivor.

Yet, the needs of the cancer survivor with pain are unique, and are different from the chronic pain patient. Worsening pain may be the only sign of the very real risk of disease recurrence or development of a second primary cancer. The new complaint of pain must be addressed thoughtfully and proactively, and not assumed that it is simply a benign exacerbation.

Nurses have a key role in assessment, management, and advocacy for cancer-related pain in the survivor. This includes educating the patient and caregivers, and exploring concerns about recurrent disease.

Case Study

Jean is a 48-year-old Pacific Islander woman with a history of Stage I lung cancer diagnosed and treated 1 year ago. She has no evidence of active cancer. Her primary pain complaint is on her right chest wall at the site of a thoracotomy incision for removal of lung cancer over a year ago. While recovering from surgery, she developed herpes zoster ("shingles") in a T-5 dermatome, much of it following along the line of the incision.

Jean reports the pain is of moderate intensity, and the skin sensitivity makes it difficult to wear a bra and clothing. The pain keeps her from enjoying her favorite activity of kayaking. She tried gabapentin, which was started at 300 mg three times a day, but was too sleepy from the drug, and quit it after 3 days, reporting that "it didn't work." Opioids help the pain but make her too sleepy as well as constipated. She declined to try an antidepressant, and has not tried a topical agent. Examination reveals a large, well-healed thoracotomy incision on the right side, with classic scars from herpes zoster in the same region. She has allodynia (sensitivity to light touch) and hyperalgesia (marked pain from pinprick).

Questions to Consider

1. What major classification is Jean's pain?
2. What is the primary diagnosis of her pain?
3. What do you think of the starting dose of gabapentin 300 mg TID and the length of the trial?
4. What other options for treatment should be considered?

REFERENCES

Alvarez, N., Galer, B., & Gammaitoni, A. (2006). Postherpetic neuralgia in the cancer patient. In O. de Leon-Casasola (Ed.), *Cancer pain: Pharmacological, interventional and palliative care approaches* (pp. 123–137). Philadelphia, PA: Saunders.

Baehring, J., & Wollmann, G. (2010). Neurologic sequelae of cancer therapy. In K. Miller (Ed.), *Medical and psychosocial care of the cancer survivor* (pp. 323–339). Boston, MA: Jones & Bartlett.

Ballantyne, J. (2007). Opioid misuse in oncology pain patients. *Current Pain and Headache Reports, 11,* 276–282.

Basen-Engquist, K., & Bodurka, D. (2007). Medical and psychosocial issues in gynecologic cancer survivors. In P. Ganz (Ed.), *Cancer survivorship: Today and tomorrow* (pp. 114–121). New York, NY: Springer.

Bruera, E. D., & Portenoy, R. K. (Eds.). (2010). *Cancer pain: Assessment and management* (2nd ed.). New York, NY: Cambridge University Press.

Burton, A., Fanciullo, G., Beasley, R., & Fisch, M. (2007). Chronic pain in the cancer survivor: A new frontier. *Pain Medicine, 8*(2), 189–198.

Campbell, S., Sun, C., Kurian, S., Francisco, L., Carter, A., Kulkarni, S., . . . Bhatia, S. (2009). Predictors of avascular necrosis of bone in long-term survivors of hematopoietic cell transplantation. *Cancer, 115*(18), 4127–4135.

Chou, R., Qaseem, A., Snow, V., Casey, D., Cross, T., Shekelle, P., & Owens, D. K. (2007). Diagnosis and treatment of low back pain: A joint clinical practice guideline from the American College of Physicians and the American Pain Society. *Annals of Internal Medicine, 147,* 478–491.

Cohen, S., Gambel, J., Raja, S., & Galvagno, S. (2011). The contribution of sympathetic mechanisms to postamputation phantom and residual limb pain: A pilot study. *Journal of Pain, 12*(8), 859–867.

D'Andrea, G. (2005). Use of antioxidants during chemotherapy and radiotherapy should be avoided. *CA: A Cancer Journal for Clinicians, 55*(5), 319–321.

Davis, M., Glare, P., & Hardy, J. (Eds.). (2005). *Opioids in cancer pain.* Oxford, England: Oxford University Press.

de Leon-Casasola, O. A. (Ed.). (2006). *Cancer pain: Pharmacologic, interventional, and palliative approaches.* Philadelphia, PA: Elsevier.

Deimling, G., Sterns, S., Bowman, K., & Kahana, B. (2005). The health of older-adult, long-term cancer survivors. *Cancer Nursing, 28*(6), 415–424.

Dent, S., Gaspo, R., Kissner, M., & Pritchard, K. (2011). Aromatase inhibitor therapy: Toxicities and management strategies in the treatment of postmenopausal women with hormone-sensitive early breast cancer. *Breast Cancer Research & Treatment, 126,* 295–310.

Din, O., Dodwell, D., Wakefield, R., & Coleman, R. (2010). Aromatase inhibitor-induced arthralgia in early breast cancer: What do we know and how can we find out more? *Breast Cancer Research & Treatment, 120,* 525–538.

Dizon, D. (2009). Quality of life after breast cancer: Survivorship and sexuality. *Breast, 15*(5), 500–504.

Driver, L., Cata, J., & Phan, P. (2006). Peripheral neuropathy due to chemotherapy and radiation therapy. In O. de Leon-Casasola (Ed.), *Cancer pain: Pharmacological, interventional and palliative care approaches* (pp. 107–121). Philadelphia, PA: Saunders.

Dworkin, R., & Schmader, K. (2001). The epidemiology and natural history of herpes zoster and postherpetic neuralgia. In C. Watson, & A. Gershon (Eds.), *Herpes zoster and postherpetic neuralgia* (2nd ed., pp. 39–64). New York, NY: Elsevier.

Elvir-Lazo, O., & White, P. (2010). The role of multimodal analgesia in pain management after ambulatory surgery. *Current Opinions in Anesthesia, 23,* 697–703.

Erb, C. (2011, September/October). CIPN: Treatment preservation and prevention are the goals. *Oncology Nurse Advisor,* 16–20.

Fassoulaki, A., Triga, A., Melemeni, A., & Sarantopoulos, C. (2005). Multimodal analgesia with gabapentin and local anesthetics prevents acute and chronic pain after breast surgery for cancer. *Anesthesia and Analgesia, 101*, 1427–1432.

Fitzgibbon, D. R., & Loeser, J. D. (2010). *Cancer pain: Assessment, diagnosis, and management.* Philadelphia, PA: Wolters Kluwer/Lippincott, Williams & Wilkins.

Fossa, S., Travis, L., & Dahl, A. (2007). Medical and psychosocial issues in testicular cancer survivors. In P. Ganz (Ed.), *Cancer survivorship: Today and tomorrow* (pp. 101–113). New York, NY: Springer.

Fu, M., & Smith, J. (2010). Lymphedema management. In B. Ferrell & N. Coyle (Eds.), *Oxford textbook of palliative nursing* (3rd ed., pp. 341–358). New York, NY: Oxford University Press.

Ganz, P. (Ed.). (2007). *Cancer survivorship: Today and tomorrow.* New York, NY: Springer.

Gebhardt, R. (2006). Pain following extremity amputation. In O. de Leon-Casasola (Ed.), *Cancer pain: Pharmacological, interventional and palliative care approaches* (pp. 103–105). Philadelphia, PA: Saunders.

Goss, P., Ingle, J., Martino, S., N.J., R., Muss, H., . . . Pater, J. L. (2003). A randomized trial of letrozole in postmenopausal women after five years of tamoxifen therapy for early-stage breast cancer. *New England Journal of Medicine, 349*(19), 1793–1802.

Harrington, C., Hansen, J., Moskowitz, M., Todd, B., & Feuerstein, M. (2010). It's not over when it's over: Long-term symptoms in cancer survivors-a systematic review. *International Journal of Psychiatric Medicine, 40*(2), 163–181.

Hewitt, M., Greenfield, S., & Stovall, E. (Eds.). (2006). *From cancer patient to cancer survivor: Lost in transition. Improving care and quality of life. Committee on Cancer Survivorship. National Cancer Policy Board.* Washington, DC: National Academy of Sciences.

Kaplan, B. (2011, September/October). Vitamin D regimen is effective in resolving bone pain related to aromatase-inhibitor therapy. *Oncology Nurse Advisor*, 36–38.

Kerns, R. (2010). Symptom burden in cancer survivorship: Managing mood, pain, fatigue, and sleep disturbances. In K. Miller (Ed.), *Medical and psychosocial care of the cancer survivor* (pp. 23–30). Boston, MA: Jones & Bartlett.

Lee, J. (2011). Sexual dysfunction after hematopoietic stem cell transplantation. *Oncology Nursing Forum, 38*(4), 409–412.

Levy, M., Chwistek, M., & Rohtesh, R. (2008). Management of chronic pain in cancer survivors. *Cancer Journal, 14*(6), 401–409.

Lintermans, A., & Nevena, P. (2011). Pharmacology of arthralgia with estrogen deprivation. *Steroids, 76*, 781–785.

Lyne, M., Coyne, P., & Watson, A. (2002). Pain management issues for cancer survivors. *Cancer Practice, 10*(Suppl. 1), S27–S32.

Mao, J., Armstrong, K., Bowman, M., Xie, S., Kadakia, R., & Farrar, J. (2007). Symptom burden among cancer survivors: Impact of age and comorbidity. *Journal of the American Board of Family Medicine, 20*(5), 434–443.

McWhinney, S., Goldberg, R., & McLeod, H. (2009). Platinum neurotoxicity pharmacogenetics. *Molecular Cancer Therapies, 8*(1), 10–16.

Melisko, M., Goldman, M., & Rugo, H. (2010). Amelioration of sexual adverse effects in the early breast cancer patient. *Journal of Cancer Survivorship, 4*(3), 247–255.

Miller, K. (2010a). Cancer survivorship today. In K. Miller (Ed.), *Medical and psychosocial care of the cancer survivor* (pp. 9–19). Boston, MA: Jones & Bartlett.

Miller, K. (Ed.). (2010b). *Medical and psychosocial care of the cancer survivor.* Boston, MA: Jones & Bartlett.

Mullen, F. (1985). Seasons of survival: Reflections of a physician with cancer. *New England Journal of Medicine, 313*(4), 270–273.

Nail, L. (2001). Long-term persistence of symptoms. *Seminars in Oncology Nursing, 17*(4), 249–254.

National Cancer Institute (NCI). (2006, September 20). *About cancer survivorship: Definitions.* Retrieved from http://cancercontrol.cancer.gov/ocs/definitions.html

National Cancer Institute (NCI). (2010, May 17). *Follow-up care after cancer treatment.* Retrieved from http://www.cancer.gov/cancertopics/factsheet/Therapy/followup#q10

National Cancer Institute (NCI). (2011, June 2). *Estimated U.S. cancer prevalence counts: Who are our cancer survivors in the U.S.?* Retrieved from http://cancercontrol.cancer.gov/ocs/prevalence/index.html

Paice, J. (2011). Chronic treatment-related pain in cancer survivors. *Pain, 152*(Suppl. 3), S84–S89.

Park, S., Bae, D., Nam, J., Park, C., Cho, C.-H., Lee, J., . . . Yun, Y. H. (2007). Quality of life and sexual problems in disease-free survivors of cervical cancer compared with the general population. *Cancer, 110*(12), 16–25.

Pavlakis, N., Schmidt, R., & Stockler, M. (2005). Bisphosphonates for breast cancer. *Cochrane Database of Systematic Reviews, 20*(3: CD003474).

Polomano, R., & Farrar, J. (2006). Pain and neuropathy in cancer survivors. *American Journal of Nursing, 106*(Suppl. 3), 39–46.

Polomano, R., Ashburn, M., & Farrar, J. (2010). Pain syndromes in cancer survivors. In E. Bruera & R. Portenoy (Eds.), *Cancer pain: Assessment and management* (2nd ed., pp. 145–163). New York, NY: Cambridge University Press.

Quill, T. E., Holloway, R. G., Shah, M. S., Caprio, T. V., Olden, A. M., & Storey, J. C. (2010). *Primer of palliative care* (5th ed.). Glenview, IL: American Academy of Hospice and Palliative Medicine.

Rastelli, A., Taylor, M., Gao, F., Armamento-Villareal, R., Jamalabadi-Majidi, S., Napoli, N., & Ellis, M. J. (2011). Vitamin D and aromatase inhibitor-induced musculoskeletal symptoms (AIMSS): A phase II, double-blind, placebo-controlled, randomized trial. *Breast Cancer Research & Treatment, 129*(1), 107–116.

Reddy, S. (2006). Pain following mastectomy, thoracotomy, and radical neck dissection. In O. de Leon-Casasola (Ed.), *Cancer pain: Pharmacological, interventional and palliative care approaches* (pp. 97–101). Philadelphia, PA: Saunders.

Rowland, J. (2008). What are cancer survivors telling us? *Cancer Journal, 14*(6), 361–368.

Sarna, L., Grannis, F., & Coscarelli, A. (2007). Physical and psychosocial issues in lung cancer survivors. In P. Ganz (Ed.), *Cancer survivorship: Today and tomorrow* (pp. 157–176). New York, NY: Springer.

Sehbai, A., Mirza, A., Ericson, S., Marano, G., Hurst, M., & Abraham, J. (2007). Osteonecrosis of the jaw associated with bisphosphonate therapy: Tips for the practicing oncologist. *Community Oncology, 4*(1), 47–52.

Sen, R. K. (2009). Management of avascular necrosis of femoral head at pre-collapse stage. *Indian Journal Orthopaedics, 43*(1), 6–16.

Smith, S., Alexander, C., & Singh-Carlson, S. (2011). Caring for survivors of breast cancer: Perspective of the primary care physician. *Current Oncology, 18*(5), e218–e226.

Sreih, A., & Obedid, E. (2010). Rheumatic problems in cancer survivors. In K. Miller (Ed.), *Medical and psychosocial care of the cancer survivor* (pp. 389–400). Boston, MA: Jones & Bartlett.v

Stavraka, C., Ford, A., Ghaem-Maghami, S., Crook, T., Agarwal, R., Gabra, H., & Blagden, S. (2011, December 8). A study of symptoms described by ovarian cancer survivors. *Gynecologic Oncology, 125*(1), 59–64.

Stein, K., Syrjala, K., & Andrykowski, M. (2008). Physical and psychological long-term and late effects of cancer. *Cancer, 112*(Suppl. 11), 2577–2592.

Sun, V., Borneman, T., Piper, B., Koczywas, M., & Ferrell, B. (2008). Barriers to pain assessment and management in cancer. *Journal of Cancer Survivorship, 2*(1), 65–71.

Syrjala, K., Martin, P., Deeg, J., & Boeckh, M. (2007). Medical and psychosocial issues in transplant survivors. In P. Ganz (Ed.), *Cancer survivorship: Today and tomorrow* (pp. 188–214). New York, NY: Springer.

Syrjala, K., Yi, J., Artherholt, S., Stover, A., & Abrams, J. (2010). Measuring musculoskeletal symptoms in cancer survivors who receive hematopoietic cell transplantation. *Journal of Cancer Survivorship, 4*, 225–235.

Vachon, M. (2001). The meaning of illness to a long-term survivor. *Seminars in Oncology Nursing, 17*(4), 279–283.

Visovsky, C., Collins, M., Abbott, L., Aschenbrenner, J., & Hart, C. (2007). Putting evidence into practice: Evidence-based interventions for chemotherapy-induced peripheral neuropathy. *Clinical Journal of Oncology Nursing, 11*(6), 901–913.

Vistad, I., Cvancarova, M., Kristensen, G., & Fossa, S. (2011). A study of chronic pelvic pain after radiotherapy in survivors of locally advanced cervical cancer. *Journal of Cancer Survivorship, 5*, 208–216.

Watson, C., & Gershon, A. (Eds.). (2001). *Herpes zoster and postherpetic neuralgia* (2nd ed.). New York, NY: Elsevier.

Watts, N., & Diab, D. (2010). Long-term use of bisphosphonates in osteoporosis. *Journal of Clinical Endocrinology & Metabolism, 95*(4), 1555–1565.

Wickham, R. (2007). Chemotherapy-induced peripheral neuropathy: A review and implications for oncology nursing. *Clincal Journal of Oncology Nursing, 11*(3), 361–376.

Wilkes, G. (2007). Peripheral neuropathy related to chemotherapy. *Seminars in Oncology Nursing, 23*(3), 162–173.

18

Palliative Care and Hospice: Care When There Is No Cure

Pamela Stitzlein Davies

You matter because of who you are. You matter to the last moment of your life, and we will do all we can, not only to help you die peacefully, but also to live until you die.

Dame Cicely Saunders (2005)
Founder of the modern hospice movement

Those suffering from advanced cancer need intensive symptom management and assistance in coping with the stress of a life-limiting illness. The focus of care shifts from achieving a *cure* to promoting *quality of life* and *relief of suffering*. Palliative care and hospice services are specialized in this, providing holistic care to the total being as the disease progresses toward end of life (Morrison & Morrison, 2006). Sometimes referred to as "care when there is no cure" (Horton, 2001), both palliative care and hospice are *philosophies of care,* as well as organized methods of providing that care, which aim to achieve the best possible quality of life in the setting of serious and advancing illness (National Comprehensive Cancer Network, 2011; National Consensus Project for Quality Palliative Care, 2009).

This chapter describes palliative care and hospice services, focusing on the oncology setting. Also included is a discussion on the status of end-of-life care in America, with expert panel recommendations on improving that care. Finally, communication skills with the patient with a serious illness are reviewed.

301

END-OF-LIFE CARE IN AMERICA

The seminal *Study to Understand Prognosis and Preferences for Outcomes and Risks of Treatments* (SUPPORT) was designed to improve end-of-life decision making and reduce the number of patients who die in a painful, prolonged manner in the ICU on a ventilator (The SUPPORT Principal Investigators, 1995). The study, assessing over 9,000 patients at five teaching hospitals in the United States, discovered many shortcomings in the care of seriously ill hospitalized patients. Family members reported moderate to severe pain in 50% of conscious patients. Unfortunately, efforts to improve pain management and physician communication around the topics of advance care planning, do-not-resuscitate (DNR) orders, and patient preferences for end-of-life care, did not improve from the Phase 1 (observation) to Phase 2 (intervention) portion of the study.

The Institute of Medicine (IOM) report in 1997 on *Approaching Death: Improving Care at the End of Life* highlighted the concerns raised by the SUPPORT study, as well as gaps in knowledge that contribute to poor care at end of life (Field & Cassel, 1997). It described organizational, educational, and societal contributors to "avoidable distress and suffering" at end of life (Field & Cassel, 1997, p. 4). The following four dimensions were identified as key in the care of the dying (Field & Cassel, 1997):

- Understanding the physical, psychologic, spiritual, and practical dimensions of caregiving
- Identifying and communicating diagnosis and prognosis
- Establishing goals and plans
- Fitting palliative and other care to these goals

The IOM report then went on to issue seven recommendations for improving care of the dying in America:

1. Patients and caregivers should expect and receive skillful care at end of life.
2. Health care providers should commit to improving care in the dying to relieve pain and symptoms.
3. Policymakers, insurance agencies, state agencies, consumers, and health care researchers should work together to improve care to the dying by developing better tools to measure quality care, develop strategies for financial incentives to sustain excellent care, and remove regulations that impede access to opioid medications.
4. Education should be provided to health care professionals at all levels on skillful care of the dying.

5. Palliative care should become a medical specialty with a defined area of expertise, education, and research.
6. Researchers should define priorities for enhancing the end-of-life knowledge base.
7. Continuing public discussion is essential to develop an understanding of the experience of dying, and the community obligations toward those approaching death.

Another important report that has shaped end-of-life care in America is the 2002 document written by a national coalition named Last Acts, titled *Means to a Better End: A Report on Dying in America Today* (Last Acts, 2002). In this report, state policies were scrutinized and rated for encouraging advanced care planning, promotion of good pain management at end of life, and end-of-life care in nursing homes. Rates of hospice enrollment were examined, as well as ICU stays in the last 6 months of life. This key report made recommendations for policy makers, health care leaders, and the public in general, in order to improve the quality of end-of-life care.

PALLIATIVE CARE VERSUS HOSPICE SERVICES

The term *hospice* comes from *hospitality*, and was first used in modern times by Dame Cicely Saunders, founder of the hospice movement, at St. Christopher's Hospice in London in 1967 (American Cancer Society, 2011). The word *palliative* is derived from *palliare*, a Latin term meaning to *cover* or *cloak*, as in *to provide protection* (Old & Swagerty, 2007).

The distinction between palliative care and hospice may be unclear, not only to patients but also to the medical team, because the terms are sometimes used interchangeably. *Palliative care* may be thought of as the broader "umbrella" of the two services, providing assistance at any point along the continuum of illness, from initial diagnosis, through aggressive treatment modalities, to end-of-life care. Hospice enrollment requires an anticipated prognosis of 6 months of life or less, although patients are typically allowed to remain enrolled if they live longer. Hospice enrollment and care is subject to precise rules and regulations that parallel the Medicare Hospice Benefit (Centers for Medicare and Medicaid Services, 2011; Hospice Directory, 2011). Table 18.1 describes major differences between the two services.

Table 18.1 ■ *Differentiating Palliative Care From Hospice Care*

	Palliative Care	Hospice Care
Focus of Care	Broad	Narrow, a subset of palliative care
Prognosis	Any prognosis, from curable disease to end of life	Six months or less if the disease follows its usual course
Exclusions to Care	None (limited by regular insurance rules and restrictions)	Patient generally must elect to forego life-prolonging or disease-modifying therapies. Procedures for comfort, such as paracentesis for ascites, may be allowed.
Medication Restrictions	Standard insurance program formulary and co-pays.	Restricted to hospice program formulary. Focus on lower cost drugs. All medications related to the hospice diagnosis are covered.
Billing	Standard fee-for-service with insurance co-pay. Some services may not be billable, such as nurse or social work visits.	100% of care is provided through the Hospice Medicare Benefit, a capitated care system. The hospice agency receives payment on a per diem rate.
Focus of Care	Optimize quality of life Excellent pain and symptom management Psycho–social–spiritual support Assist with determining goals of care for medical treatment decisions Assist with care coordination Advocate for patient-stated goals of care	Optimize quality of life as end of life approaches Excellent pain and symptom management Psycho–social–spiritual support Assist with determining goals of care for end-of-life care Assist with care coordination Advocate for patient-stated goals of care Support of the family/caregiver Bereavement support

Table 18.1 ▧ *Differentiating Palliative Care From Hospice Care (continued)*

	Palliative Care	Hospice Care
Services Available	Dependent on the individual palliative care program. May include a physician, nurse, nurse practitioner, physician assistant, social worker, chaplain, childlife specialist, physical therapist and others	Care primarily given by the hospice nurse and home health aide a few visits per week. Other core team members include hospice medical director, social worker, chaplaincy. Other services may be available
Location of Care	Inpatient hospital Outpatient clinic Patient home Long-term care facility	90% of care occurs in the patient's home with family members as caregivers, or at long-term care facility or inpatient hospice center
Durable Medical Equipment (DME)	DME covered if meets Medicare/Insurance requirements	DME provided as part of hospice benefit as needed, and regardless of functional level: bed, bedside commode, shower chair, oxygen

Source: Quill et al., (2010); Morrison & Morrison (2006).

Palliative Care

Palliative care evolved as a separate entity from hospice in the late 20th century when requirements of hospice enrollment, with the accompanying limitations, became a barrier to care in some cases (Morrison & Meier, 2004). Broader in its scope, patients enrolled with a palliative care service may be given aggressive life-prolonging treatment such as chemotherapy, surgery, solid organ transplant, or stem cell transplant. Unlike hospice, prognosis is not a factor in determining whether a patient may receive services: Patients may have a curable illness and still receive palliative care. The goal of palliative services is to "walk alongside" the patient/family unit in the midst of a serious illness. This includes clarifying goals of care, communicating these goals to the team, acting as an advocate for the patient and family, addressing psychosocial and spiritual needs, encouraging use of coping skills, and providing excellent symptom management (National Consensus Project for Quality Palliative Care, 2009).

Definition of Palliative Care

Palliative care is a supportive approach to care with a focus on optimizing quality of life and reducing suffering of those with life-limiting illness. The "unit" of care includes patients and their family members, significant others, and caregivers. It addresses physical concerns as well as emotional, social, and spiritual needs. There are a number of formal definitions of palliative care; the World Health Organization (WHO) definition is listed in the following box.

WORLD HEALTH ORGANIZATION DEFINITION OF PALLIATIVE CARE

Palliative care is an approach that improves the quality of life of patients and their families facing the problem associated with life-threatening illness, through the prevention and relief of suffering by means of early identification and impeccable assessment and treatment of pain and other problems, physical, psychosocial, and spiritual. Palliative care:

- provides relief from pain and other distressing symptoms;
- affirms life and regards dying as a normal process;
- intends neither to hasten or postpone death;
- integrates the psychological and spiritual aspects of patient care;
- offers a support system to help patients live as actively as possible until death;
- offers a support system to help the family cope during the patients illness and in their own bereavement;
- uses a team approach to address the needs of patients and their families, including bereavement counseling, if indicated;
- will enhance quality of life, and may also positively influence the course of illness;
- is applicable early in the course of illness, in conjunction with other therapies that are intended to prolong life, such as chemotherapy or radiation therapy, and includes those investigations needed to better understand and manage distressing clinical complications.

Reprinted with permission. Retrieved from http://www.who.int/cancer/palliative/definition/en/

Ideally, palliative care services are begun early in the trajectory of care for a life-limiting illness such as cancer, dementia, or heart failure. As the disease progresses, palliative services are intensified, while less focus is given to treatments with curative intent (National Consensus Project for Quality Palliative Care, 2009). This concept is illustrated in Figure 18.1.

Palliative Care Services

Eighty five percent of large hospitals now have a palliative care program (Center to Advance Palliative Care, 2011). The types of services offered are wide ranging, depending on each center. A full-service program may utilize physicians, nurse practitioners, physician assistants, nurses, social workers, chaplains, childlife specialists, psychiatrists, psychologists, pharmacists, dieticians, physical therapists, and support staff, with 24-hour, 7-days-a-week coverage (Morrison & Meier, 2004). A small palliative program may consist of only a part-time nurse who has a physician available for case discussions. Some programs focus more on pain and symptom management; other programs center on the psychosocial aspects of coping with serious illness, legacy work, and future planning needs (such as completing durable power of attorney for health care and living will forms); larger programs can provide all of these services.

The site of care may be inpatient, an outpatient center, a long-term care facility, or in the home. Physician and other provider services are billed via fee-for-service rules as allowed by insurance. These programs are seldom self-sustaining, and are usually supported by grants or the institution (Goldsmith, Dietrich, Du, & Morrison, 2008). Many hospice agencies have recently begun expanding their programs to add palliative care as an option (Coyle, 2010). This is especially helpful for those who decline to enroll in hospice care, or want to continue to pursue chemotherapy or other therapies that the hospice benefit may not cover (Wright & Katz, 2007).

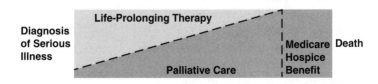

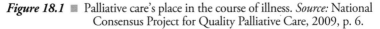

Figure 18.1 ■ Palliative care's place in the course of illness. *Source:* National Consensus Project for Quality Palliative Care, 2009, p. 6.

A sample patient brochure describing a palliative care service at an outpatient ambulatory cancer center is shown in the following box.

SEATTLE CANCER CARE ALLIANCE
SUPPORTIVE AND PALLIATIVE CARE SERVICE

WHAT IS THE SUPPORTIVE AND PALLIATIVE CARE SERVICE?

The goal of the Supportive and Palliative Care Service is to prevent and relieve suffering and to support the best possible quality of life for patients and their families, regardless of the stage of their disease. Supportive and Palliative Care Service can be delivered along with life-prolonging treatment. Our goal includes enhancing quality of life for patient and family, helping with decision making, and providing opportunities for personal growth.

- Relief from pain
- Relief from symptoms
- Relief from stress of cancer

We will work with you to better understand your condition and your choices for care, improve your ability to tolerate treatment, and carry on with everyday life.

YOU CAN BENEFIT AT ANY POINT IN YOUR CARE.

The Supportive and Palliative Care Service works with people at every stage of their illness. We will coordinate with your oncology team to provide in-depth symptom management. Your oncologist will continue to be the one that makes the decision with you about your care.

WHAT DO WE OFFER?

We will work with your oncologist to provide specialized care for:

- Controlling pain
- Controlling physical symptoms
- Coping with the stress of cancer
- Talking with your family
- Determining what is most important to you
- Preparation for the future
- Advance directives for health care

- Living Will
- Deciding when it is right to enroll in hospice
- Promoting the best quality of life possible

THE SUPPORTIVE AND PALLIATIVE CARE SERVICE IS DIFFERENT FROM HOSPICE.

Hospice care is provided to patients by specialized nurses, social workers, and chaplains. It is designed for patients in the last 6 months of life. The care is usually provided in the home with the hospice team visiting regularly. If it is time for hospice care, we assist you with the referral, and provide ongoing coordination of care with the team.

Reprinted with permission.

When introducing a palliative care referral to patients and their caregivers, the team must be especially sensitive to address potential fears that may arise. It should be emphasized that a consultation is not "giving up" on the patient. Rather, the goal is to *augment* standard care by providing intensive management of symptoms, emotions, and spiritual needs of the patient and family unit in a culturally appropriate manner (Quill et al., 2010). Adding palliative care services often involves an *intensification* of the overall care management, not a reduction, as the issues in all domains of care are addressed (Coyle, 2010).

Benefits of Palliative Care

Complementing standard oncology care with palliative services seems a logical way to meet the goal of improved quality of life in advancing illness. However, the astonishing finding of a seminal study by Temel and colleagues (2010) was that patients with metastatic non-small cell lung cancer who received early palliative care not only reported improved quality of life, but also *lived 3 months longer* than those who received standard care. Study coauthor Lynch said "If this was a drug, this would be on the front page of every paper in the country, talking about 'New advance in lung cancer!'" (Szabo, 2011). These surprising findings have highlighted the field of palliative medicine for the public, and have increased referrals by oncologists (Center to Advance Palliative Care, 2011).

Clinical Pearl	Benefits of palliative care include the following: • Better quality of life • Longer life • Lower cost of care • Fewer hospital readmissions *Source*: Temel et al. (2010); Morrison et al. (2008); Smith & Hillner (2011).

National Consensus Project for Quality Palliative Care

The National Consensus Project for Quality Palliative Care developed *Clinical Practice Guidelines* to promote the quality of care provided, reduce variability across programs, facilitate collaboration, and standardize reimbursement (National Consensus Project for Quality Palliative Care, 2009). The initial guidelines were released in 2004, and updated in 2009. Eight domains of palliative care were established, to define the specialty and differentiate it from other types of care. These domains are as follows:

- Structure and processes of care
- Physical aspects of care
- Psychosocial and psychiatric aspects of care
- Social aspects of care
- Spiritual, religious, and existential aspects of care
- Cultural aspects of care
- Care of the imminently dying patient
- Ethical and legal aspects of care
  (National Consensus Project for Quality Palliative Care, 2009)

Certification in Palliative Care

Based on these guidelines for exceptional palliative care, The Joint Commission began offering *Advanced Certification for Palliative Care* in September 2011 to hospitals "that demonstrate exceptional patient and family-centered care" with a focus on improving quality of life to those with serious illness (The Joint Commission, 2011). Certification requires a multidisciplinary program to address physical, social, and spiritual needs of patients. Consultative services must be available at all times of the day and night, every day of the week, and there should be evidence that hospital leadership supports the program. It is hoped that this important certification will motivate more hospitals to establish full-service palliative care programs.

Individual certification is available for nurses through the Hospice and Palliative Nurses Association (www.HPNA.org) as a Certified Hospice and Palliative Nurse (CHPN) or an Advanced Certified Hospice and Palliative Nurse (ACHPN; National Board for Certification of Hospice and Palliative Nurses [NBCHPN], 2011). Physicians may obtain subspecialty board certification in Hospice and Palliative Medicine through the American Board of Medical Specialties (American Academy of Hospice and Palliative Medicine [AAHPM], 2011).

Hospice Services

Hospice care is paid for by Medicare, Medicaid, private insurance, Veterans Affairs, Tricare, or Health Maintenance Organizations (Hospice Directory, 2011). The *Medicare Hospice Benefit* has strict guidelines for enrollment and services, and most agency and insurance rules parallel those of Medicare (Centers for Medicare and Medicaid Services, 2011). The most prominent requirement is the patient must have an anticipated lifespan of 6 months or less, if the disease runs the usual course. Prognosis must be determined by two attending physicians, usually the patient's primary physician for the terminal illness (oncologist, cardiologist, pulmonologist, family doctor) and the hospice medical director. Hospice eligibility should be considered a "prognosis-based" not a "needs-based" program. The prognosis requirement prevents enrollment for several chronic debilitating diseases with high-care needs, such as dementia, amyotrophic lateral sclerosis (ALS), or COPD, until very late in the disease process, due to the vagaries of predicting death in these conditions (Gazelle, 2007). Prognosis is somewhat easier to determine in advanced cancer. One tool that is helpful in prognosticating is the Palliative Performance Scale, as shown in Table 18.2 (Anderson, Downing, & Hill, 1996). This validated scale is built upon the Karnofsky Performance Scale concept, with additional items listed for level of ambulation, consciousness, oral intake, and ability for self-care. Estimated median survival in days is indicated, based on the performance scores.

All medications related to the hospice diagnosis (such as opioids, laxatives, antiemetics, and pancreatic enzymes for pancreatic cancer) are

Table 18.2 ■ Palliative Performance Scale

The Palliative Performance Scale (PPS) uses five observer-rated domains correlated to the Karnofsky Performance Scale (100-0). The PPS is a reliable and valid tool and correlates well with actual survival and median survival time for cancer patients. It has been found useful for purposes of identifying and tracking potential care needs of palliative care patients, particularly as these needs change with disease progression. Large validation studies are still needed, as is analysis of how the PPS does, or does not, correlate with other available prognostic tools and commonly used symptom scales.

%	Ambulation	Activity Level Evidence of Disease	Self-Care	Intake	Level of Consciousness	Estimated Median Survival in Days (a)	(b)	(c)
100	Full	Normal / No Disease	Full	Normal	Full			
90	Full	Normal / Some Disease	Full	Normal	Full		N/A	108
80	Full	Normal with effort / Some Disease	Full	Normal or reduced	Full	N/A		
70	Reduced	Can't do normal job or work / Some Disease	Full	As above	Full	145		

						a	b	c
60	Reduced	Cannot do hobbies or housework *Significant Disease*	Occasional assistance needed	As above	Full or confusion	29	4	41
50	Mainly sit/lie	Cannot do any work *Extensive Disease*	Considerable assistance needed	As above	Full or confusion	30	11	
40	Mainly in bed	As above	Mainly assistance	As above	Full or drowsy or confusion	18	8	
30	Bed bound	As above	Total care	Reduced	As above	8	5	
20	Bed bound	As above	As above	Minimal	As above	4	2	6
10	Bed bound	As above	As above	Mouth care only	Drowsy or coma	1	1	
0	Death	–	–	–	–	–	–	

a. Survival postadmission to an inpatient palliative unit, all diagnoses (Virik, 2002).

b. Days until inpatient death following admission to an acute hospice unit, diagnoses not specified (Anderson et al., 1996).

c. Survival postadmission to an inpatient palliative unit, cancer patients only (Morita, 1999).

Source: Anderson, F., Downing, G. M., & Hill, J. (1996). Palliative Performance Scale (PPS): A new tool. *Journal of Palliative Care, 12*(1), 5–11 and Ho, F., Lau, F., Downing, M., & Lesperance, M. (2008). A reliability and validity study of the Palliative Performance Scale. *BMC Palliative Care, 7*(10), 1–10.

provided at minimal to no cost. Hospice agencies are reimbursed by Medicare on a capitated *per diem* rate for each patient; therefore, cost control is a major concern for hospice medical directors. For this reason, most hospice agencies will switch a patient's opioid medications to less expensive options (such as morphine or methadone) from more costly prescriptions (such as oxycodone SR [OxyContin]).

Services and Sites of Hospice Care

Ninety percent of hospice care in the United States is provided in the home (American Cancer Society, 2011). Family members and friends act as the primary caregivers, with scheduled hospice nurse visits once a week or more often as needed. A nurse is available by phone at all times, with unscheduled visits made for urgent needs that may arise, such as uncontrolled pain, dyspnea, bleeding, or anxiety. Core services also include a home health aide visit several times a week to help change bedsheets and provide safety in bathing. Intensive EOL psychosocial and spiritual counseling is available to the patient and caregivers through social workers and chaplain services. All hospices offer bereavement counseling for 13 months after patient death as part of the hospice benefit (Gazelle, 2007). Other services that may be available, depending on the individual hospice system, include complementary therapies such as massage, Reiki, pet therapy, aromatherapy, meditation, hypnotherapy, and music therapy. Additionally, volunteers provide companion services to give family members a few hours' break.

Most patients report a desire to die at home (Steinhauser et al., 2000). However, full-time care of a dying person is difficult, and places a tremendous burden on the spouse, parents, adult children, or other caregivers. The work is both physically and emotionally exhausting. As symptoms escalate in the last days to week of life, caregivers must give full attention to their loved one, typically getting little sleep, and often feeling overwhelmed by the experience. The hospice benefit includes *respite care* to give family members a 5-day break from caregiving (American Cancer Society, 2011).

Other sites of hospice care include specialized free-standing hospice centers, a dedicated unit in an acute care hospital, or long-term care facilities, some of which have specialized hospice wings. Unfortunately, access to these sites of care may be limited by the hospice benefit. Hospice community nurse liaisons may be available in some areas to visit patients in a standard acute care hospital (Kuehn, 2007). They work closely with the inpatient staff to facilitate hospice enrollment, and assist with transfer arrangements to a private home, a nursing home, or an inpatient hospice center (American Cancer Society, 2011).

Treatments with the purpose of cure or extending life are not consistent with the goals of hospice care. Therefore, standard oncology treatments are generally not allowed, although a short course of palliative radiation for pain and symptom control may be permitted. Some larger hospice agencies offer "dual enrollment," also referred to as "open access" care, which allows enrollment in hospice while continuing to receive palliative antineoplastic chemotherapy or expensive therapies such as total parenteral nutrition (Wright & Katz, 2007). However, this option is more the exception than the rule, and depends on insurance and local hospice policies. Most patients must make what Casarett et al. refer to as "the terrible choice" between the many benefits of hospice care and palliative chemotherapy that may keep the tumor at bay for a period of time (2008).

Timing of Hospice Referral

Consideration should be given to a hospice referral in the oncology patient who meets the following criteria:

- Low performance status
  - Eastern Cooperative Oncology Group (ECOG) Score >2
  - Karnofsky Performance Score (KPS) <50
  - Palliative Performance Score (PPS) <50
- Tumor characteristics
  - Distant metastasis
  - Liver metastasis
  - Malignant complication, such as bowel obstruction, pericardial or pleural effusion, or hypercalcemia
  - Multiple tumor sites (≥5)
  - Carcinomatous meningitis

(Anderson et al., 1996; Casarett & Quill, 2007; Harrington & Smith, 2008; Weckmann, 2008; Younis et al., 2007)

What Patients Want at End of Life

Steinhauser and colleagues (2000) sought to define key attributes that patients, family members, and health care providers consider important at end of life, with the goal of improving care of the dying.

"Freedom from pain" was the most important item in all groups. Other items, in order of importance, include the following:

1. Freedom from pain
2. At peace with God
3. Presence of family
4. Mentally aware
5. Treatment choices followed
6. Finances in order
7. Feel life was meaningful
8. Resolve conflicts
9. Die at home

Tasks at End of Life

Ira Byock, a palliative and hospice physician, has written extensively about the concept of *dying well* (Byock, 1997, 2002, 2004). He suggests four statements that the dying person is encouraged to communicate to loved ones. Completing "tasks" such as those in the following list is part of the process of finding peace and meaning in the face of death:

■ Please forgive me
■ I forgive you
■ Thank you
■ I love you

By saying these words to loved ones, Byock proposes that the terminally ill person may come to closure, which can lead to a peaceful death.

COMMUNICATION SKILLS IN THE SETTING OF A LIFE-LIMITING ILLNESS

Communication skills form a core aspect of nursing care of the patient with advanced cancer (Dahlin, 2010). In 1998, the American Association of Colleges of Nursing (AACN) together with the Robert Wood Johnson Foundation issued a document titled *Peaceful Death: Recommended Competencies and Curricular Guidelines for End-of-Life Nursing Care* (AACN, 1998). Among other competencies, they urged education for all nurses on communication skills at end of life. This is especially important for nurses in the fields of oncology, critical care, palliative and hospice care, because they are faced with death and dying on a daily basis (Dahlin, 2010). One of the key outcomes of this summit was development of the *End of Life Nursing Education Consortium* (ELNEC, www.aacn.nche.edu/elnec).

This excellent program provides in-depth instruction to nurses over several days on end-of-life topics including pain, symptoms, communication, spirituality, ethics, cultural aspects, and care in the final hours of life. Specialized ELNEC programs focus on oncology, critical care, pediatrics, geriatrics, veterans' care and international issues.

Perceiving the Unspoken Message

The ability to assess the psychological, spiritual, and cultural domains related to illness will help the nurse to recognize "hidden messages" from the patient. For example, on the surface, a conversation about worsening pain in a patient with metastatic prostate cancer may appear to be purely about pain medications. However, the astute nurse will recognize there may be many "unspoken" concerns that are not verbalized, such as the following:

- Does worsening pain mean my cancer is worse?
- Am I going to die?
- Will I die in unbearable pain?
- I'm afraid! Help me!

By attending to these unexpressed worries and fears, the nurse will provide holistic care to the patient with advanced illness. This will help to reduce anxiety, improve coping, and may decrease the overall pain complaint.

In an investigation titled *Coping With Cancer*, Wright and colleagues (2008) assessed 332 patients with terminal cancer, and their caregivers, in a multi-site prospective study assessing whether end-of-life discussions impacted quality of life, futile aggressive interventions, and psychologic well-being of patients and caregivers. Of the 123 patients who had end-of-life discussions, they received less inappropriately aggressive medical care in the terminal phase. The results were that these patients were 8.3 times less likely to be resuscitated; 6.9 times less likely to be on a ventilator; and 3 times less likely to be admitted to the ICU. These discussions were not associated with worsening depression or more worry. Importantly, end-of-life discussions were associated with better quality of life in the final days, earlier hospice referrals, and better bereavement adjustment for caregivers after death.

Difficult Conversations

Nurses often find themselves participating in "difficult" discussions related to sharing bad news (Schulman-Green et al., 2005). Back, Arnold, Baile, Tulsky, and Fryer define *bad news* as "any information that adversely alters one's expectations for the future" (2005, p. 169). In oncology, these conversations center on the following:

■ A new cancer diagnosis
■ Disease recurrence after a period of being disease free
■ Progression of cancer on current treatment regimen
■ Change from *curative* focus of treatment to *palliative* focus (defined as symptom management without hope of a cure)
■ Time to stop chemotherapy, no further useful treatments available
■ Time to enroll in hospice, preparation for death
■ Do-not-resuscitate and do-not-intubate (DNR/DNI) orders

The decision to end anticancer treatment and transition to palliative care or hospice is stressful on the patient and family as well as the oncologist and medical team. Good communication skills are essential to aid in this difficult discussion (Morita et al., 2004). Nurses can assist with this challenging time of transition by providing support to the patient and family, while exploring and addressing concerns they may have (Duggleby & Berry, 2005). Many patients express a sense of abandonment when therapy is terminated (Coyle, 2010). However, use of excellent communication skills in the setting of difficult conversations may decrease psychologic suffering and existential distress, and lessen this sense of abandonment (Back et al., 2005).

Words to Use

How can the nurse help when bad news is conveyed? These discussions may occur in a scheduled family meeting with the oncologist and other team members, on the phone in an outpatient oncology clinic, or on the inpatient unit in the middle of the night in follow up to the oncologist's conversation earlier in the day. Difficult conversations can be quite challenging, but may also be tremendously rewarding. Having a few basic communication tools can help significantly. Open-ended questions are useful in gently exploring the patient's concerns related to the bad news. Examples include the following:

■ What is your understanding of your situation?
■ How is the treatment going for you?
■ What have you found to be the most difficult thing about having cancer?
■ What are you hoping for?
■ What are you fearful of?
■ (Patient or caregiver starts crying): Tell me about the tears.
■ This must be very difficult for you.
■ It must be hard to watch your loved one suffer from pain.

(Back et al., 2005; Buckman, 2001; Evans, Tulsky, Back, & Arnold, 2006; Farber & Farber, 2006; Morrison & Morrison, 2006)

These conversations take skill and practice, and they also take time. As Duggleby and Berry point out: "The adjustment to death is a process and cannot be rushed" (2005, p. 427).

Silence

Appropriate use of silence is a key communication technique (Evans et al., 2006). During a difficult conversation about end-of-life issues, allow periods of silence in the discussion. Ten to 60 seconds of quiet, active presence, with engaged body language, may allow the conversation to open up to areas of fear and worry that have not yet been expressed. This empathetic presence can be a form of *witness* to the suffering that is being endured (Farber, Thomas Egnew, & Farber, 2004). Silence can help the patient and caregiver to start to attend to the difficult issues at hand, and help them find ways to cope in the face of a serious illness.

It takes regular practice and self-awareness for nurses to become comfortable with periods of silence. After a prolonged pause, if you are becoming uncomfortable, helpful statements to break the silence are: "What were you thinking about just then?" or, "What is making you pause?" (Buckman, 2001). Also, be aware that the patient may be fatigued from the conversation, and simply needs to rest.

Communication Continuers

Patients learn quickly that medical personnel tend to be in a hurry and do not take the time to listen for very long. Hence, they may offer short "sound bites" for answers. *Communication continuers* can be helpful to let the patient know that you desire to know more, and have the time to listen to them. Examples include "tell me more," "mmm hmmm," or mirror techniques (repeating back a patient's statement) such as "that pain made you feel like giving up," or "you aren't sure if you can take chemotherapy anymore" (Buckman, 2001). Body language such as nodding, empathetic expression, or appropriate use of eye contact will also facilitate the conversation. Also be aware of *conversation terminators*, either by the medical team or the patient and family (Farber, 2011). These may include "closed" body language (arms crossed, turned away), repeatedly changing the topic, or blunt statement of "I don't want to talk about this anymore" (Buckman, 2001). Don't try to force a "difficult" conversation if there are multiple conversation terminators present. Instead, try to learn more about their point of view by utilizing the guided narrative approach provided in the next section.

Guided Narrative

Farber (2011) has proposed a technique called *guided narrative* to help the team gain understanding of the patient and caregiver perspective. This is especially helpful with challenging situations, such as complex family dynamics, that are affecting medical decision making. Examples include the patient/caregiver insisting on aggressive medical therapies (full resuscitation, intubation with ventilation) when counseled that it would be medically futile, or pressing for more chemotherapy when the oncologist has explained that the patient is actively dying. The context for a guided narrative approach to a family meeting starts with questions such as "I would like to hear your perspective on how things are going right now" (Farber, 2011). See the following box for examples of this approach to difficult conversations.

Guided Narrative for Difficult Discussions in a Palliative Care Setting (Farber, 2011)

- What do you already know?
  - What is your understanding of your situation?
  - How do you see things?
- What is important to you right now?
  - What is important to discuss today?
  - What do you see as your future?
- What are your experiences?
  - Have you ever cared for someone who is seriously ill?
  - What are your experiences with loss?
- Goals of care
  - What are you hoping for?
  - What are you concerned (worried, afraid) about?
- What else do you want me to know about who you are or what you believe to help me take better care of you?

© Lu and Stu Farber/Tyler Associates, 2011. Reprinted with permission.

TOTAL PAIN

The concepts of *meaning* and *closure* at the end of life are essential not only for spiritual well-being, but may impact the report of pain. This has a bearing on nursing assessment and management of pain. When facing death, an acute existential crisis develops, which impacts all areas of our being: physical, psychosocial, and spiritual (Ong, 2005). Dame Cicely Saunders, founder of the modern hospice movement, coined the term *total pain* to describe this crisis, and how it influences our use of the word "pain." Describing Saunders's work, Clark (2000) writes:

> Total pain was tied to a sense of narrative and biography, emphasizing the importance of listening to the patient's story and of understanding the experience of suffering in a multifaceted way. This was an approach that saw pain as a key to unlocking other problems and as something requiring multiple interventions for its resolution. Thus was formulated the idea of total pain as incorporating physical, psychological, social, emotional, and spiritual elements. (p. 1)

By practicing the communication techniques described earlier, the nurse may utilize narrative to explore sources of unrelieved pain that no opioid could ever touch.

Clinical Pearl | It is important for the nurse to recognize that *pain* is a complex and multifactorial experience. Skilled use of communication techniques will help the nurse to uncover and address profound psychosocial, spiritual, or existential sorrow that may be amplifying the report of pain.

Betty Ferrell is a leader in nursing research in pain management, palliative care, and quality-of-life issues. Building on Saunders's concept of *total pain,* she created a model showing the impact pain has on the various dimensions of quality of life. See Figure 18.2. It is important for the nurse to recognize that *pain* is a complex and multifactorial experience (Ferrell, Grant, Padilla, Vemuri, & Rhiner, 1991).

Pain Impacts the Dimensions of Quality of Life

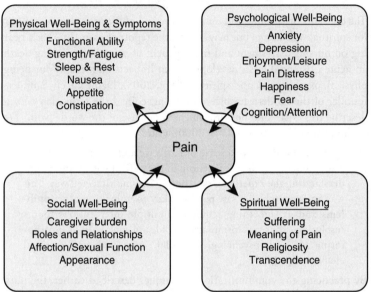

Figure 18.2 ■ Pain impacts the dimensions of quality of life.
Source: © Betty Ferrell, PhD, RN, and Marcia Grant, DNSc, RN, City
of Hope Medical Center, Duarte, CA. Reprinted with permission. From
http://prc.coh.org/pdf/pain_QOL_model.pdf

Denial

It is not uncommon to receive a verbal palliative care referral stating something along the lines of: "This patient is in denial. Please see them and get a no code order." Or, "The patient and family are refusing a hospice referral, they want more chemo. Please help us manage their denial." In practice, we may hear medical personnel expressing frustration about dealing with a patient "in denial." Nurses need to better understand the process of denial, so that we can assist patients as they move along the continuum toward death.

In her excellent article *Understanding Denial*, Stephenson (2004) explores this concept. She points out that denial may be adaptive or maladaptive, and there are different echelons of denial, some more disruptive than others. Use of denial may allow time to mobilize internal resources to help individuals cope with an unbearable situation, preserve a sense of control, or maintain internal integrity. Denial is a complex and fluid process that fluctuates over time. Stephenson describes *windows of opportunity* when "the resilience of denial may appear temporarily weakened" and the patient acknowledges the possibility of the worst happening (2004, p. 986). These *windows of opportunity* commonly occur in the middle of the night when the patient cannot sleep. Inpatient nurses are uniquely positioned to gently explore patients' fears and the motivations for taking a certain position about treatment options. By facilitating communication in this manner, the nurse can provide support to help the patient move from maladaptive patterns of coping to more adaptive patterns.

SUMMARY

Palliative care and hospice services are part of the spectrum of care in nursing. Indeed, it is one of the few specialties that impacts every patient we see, because we all die. The nurse who cares for oncology patients, in whatever setting, needs to understand some of the unique issues related to palliative care and hospice services. The challenge is to move referrals to palliative care and hospice "upstream"; that is, encouraging earlier referrals in the course of a life-limiting illness (National Consensus Project for Quality Palliative Care, 2009). More timely involvement of palliative care and hospice services has been shown to result in improved quality of life and even longer length of life (Temel et al., 2010).

Providing quality pain management in advanced cancer is essential knowledge for nurses. Therefore, the concept of *total pain* is important to understand, because multiple dimensions of the being will impact upon the pain report. These dimensions include not only the physical, but also psychologic, spiritual, and social domains. The nurse must consider what other domains may be fueling the pain report, especially if it is not improved with standard therapies. Use of narrative to explore these other dimensions will help the medical team understand the patient's perspective, improve quality of life, and decrease overall suffering (Ferrell et al., 1991).

Case Study

Jim is a 66-year-old male with non-Hodgkin's lymphoma diagnosed 6 months ago. His disease was refractory to multiple chemotherapy regimens. Plans for a stem cell transplant were aborted due

(continued)

to inability to get his disease into remission. He recently completed a short course of radiation therapy to control severe pain in the neck related to bulky disease. The oncologist, Dr. Smith, arranges a family conference and told Jim and his wife that there are no more chemotherapy regimens to try, explains that Jim's prognosis is 3 months, and proposes immediate hospice enrollment. Jim seems genuinely shocked to hear this news. His neck tumors have been shrinking from radiation therapy, and he insists "I'm going to beat this! I'm already getting better!" He appears offended, and adamantly refuses hospice enrollment. Jim deflects all further attempts at discussion with tales of the job he hopes to get, money he plans to make, and the house he will build over the next few years.

Later that day, he presents to the emergency department in a full-blown panic attack and complains of severe neck pain, which require high doses of intravenous opioid and benzodiazepine to control. Palliative care services are consulted because he refuses to agree to a DNR (do-not-resuscitate) order and hospice care. After his assessment the next day, the palliative care nurse practitioner reports that Jim understands what Dr. Smith told him, but just cannot believe it because he is feeling better after radiation treatment. He remains "extremely hopeful" for a cure, and feels traumatized by what Dr. Smith told him. The NP recommends a psychiatry consult for management of panic disorder, and encourages the oncology team not to press Jim with issues related to his poor prognosis, hospice referral, or code status for the next day or two.

Questions to Consider

1. Jim's pain has been markedly improved with the radiation therapy. What probably triggered this sudden report of severe pain?
2. Why did the palliative care nurse practitioner suggest not pressing Jim on his code status and prognosis at this time? What needs to happen to move these discussions forward?
3. Do you think Jim is "in denial"? Is his coping adapative or maladaptive?
4. Jim rings his call bell at 3 a.m. He says he cannot sleep and is really afraid of what is happening. "I'm afraid I'm going to die!" What do you say next?

REFERENCES

American Association of Colleges of Nursing (AACN). (1998, February). *Peaceful death: Recommended competencies and curricular guidelines for end-of-life nursing care.* Retrieved from http://www.aacn.nche.edu/elnec/peaceful-death

American Academy of Hospice and Palliative Medicine (AAHPM). (2011). *ABMS Certification.* Retrieved from http://www.aahpm.org/certification/default/abms.html#individual1

American Cancer Society. (2011). *Hospice care.* Retrieved from http://www.cancer.org/Treatment/FindingandPayingforTreatment/ChoosingYourTreatmentTeam/HospiceCare

Anderson, F., Downing, G., & Hill, J. (1996). Palliative Performance Scale (PPS): A new tool. *Journal of Palliative Care, 12*(1), 5–11.

Back, A., Arnold, R., Baile, W., Tulsky, J., & Fryer-Edwards, K. (2005). Approaching difficult communication tasks in oncology. *CA: A Cancer Journal for Clinicians, 55*, 164–177.

Buckman, R. (2001). Communication skills in palliative care: A practical guide. *Neurologic Clinics, 19*(4).

Byock, I. (1997). *Dying well: Peace and possibilities at the end of life.* New York, NY: Riverhead Books.

Byock, I. (2002). The meaning and value of death. *Journal of Palliative Medicine, 5*(2), 279–288.

Byock, I. (2004). *The four things that matter most: A book about living.* New York, NY: Free Press.

Casarett, D., & Quill, T. (2007). "I'm not ready for hospice": Strategies for timely and effective hospice discussions. *Annals of Internal Medicine, 146*, 443–449.

Casarett, D., Fishman, J., Lu, H., O'Dwyer, P., Barg, F., & Naylor, M. (2008). The terrible choice: Re-evaluating hospice eligibility criteria for cancer. *Journal of Clinical Oncology, 27*(6), 953–959.

Center to Advance Palliative Care (CAPC). (2011). *Palliative care in hospitals continues rapid growth for 10th straight year, according to latest analysis.* Retrieved from http://www.capc.org/news-and-events/releases

Centers for Medicare & Medicaid Services. (2011, August). *Medicare hospice benefits.* Retrieved from http://www.medicare.gov/Publications/Pubs/pdf/02154.pdf

Clark, D. (2000, July/August). *Total pain: The work of Cicely Saunders and the hospice movement.* Retrieved from http://www.ampainsoc.org/library/bulletin/jul00/hist1.htm

Coyle, N. (2010). Introduction to palliative nursing care. In B. Ferrell & N. Coyle (Eds.), *Oxford textbook of palliative nursing* (3rd ed., pp. 3–11). New York, NY: Oxford University Press.

Dahlin, C. (2010). Communication in palliative care: An essential compentency for nurses. In B. Ferrell & N. Coyle (Eds.), *Oxford textbook of palliative nursing* (3rd ed., pp. 107–133). New York, NY: Oxford University Press.

Duggleby, W., & Berry, P. (2005). Transitions and shifting goals of care for palliative patients and their families. *Clinical Journal of Oncology Nursing, 9*(4), 425–428.

Evans, W., Tulsky, J., Back, A., & Arnold, R. (2006). Communication at times of transitions: How to help patients cope with loss and re-define hope. *The Cancer Journal, 12*, 417–424.

Farber, A., & Farber, S. (2006). A respectful death: The power of relationship in end-of-life care. In R. Katz & T. Johnson (Eds.), *When the healing professional weeps* (pp. 221–237). New York, NY: Routeledge.

Farber, S. (2011). Words that work: Narrative strategies for difficult conversations. *End-of-Life Nursing Education Consortium. Lecture.* Seattle, WA.

Farber, S., Thomas Egnew, T., & Farber, A. (2004). A respectful death. In J. Borzoff & P. Silverman (Eds.), *Living with dying* (pp. 102–107). New York, NY: Columbia University Press.

Ferrell, B., Grant, M., Padilla, G., Vemuri, S., & Rhiner, M. (1991). The experiences of pain and perceptions of quality of life: Validation of a conceptual model. *The Hospice Journal, 7*(3), 9–24.

Field, M., & Cassel, C. (1997). *Approaching death: Improving care at the end of life.* Retrieved from http://www.nap.edu/catalog/5801.html

Gazelle, G. (2007). Understanding hospice—An underutilized option for life's final chapter. *New England Journal of Medicine, 357*(4), 321–324.

Goldsmith, B., Dietrich, J., Du, Q., & Morrison, R. (2008). Variability in access to hospital palliative care in the United States. *Journal of Palliative Medicine, 11*(8), 1094–1102.

Harrington, S., & Smith, T. (2008). The role of chemotherapy at the end of life: "When is enough, enough?" *Journal of the American Medical Association, 299,* 2667–2678.

Ho, F., Lau, F., Downing, M., & Lesperance, M. (2008). A reliability and validity study of the Palliative Performance Scale. *BMC Palliative Care, 7*(10), 1–10.

Horton, J. (2001). Hospice: Care when there is no cure. *North Carolina Medical Journal, 62*(2), 86–90.

Hospice Directory. (2011). *Paying for hospice: Medicare/Medicaid/More Options.* Retrieved from http://www.hospicedirectory.org/cm/about/paying

Kuehn, B. (2007). Hospitals embrace palliative care. *Journal of the American Medial Association, 298*(11), 1263–1265.

Last Acts. (2002). *Means to a better end: A report on dying in America today.* Retrieved from http://www.rwjf.org/pr/product.jsp?id=15788

Morita, T., Akechi, T., Ikenaga, M., Kizawa, Y., Kohara, H., Mukaiyama, T., . . . Uchitomi, Y. (2004). Communication about the ending of anticancer treatment and transition to palliative care. *Annals of Oncology, 15,* 1551–1557.

Morita, T., Tsunoda, J., Inoue, S., & Chihara, S. (1999). Validity of the Palliative Performance Scale from a survival perspective. *Journal of Pain and Symptom Management, 18*(1), 2–3.

Morrison, L., & Morrison, R. (2006). Palliative care and pain management. *Medical Clinics of North America, 90,* 983–1004.

Morrison, R., & Meier, D. (2004). Palliative care. *New England Journal of Medicine, 350,* 2582–2590.

Morrison, R., Penrod, J., Cassel, J., Caust-Ellenbogen, M., Litke, A., Spragens, L., …Meier, D. E. (2008). Cost savings associated with U.S. hospital palliative care consultation programs. *Archives of Internal Medicine, 168*(16), 1783–1790.

National Consensus Project for Quality Palliative Care. (2009). *Clinical practice guidelines for quality palliative care.* Retrieved from http://www.nationalconsensusproject.org

National Board for Certification of Hospice and Palliative Nurses (NBCHPN). (2011). Retrieved from http://www.nbchpn.org

National Comprehensive Cancer Network (NCCN). (2011). *Clinical practice guidelines in oncology: Palliative care.* Retrieved from http://www.nccn.org/professionals/physician_gls/pdf/palliative.pdf

Old, J., & Swagerty, D. (2007). *A practical guide to palliative care.* Philadelphia, PA: Wolters Kluwer.

Ong, C.-K. (2005). Embracing Cicely Saunders's concept of total pain. *British Medical Journal, 331,* 5.

Quill, T. E., Holloway, R. G., Shah, M. S., Caprio, T. V., Olden, A. M., & Storey, J. C. (2010). *Primer of palliative care* (5th ed.). Glenview, IL: American Academy of Hospice and Palliative Medicine.

Saunders, C. (2005). Foreword. In D. Doyle, G. Hanks, N. Cherny, & K. Calman (Eds.), *Oxford textbook of palliative medicine* (3rd ed., pp. xvii–xx). Oxford: Oxford University Press.

Schulman-Green, D., McCorkle, R., Cherlin, E., Johnson-Hurzeler, R., Bradley, E., & Thompson, J. (2005). Nurses' Communication of prognosis and implications for hospice referral: A study of nurses caring for terminally ill hospitalized patients. *American Journal of Critical Care, 14,* 64–70.

Smith, T., & Hillner, B. (2011). Bending the cost curve in cancer care. *New England Journal of Medicine, 364*(21), 2060–2065.

Steinhauser, K., Christakis, N., Clipp, E., McNeilly, M., McIntyre, L., & Tulsky, J. (2000). Factors considered important at the end of life by patients, family, physicians, and other care providers. *Journal of the American Medical Association, 284,* 2476–2482.

Stephenson, P. (2004). Understanding denial. *Oncology Nursing Forum, 31*(5), 985–988.

Szabo, L. (2011). Palliative care focuses on life. *USA Today,* pp. 1–2 D.

Temel, J., Greer, J., Muzikansky, A., Gallagher, E., Admane, S., Jackson, V., …Lynch, T. J. (2010). Early palliative care for patients with metastatic non–small-cell lung cancer. *New England Journal of Medicine, 363,* 733–742.

The Joint Commission. (2011). *Advanced certification for palliative care programs.* Retrieved from http://www.jointcommission.org/certification/palliative_care.aspx

The SUPPORT Principal Investigators. (1995). A controlled trial to improve care for seriously ill hospitalized patients: The study to understand prognoses and preferences for outcomes and risks of treatments (SUPPORT). *Journal of the American Medical Association, 274,* 1591–1598.

Virik, K., & Glare, P. (2002). Validation of the palliative performance scale for inpatients admitted to a palliative care unit in Sydney, Australia. *Journal of Pain and Symptom Management, 23*(6), 455–457.

Weckmann, M. (2008). The role of the family physician in the referral and management of hospice patients. *American Family Physician, 77*(6), 807–812, 817–818.

World Health Organization. (n.d.). *WHO definition of palliative care.* Retrieved from http://www.who.int/cancer/palliative/definition/en/

Wright, A., & Katz, I. (2007). Letting go of the rope—Aggressive treatment, hospice care, and open access. *New England Journal of Medicine, 357*(4), 324–327.

Wright, A., Zhang, B., Ray, A., Mack, J., Trice, E., Balboni, T., ... Prigerson, H. G. (2008). Associations between end-of-life discussions, patient mental health, medical care near death, and caregiver bereavement adjustment. *Journal of the American Medical Association, 300*(14), 1665–1673.

Younis, T., Milch, R., Abul-Khoudoud, K., Lawrence, D., Mirand, A., & Levine, E. (2007). Length of survival of patients with cancer in hospice: A retrospective analysis of patients treated at a major cancer center versus other practice settings. *Journal of Palliative Medicine, 10*(2), 381–389.

19

Pain Management at the End of Life

Pamela Stitzlein Davies

Uncontrolled pain at the end of life is nearly a universal fear (Steinhauser et al., 2000). Fortunately, the vast majority of cancer pain can be controlled in the final days, especially under the expert care of an experienced nurse. In this chapter, we will review strategies for pain management in the final days and hours of life, the principle of *double effect,* and the management of refractory symptoms with proportionate palliative sedation.

PAIN AT THE END OF LIFE

Cancer-related pain may arise throughout the course of the illness, but occurs most commonly as the disease progresses. Approximately one-third of patients in active cancer treatment report pain. In advanced cancer, the incidence of pain increases to two-thirds (Paice, 2010). In a review of 64 studies by Higginson and Murtagh (2010), the mean prevalence of pain in advanced cancer was estimated at 75%, with a range of 53% to 100%. Some tumor types are more likely to cause pain in advanced cancer, including the following (Higginson & Murtagh, 2010):

- Sarcoma (100%)
- Multiple myeloma (100%)
- Head and neck cancers (80%)
- Genitourinary (77%)
- Esophagus (74%)
- Prostate (64%)
- Pancreas (72% to 100%)

- Ovary (46% to 71%)
- Breast (40% to 89%)
- Lung (17% to 74%)

Leukemias are the least likely to have late-stage pain, at 5% prevalence. However, incidence of pain in another common liquid tumor, lymphoma, may range from 20% to 78% (Higginson & Murtagh, 2010).

> *Clinical Pearl*   Pain at end of life is a common fear of patients and caregivers. Seventy-five percent of those with advanced cancer will experience pain. The tumor types most commonly associated with pain at end of life are: sarcoma, multiple myeloma, and head and neck, genitourinary, esophagus, and pancreas cancers.

Physiologic Causes of Worsening Pain at the End of Life

Patients commonly experience an escalation of pain in the final weeks of life (Berry & Griffie, 2010). Previously well-controlled pain may become out of control. Each opioid dose increase may help for a few days or weeks, then may require further increases to maintain comfort. It can be a challenge for the family or nurse to "stay ahead" of the pain. As noted in Chapter 14 in the section on management of a *pain crisis,* the nurse must first try to determine the *cause* of the worsening pain in order to create a treatment strategy (Mercadante, 2007).

The most common etiology for worsening pain is progression of the disease, which leads to tumor compression on the tissues, nerves, and organs. Disease progression at the end of life causes diverse and profound effects on the body leading to severe pain. Examples include the following:

- Bowel perforation causing severe abdominal pain
- Ureteral obstruction causing severe flank pain
- Tumor mass effect in the brain causing severe headache
- Pathologic fracture causing severe limb or back (vertebral) pain
- Tumor mass effect in the pelvis with pressure on the sciatic nerve causing severe sciatica
- Abscesses or cutaneous (fungating) spread of the tumor causing wound pain

Other physiologic causes of worsening pain at end of life include obstipation, urinary retention, candidiasis, wounds, or ulcers (Furst & Doyle, 2005). Unfortunately, worsening pain may also be caused by failure of the caregiver to administer proper doses of opioids due to fear of overdose or even a concern for addiction in the dying patient (Doyle, 2005). Once the patient is confined to bed, and is within days to 1 to 2 weeks of death, tumor-specific treatments (chemotherapy, radiation, surgery) are not typically used (Furst & Doyle, 2005). The primary therapies for pain control in the actively dying patient are opioids and steroids.

It is important for the nurse to anticipate and recognize the phenomenon of pain intensification in the final days of life (Moryl, Coyle, & Foley, 2008). See Chapter 14, "Treatment of a Cancer Pain Crisis," for a detailed example of dose titration for worsening pain. Careful inquiry should be made as to how often the pain medicines are given, in what dose, and any concerns the caregiver may have about use of opioids (Doyle, 2005).

Psychosocial and Spiritual Causes of Worsening Pain

A pain crisis may be precipitated by acute distress from psychologic, social, cultural, or spiritual concerns. Severe death anxiety, fear of "nonbeing," and existential suffering related to imminent demise will escalate the pain report (Roth & Massie, 2009). As shown in Figure 18.2, the impact of these dimensions on pain is depicted. Close coordination with the hospice or palliative care team social worker, chaplain, or psychologist will assist in identification and management of such crises.

According to Roth and Massie (2009), the focus of psychotherapy in this advanced disease setting is on helping the patient to *contain* the anxiety, rather than gain insight into the causes. Use of active listening and occasional supportive instructions are helpful for the patient facing death (Wilson et al., 2009). Medication management primarily involves use of anxiolytics (benzodiazepines) as well as antipsychotics. Initiation of an antidepressant may be considered if it is felt the patient still has several weeks of life left (as it takes 2 to 4 weeks for these drugs to become effective), because they are excellent at managing anxiety as well as depression (Wilson, Lander, & Chochinov, 2009). It is important to review the entire medicine list for anything that may be contributing to anxiety. Dexamethasone (Decadron) and methylphenidate (Ritalin) are two agents commonly used near the end of life that may worsen symptoms of anxiety. Discontinuation or dose reduction may be needed.

Terminal Delirium

Delirium is extremely common in the last days to weeks of life, occurring in 85% of cancer patients (Breitbart, Lawlor, & Friedlander, 2009). It may mimic a pain crisis, but responds to antipsychotics/neuroleptics (such as haloperidol) or benzodiazepines (such as lorazepam), rather than increasing doses of opioids (O'Leary, Stone, & Lawlor, 2010). Symptoms of delirium are restlessness, anxiety, irritability, hallucinations, delusions, sleep disturbances, tremors, and myoclonus. It is usually worse at night. In the final days, terminal delirium is attributed to the accumulation of metabolites from multiorgan failure (Quill et al., 2010). Other causes include dehydration, metabolic and infectious sources, paraneoplastic syndromes, and medications.

The astute nurse will always keep terminal delirium in the differential diagnosis as a possible cause of complaints of worsening pain in the dying patient (Heidrich & English, 2010). If escalating doses of opioids seem to have little effect, a trial of an antipsychotic or benzodiazepines may yield a response. These drugs are included on standard hospice and comfort care order sets (see the next section).

Clinical Pearl	The most common causes of worsening pain in the final days of life are (Paice, 2010; O'Leary et al., 2010): • Progression of the disease causing worsening pain from tumor compression of nerves and organs • Inability to swallow or lack of absorption of pain medicines • Death anxiety, which contributes to report of pain • Terminal delirium, which may present as pain complaints and pain behaviors

---

SYMPTOMS IN THE FINAL DAYS AND HOURS OF LIFE

Multiple new symptoms arise in the final days, which herald that death is imminent. These symptoms include the following (Quill et al., 2010; Berry & Griffie, 2010):

- Dyspnea
- Changes in respiratory pattern
  - Shallow breathing
  - Cheyne-Stokes respirations: Periods of rapid, deep breathing followed by long apneic periods lasting 30 seconds to 2 minutes

- Moist, noisy respirations ("death rattle")
- Fever
- Inability to swallow
- Incontinence of bowel and bladder
- Profound weakness
- Mottling (dusky bluish color) and coolness of fingers, elbows, knees, feet
- Restlessness, agitation, delirium
- Decreased level of consciousness, coma

Family education and reassurance by the nurse are essential to help them cope with this difficult time, and with the frightening symptoms that occur in the days prior to death (von Gunten, 2009).

Management of Terminal Symptoms

Home hospice and inpatient comfort-care order sets include medications that are standard for symptom control at end of life. These include the following drugs, with sample orders such as the following (Quill et al., 2010):

- Opioids (morphine, oxycodone, hydromorphone): To control pain and dyspnea
  - Note: Morphine is commonly used, but should be avoided in renal and hepatic impairment (Miaskowski et al., 2008).
  - Oxycodone 5 mg tablet, 5 to 20 mg every hour PO/SL (may crush tablet) prn for pain, dyspnea, shortness of breath (SOB)
- Benzodiazepine (lorazepam, diazepam, midazolam): For control of anxiety, nausea, dyspnea insomnia, agitation, seizure
  - Note: Occasionally, benzodiazepines may contribute to worsening agitation and depression, especially at higher doses (Quill et al., 2010).
    - Lorazepam 0.5 to 1 mg PO/SL/pr/SC/IV every hour prn for anxiety, nausea, dyspnea, agitation, seizure
    - Maximum 6 mg/8 hr
- Antipsychotic (haloperidol [Haldol]), chlorpromazine [Thorazine], olanzapine [Zyprexa]): For control of agitation and nausea
  - Note: Use of haloperidol is preferred over a benzodiazepine for control of delirium and agitation (Heidrich & English, 2010).
    - Haloperidol 0.5 to 2 mg PO/SL/pr q30 to 60 minutes, or 0.5 to 1 mg IV/SC q30 to 60 minutes, prn for anxiety, nausea, agitation, hallucinations, paranoia; maximum 6 mg/8 hr
- Steroid (dexamethasone [Decadron]): For management of pain from tumor compression of nerves, nausea
  - Note: In the last few days of life, glucose fingerstick monitoring is not typically performed (Paice, 2010).
  - Dexamethasone 4 mg PO/SL/IV every morning for neuropathic pain.

- Anticholinergic agent (atropine, glycopyrrolate [Robinul], scopolamine [Transderm Scop]: To dry excess pulmonary and oral secretions
  - Atropine 1% ophthalmic solution; give 4 drops SL every 4 hours for excess secretions
- Other medications included in standard comfort-care order sets for as-needed use include: acetaminophen for pain or fever, prochlorperazine suppositories for nausea, bisacodyl suppository or sodium phosphate (Fleets) enema for constipation (Quill et al., 2010).

ALTERNATE ROUTES OF MEDICATION ADMINISTRATION

As the patient approaches the final days of life, decreased consciousness and loss of the ability to swallow pills is common. Oral medications will need to be given by other routes to manage pain, anxiety and delirium. In a retrospective chart review of 90 patients in the last 4 weeks of life, Coyle, Adelhardt, Foley, and Portenoy (1990) found that 62% of patients could take oral feedings 4 weeks prior to death; this decreased to 43% in the week prior to death; and only 20% in the last 24 hours of life.

Alternate nonoral routes of drug delivery include the following (Miaskowski et al., 2008; Paice, 2010; Radbruch, Trottenberg, Elsner, Kaasa, & Caraceni, 2011):

- Subcutaneous
- Intravenous
- Sublingual
- Transmucosal/buccal
- Rectal
- Transdermal
- Intraspinal/epidural
- Less commonly used routes include the following:
  - Nasal
  - Transdermal iontophoretic PCA
  - Nebulization
  - Vaginal
  - Stoma
  - Enteral feeding tube

Sublingual, subcutaneous, and rectal routes are the most commonly used in the home hospice setting. See Chapter 4 for additional information on opioids, and Chapter 8 for information on neuraxial administration.

Sublingual Route of Medication Administration

Many opioids can be given by the sublingual (SL) route. All *rapid-acting* oral opioid tablets may be crushed and given SL. This includes immediate-release morphine, oxycodone, and hydromorphone tablets. Hospice nurses teach caregivers to crush the tablets between two spoons, add a few drops of vanilla-flavored syrup (sweetened), to make approximately 0.4 mL of fluid. The solution is drawn up in a 1 mL syringe and instilled under the tongue. This method is well tolerated by semiconscious and comatose patients, as there is minimal fluid used. Commercially produced opioid solutions are available for immediate-release morphine, oxycodone, and hydromorphone, which can be given orally or sublingually. However, depending on the dose and concentration, these solutions may result in a larger quantity of liquid being administered, which could trickle down the throat and cause choking in the unconscious patient. For example, if the patient requires 10 mg morphine every 2 hours for comfort, and morphine solution 2 mg/mL is used, this results in 5 mL given SL, which is too much fluid for this route. Changing the solution to morphine concentrate (20 mg/mL) will decrease the quantity of liquid to 0.5 mL, which is acceptable in this setting. Methadone is also available in a solution, which may be given by SL administration. See Chapter 4 for specific issues related to use of methadone.

Controlled-release (CR), extended-release (ER), or sustained-release (SR) tablets, capsules, or sprinkles, such as morphine CR (MS Contin), morphine ER (Kadian ER), morphine SR (Oramorph SR), oxycodone CR (OxyContin), and oxymorphone (Opana ER), should *not* be crushed, as this will convert them to immediate release, which could potentially cause accidental overdose (Miaskowski et al., 2008).

Rectal Route of Medication Administration

Referred to as the "forgotten" route, rectal administration of medication was used as far back as Hippocrates, but has been bypassed due to cultural and social factors (Cole & Hanning, 1990; Davis, Walsh, LeGrand, & Naughton, 2002). In the home hospice setting, the rectal route is an excellent option for obtaining systemic drug levels of opioids and other drugs, when intravenous or subcutaneous access is not available. This is especially useful when there is a sudden loss of swallowing ability due to debility, tumor, or seizure. Opioid administration by rectum results in faster and longer maintained pain relief when compared to the oral route (Radbruch,

Trottenberg, Elsner, Kaasa, & Caraceni, 2011). This is because the rectal route is theorized to partially bypass the "first-pass effect" in the liver, and therefore may achieve higher blood levels more rapidly (McQuay, 1990).

Some oral medicines can be given rectally, in tablet or capsule form, although this is not an FDA-approved route. The tablets or capsules can be inserted directly into the rectum with a small amount of lubricant jelly, or they may be placed in an empty gel capsule (size 0 or 00), which are available over the counter at larger pharmacies. However, small studies show there is high interindividual variation in bioavailability of sustained-release morphine tablets when given rectally (Walsh & Tropiano, 2002). Dehydration and other factors may account for variability.

It is best to consult a hospice pharmacist prior to rectal administration of an oral drug, as not all are absorbed. For example, gabapentin requires *active* transport for absorption, but drugs given rectally are absorbed by *passive* transport (Davis, Walsh, LeGrand, & Naughton, 2002). However, other drugs for neuropathic pain, such as tricyclic antidepressants (amitriptyline) and the anticonvulsants lamotrigine and carbamazepine are absorbed rectally (Davis et al., 2002). Tablets are crushed and put in an empty gel capsule or mixed with a vehicle solution. Ideally, if utilized for any length of time, medications should be changed to suppositories that are specifically formulated for rectal administration and absorption or professionally prepared by a compounding pharmacist.

Rectal administration should be avoided in rectal cancer, tumors invading the perineum, or prior abdominoperineal resection (Davis et al., 2002). Stool impaction must be resolved prior to rectal administration of drugs. Diarrhea will likely result in expulsion of the medicine (Nee, 2006). Rectal administration should be avoided in patients with severe thrombocytopenia (e.g., less than 20,000) due to risk of bleeding. Neutropenia of less than 500/mL is often listed as a contraindication of rectal administration, although risk of infection is unlikely to be a major consideration in the last few days of life. Occasionally patients have local reactions of the rectal mucosa (inflammation or pruritis), which prevent use of this route (Radbruch et al., 2011). Lastly, if turning the patient for the purpose of rectal administration is too painful, other routes should be explored.

Subcutaneous Route of Medication Administration

A systematic review of 72 studies comparing various alternative routes of opioid administration found the subcutaneous route had the best evidence base (Radbruch et al., 2011). This route is commonly used in hospice settings when parenteral drugs are required for pain and symptom control, since maintaining intravenous access can be difficult in the home, and is associated with more complications (Paice, 2010). Intravenous and subcutaneous routes have comparable steady state serum levels, although the subcutaneous route has lower peak effect and longer offset after opioid bolus (Miaskowski et al., 2008). Drugs can be given either as an intermittent injection, or a continuous infusion, via special indwelling subcutaneous needle and catheter sets. Drugs should be concentrated as much as possible to minimize the fluid volume delivered. Amounts over 2 to 3 mL/hr are difficult to absorb in the subcutaneous tissue. Hydromorphone (Dilaudid) is popular for subcutaneous infusion, as it is available in more concentrated injectable form.

Pain at the injection site is the most common adverse reaction from subcutaneous administration, especially with higher volumes of infusion. The injection site needs to be rotated every 2 to 3 days. Morphine, in particular, may cause issues when given subcutaneously, as it is less soluble; and local histamine release may cause problems, especially in more concentrated forms (Miaskowski et al., 2008).

Other Routes of Medication Administration

Intranasal

Intranasal administration of opioids for breakthrough cancer pain (BTCP) is an ideal option due to ease of administration and rich blood supply in the nasal mucosa (Vascello & McQuillan, 2006). Fentanyl (Lazanda) nasal spray was FDA approved in 2011 for BTCP under the Risk Evaluation and Mitigation Strategy (REMS) program. It is available in 100 mcg or 400 mcg per spray, and 1 to 2 sprays are given every 2 hours as needed for BTCP (Lazanda Package Insert, 2011). In a comparison of morphine sulfate-immediate release (MSIR) versus fentanyl nasal spray in 106 patients with BTCP, the nasal spray was found to work more quickly than MSIR, with onset of clinically meaningful pain relief at 10 minutes after dosing (Davies et al., 2011). Patient acceptability of the nasal route was reported to be high. The authors report ease of caregiver administration of the nasal spray for BTCP, which is advantageous in the final days of life. As this product is available by brand name only, cost will be a major consideration in its use.

Nebulization

Nebulized opioids for BTCP management has long been considered, due to the theorized rapid absorption from the lung, but no controlled studies have been performed in cancer pain (Vascello & McQuillan, 2006). However, several small studies have been done on management of dyspnea (DiSalvo, Joyce, Tyson, Culkin, & Mackay, 2007). Nebulized morphine was not superior to subcutaneous morphine in 12 patients with cancer-related dyspnea (Bruera et al., 2005). Other small studies on nebulized morphine, hydromorphone, or fentanyl for dyspnea or acute noncancer pain show promise, but the results are mixed (Ben-Aharon, Gafter-Gvili, Paul, Leibovici, & Stemmer, 2008; Pasero & McCaffery, 2011).

Enteral

Enteral administration of the long-acting morphine (Kadian ER) is an option when a 16 Fr or larger gastrostomy tube is present. Kadian ER capsules are filled with pellets. The capsules are opened and mixed into 10 mL of water. This is poured into the gastrostomy tube through a funnel, followed by a 10 mL flush of water (Kadian Package Insert, 2010). Both Kadian ER and Avinza ER pellets may also be sprinkled onto applesauce if the patient can swallow some food. These brand-name formulations are more expensive.

Vaginal

Vaginal delivery of drugs is an alternative to rectal administration. This requires use of a plug, as the vagina has no sphincter. Paice (2010) suggests use of a tampon covered with a condom, or a urinary catheter placed in the vagina with the balloon inflated.

Topical

Caregivers are sometimes curious about the use of compounded topical agents for pain when a patient can no longer swallow pills. There are several commercially available topical agents for pain, including lidocaine (Lidoderm) 5% patch, capsaicin (Zostrix), and diclofenac (Voltaren) gel (see Chapter 5). However, these have limited use in the management of end-stage cancer pain. Compounded opioids may be helpful for management of wound pain or mucositis, but otherwise would not reach the systemic effect that is required for pain management at end of life (Coyne, Hansen, & Watson, 2006; Jacobsen, 2009).

Intramuscular

Ongoing management of pain and other symptoms by the intramuscular route is considered inappropriate in the palliative care setting, due to pain associated with injections as well as poor absorption at end of life (Paice, 2010; Radbruch et al., 2011).

THE PRINCIPLE OF *DOUBLE EFFECT*

The principle of *double effect* refers to the risk of hastening death while in pursuit of pain control in the dying patient (Knight & Espinosa, 2010). Based in Roman Catholic moral theology, ethical principles maintain that the potential "bad" effect (hastening death) is outweighed by a known "good" effect (pain control) if the intent is for relief of distressing pain (Fohr, 1998). Patterson and Hodges (1998) refer to it as "the leading ethical principle by which we can ethically and legally relieve the suffering of dying patients" (p. 1389). Although this topic is much debated in the fields of medicine, ethics, law, and philosophy (Jansen, 2010), clinicians who manage pain at end of life know that it is actually quite *difficult* to hasten death with opioids once a patient is tolerant to them (Manfredi, Morrison, & Meier, 1998; Mercadante, 2007). In fact, relieving pain with opioids at end of life likely *prolongs* life rather than shortens it (Fohr, 1998).

Nurses should be confident in their approach to pain management at the end of life without being fearful of "killing" the patient with pain medicines. The American Nurses Association's *Code of Ethics* (2001) is unambiguous on the principle of double effect, stating:

"The nurse should provide interventions to relieve pain and other symptoms in the dying patient even when those interventions entail risks of hastening death. However, nurses may not act with the sole intent of ending a patient's life even though such action may be motivated by compassion...and quality of life considerations." (Provision 1.3)

If a nurse is concerned about this issue, she should speak to the supervisor, the prescribing clinician, and/or initiate an ethics consult for review.

The Last Dose

For the patient receiving opioids to relieve end of life pain, there will always be a "last dose" of medicine given before the patient dies. This may be in close temporal proximity to the death (e.g., within minutes), leaving the nurse or family member with the impression that they *caused* the death.

Such concerns can produce great distress, haunting someone for years, even decades. However, when the situation is analyzed, it is often the case that there was not enough time for the medicine to be absorbed, must less cause harm. Clinicians must educate the caregivers, and sometimes their colleagues, that the death was from the illness, not from the "last dose" of prescribed opioid.

Mercadante (2007) reviewed drug titration for cancer pain in the opioid-naïve and opioid-tolerant patient. He recommends a step-wise approach, with frequent dose increases as needed for comfort and close observation. He concludes that it is safe to rapidly titrate drugs to manage uncontrolled pain in a supervised setting. Sedation nearly always precedes respiratory depression, and uncontrolled pain is a strong driver of respiration and arousal (Quill et al., 2010). As noted earlier, a fatal overdose is unlikely.

PROPORTIONATE PALLIATIVE SEDATION

Proportionate palliative sedation (also termed *sedation for refractory symptoms*), refers to "the use of progressively higher levels of sedation for the relief of intractable and distressing physical symptoms at the end of a patient's life" (Quill et al., 2010, p. 139). The goal is to relieve physical and emotional suffering not managed with other standard therapies. Hastening death is not the purpose of palliative sedation, and its use is typically considered only in the imminently dying patient (e.g., within days of death). Current authors favor using the term "*proportionate* palliative sedation" to reflect the use of progressively higher drug doses, as needed, to properly control symptoms. Unconsciousness is not the goal of palliative sedation, but may be required for uncontrollable symptoms (Quill et al., 2010).

Sedation for refractory symptoms is performed when standard therapies fail to control intractable conditions such as (Knight & Espinosa, 2010; Muller-Busch, Andres, & Jehser, 2003; Quill et al., 2010):

- Pain
- Dyspnea
- Nausea and vomiting
- Seizures
- Bleeding
- Anxiety/panic
- Agitated terminal delirium

Before instituting sedation for refractory symptoms, the patient (if he or she still retains capacity for decision making) and surrogate decision maker should be counseled regarding the purpose and goals of therapy. Many facilities require signed consent before instituting palliative sedation. A written do not resuscitate (DNR) order must be confirmed or obtained, and decisions regarding use of artificial hydration and feeding should be reviewed. Unnecessary nursing care and monitoring should be discontinued, such as frequent vital sign checks, labs, ECG monitoring, and continuous pulse oximeter monitoring. Monitor alarms should be silenced. Every effort should be made to move the patient to a private room, with a quiet and peaceful setting (Salacz & Weissman, 2009). Consultation with the pain and palliative care service should be considered to assist with complex symptom management, and social work and chaplain referrals should be offered to assist the patient and family/caregiver. An urgent ethics consult should be considered if there is significant conflict or uncertainty about the appropriateness of the plan of care between the staff or family members. Detailed documentation of these discussions and plans of care is essential.

Use of proportionate palliative sedation is occasionally considered for extreme existential distress alone. However, this is controversial in nature. Such nonphysical symptoms may include a sense of meaninglessness, being a burden, death anxiety, panic, or other severe psychologic or spiritual distress (Knight & Espinosa, 2010).

The drug classes used for palliative sedation are benzodiazepines and barbiturates. Dose examples include (Knight & Espinosa, 2010; Quill et al., 2010):

- Lorazepam (benzodiazepine):
  - Bolus dose: 0.5 to 2 mg slow IV push
  - Maintenance infusion: 0.01 to 0.1 mg/kg/hr IV
  - Other routes: subcutaneous, oral, buccal
- Phenobarbitol (barbiturate)
  - Bolus: 200 mg slow IV push; repeat every 10 to 15 minutes until comfortable
  - Maintenance infusion: 0.5–1 mg/hr IV
  - Other routes: subcutaneous, rectal suppository

It is important to continue opioid therapy for management of pain and dyspnea after the sedative therapy is initiated.

Clinical Pearl	It is important to continue opioid therapy for management of pain and dyspnea after the sedative therapy is initiated.

Mean survival after institution of sedation for refractory symptoms is 2-½ days, with a range of less than 1 day to 6 days (Muller-Busch et al., 2003). Experts do not believe palliative sedation hastens death. The Knight and Espinosa (2010) reference contains a sample policy and procedure and physician orders for palliative sedation in the intensive care unit.

SELF-CARE

Nursing care of the dying patient is highly rewarding, but also emotionally demanding. Managing the patient with rapidly escalating pain and symptoms can be disconcerting and exhausting. In care of the dying, we experience the very essence of life and death on a daily basis. Exposure to death, grief, and loss causes us to confront our own mortality and brings up memories of past losses. We may, at times, be filled with sadness, despair, and hopelessness, putting us at risk for burnout and compassion fatigue (ANA Board of Directors, 2010).

Signs and symptoms of burnout include (Meier, Back, & Morrison, 2001; Old & Swagerty, 2007):

- Work is no longer rewarding
- Feeling emotionally exhausted
- Anger
- Depersonalization of the patient
- Cynicism
- Avoiding challenging paitents *or* increasing contact with them
- Sense of failure
- Depression
- Physical symptoms: aches and pains, muscle tension, sleep changes

If job stressors are escalating, and you find yourself "crying in the stairwell" too often (Kirklin, 2005), these steps have been found to be helpful (Meier et al., 2001):

- Name the feeling (e.g., anger, guilt, frustration).
- Accept that these feelings are normal human emotions.
- Step back and reflect on the emotion and get perspective on how it is impacting your care of the patient.
- Talk to a trusted collegue. (p. 3012)

Talking about these feelings can be most helpful in exploring these issues. Colleagues, such as a coworker, supervisor, social worker, chaplain, or human resources staff can help. Many worksites have employee assistance programs (EAP) that provide free professional counseling. The important issue is to recognize the problem and seek assistance before it becomes so severe that burnout begins to interfere with personal or professional life.

Regular practice of self-care exercises becomes *essential* to our overall emotional, physical, and mental well-being, not just a good suggestion (ANA Board of Directors, 2010). Use of a consistent wellness strategy can improve empathy, coping, and job satisfaction (Vachon & Huggard, 2010). Self-care may take on many forms, such as regular exercise, yoga, relaxation and breathing techniques, massage, acupuncture, hobbies, time with friends or family, journaling, reading poetry, singing in choirs, enjoying fine art, meditation, prayer, or pursuing religion and spirituality. The workplace can support self-care by creating opportunites to discuss and reflect on challenging cases with colleagues in a "safe" setting. Whatever strategies are chosen, the key is to give wellness care high priority in our busy lives, and take time to practice it regularly. This will help promote satisfaction and health in our work and personal life, and prevent compassion fatigue and burnout (Vachon & Huggard, 2010).

SUMMARY

The essential role of the nurse in managing pain and symptoms in the final hours cannot be overemphasized. It is the *nurse* who spends the most time with the dying patient and his or her family, both at the bedside and on the phone. Physicians and advanced practice nurses rely on the assessment of the home hospice nurse when writing orders.

Caring for the dying patient takes specialized skills and knowledge in pain and symptom management. The American Nurses Association Position Statement on end of life care states that nurses have an obligation to acquire competencies in end of life care of the patient and family (ANA Board of Directors, 2010). Baccalaureate nursing education is beginning to include this content. An excellent educational option for practicing nurses is the End-of-Life Nursing Education Consortium (ELNEC). This program provides excellent educational content on end of life topics. (For more information, see: www.aacn.nche.edu/ELNEC.)

Whether in the home, acute care hospital, ICU, skilled nursing facility, or inpatient hospice center, care at the end of life can be extremely gratifying work. A talented nurse can make all the difference for the patient and caregivers. Berry and Griffie (2010) point out that we "only have one chance to 'get it right' when it comes to caring for the dying persons and their families as death nears" (p. 630). We can do this by learning the skills needed for exemplary end-of-life pain and symptom management.

Case Study

Constance is a 56-year-old Caucasian female with end-stage abdominal leiomyosarcoma. She recently enrolled in hospice when she became too ill to come to the clinic for further chemotherapy. Prior to diagnosis 4 years ago, she was on moderate-dose opioid therapy for chronic neck and back pain and fibromyalgia. The sarcoma caused significant pain, and required escalating doses of opioids throughout the course of the disease.

For the last 2 years, she was on high doses of opioids but reported only "adequate" pain control, with a typical pain report of 6 to 7 on a 0 to 10 scale. Multiple opioid rotations were performed in an effort to provide better pain control and contain the side effects from high-dose opioid therapy. Immediately prior to hospice enrollment, she was on methadone 30 mg TID; oxycodone 15 mg tab, taking 22 tablets per day; gabapentin (Neurontin) 1,200 mg TID, duloxetine (Cymbalta) 30 mg BID, cyclobenzaprine (Flexeril) 10 mg TID, lidocaine (Lidoderm) 5% patches, and celecoxib (Celebrex) 200 mg BID.

Constance suffered from anxiety and depression, and had a history of childhood trauma. She brought these topics up frequently to her oncologist, team nurse, and infusion nurse during clinic visits, but always declined counseling. She is no longer is able to work as a computer technician. Her supportive husband Joe accompanies her to each visit, and she appears to gain a lot of strength from his comforting presence. She has an adult son from a prior marriage. Previously, they had an estranged relationship, but this has been mended since she became ill. Her son lives with, and helps care for, Constance while Joe is at work. Constance's mother is older and frail, but lives in the area. Her father is deceased. She is out of touch with her siblings and ex-husband despite her terminal illness. The patient and husband decline a chaplain visit for spiritual support. They also decline the social worker's offer to contact family members regarding Constance's situation.

As Constance approached her final days of life, the abdominal and pelvic pain became uncontrolled. She was unable to swallow oral medications, which included the opioids and adjuvant medications. The hospice attempted rectal and vaginal administration of the medications, but this was unsuccessful due to massive tumor bulk in the abdomen and pelvis, causing the suppositories to be expelled from the rectal or vaginal vault. She was changed to fentanyl patch 400 mcg/hr with hydromorphone 20 mg sublingual every 1 to 2 hours, but still reported severe, uncontrolled pain. She is receiving haloperidol and lorazepam sublingual for periods of delirium with episodes of severe anxiety. When alert, she repeatedly cries, "This hurts so bad, just let me die!" Joe is in tears and begs that something be done.

The hospice nurse consults with the hospice medical director, regarding options for pain and anxiety management. Constance is started on a patient-controlled analgesia morphine intravenous infusion (IV PCA) at 10 mg/hr with 5 mg bolus every 15 minutes as needed. This is rapidly titrated up to 40 mg/hr with 40 mg bolus every 10 minutes. Due to ongoing, severe pain, the hospice medical director, nurse, and social worker meet with the patient and family to discuss admission to the small local community hospital for palliative sedation. Unfortunately, they are not sure the inpatient attending will agree to this option. Ultimately, the husband decides to take his wife to the emergency department of the major medical center 60 miles away, where she has been receiving her cancer care. He requests inpatient admission for pain control and sedation for refractory symptoms.

The pain and palliative care team assesses Constance, and palliative sedation is instituted. She is started on IV midazolam infusion at 1 mg/hr and morphine 50 mg/hr, with haloperidol 1 mg IV push QID. The drugs are rapidly escalated over the next 5 days to midazolam 18 mg/hr, morphine 150 mg/hr, and haloperidol 4 mg QID. The hospital chaplain visits Constance and reports that she was raised in the Mormon faith, but left the church as a teenager. She says she is fearful of dying because she is not sure she will go to heaven since she is no longer practicing.

Constance becomes sleepier but remains arousable. She reports being more comfortable, but still has severe pain. She develops myoclonus (jerking). Ketamine is started, but stopped within 12 hours due to worsening agitation.

(*continued*)

Three days later, she is somnolent and minimally arousable on midazolam 22 mg/hr, morphine 50 mg/hr, and haloperidol 5 mg QID. She appears comfortable. She dies on the 10th hospital day with her husband, son, and mother at her side. Joe expresses his great appreciation for the option of proportionate palliative sedation to manage her uncontrolled symptoms.

Questions to Consider

1. What factors (physical, genetic, psychosocial, spiritual, existential) may be contributing to the difficulty in controlling Constance's pain in the final days of life? (Also see Chapters 11, 18, and 20.
2. What is the most likely cause of the myoclonic jerks? (See Chapter 6.)

REFERENCES

American Nurses Association (ANA). (2001). *Code of ethics for nurses.* Retrieved from http://nursingworld.org/MainMenuCategories/EthicsStandards/CodeofEthicsforNurses/Code-of-Ethics.pdf

ANA Board of Directors. (2010, June 14). *Registered nurses' roles and responsibilities in providing expert care and counseling at the end of life.* Retrieved from http://www.nursingworld.org/MainMenuCategories/Policy-Advocacy/Positions-and-Resolutions/ANAPositionStatements/Position-Statements-Alphabetically/etpain14426.pdf

Ben-Aharon, I., Gafter-Gvili, A., Paul, M., Leibovici, L., & Stemmer, S. (2008). Interventions for alleviating cancer-related dyspnea: A systematic review. *Journal of Clinical Oncology, 26*(14), 2396–2404.

Berry, P., & Griffie, J. (2010). Planning for the actual death. In B. Ferrell & N. Coyle (Eds.), *Oxford textbook of palliative nursing* (3rd ed., pp. 629–644). New York, NY: Oxford University Press.

Breitbart, W., Lawlor, P., & Friedlander, M. (2009). Delirium in the terminally ill. In H. Chochinov, & W. Breitbart (Eds.), *Handbook of psychiatry in palliative care* (2nd ed., pp. 81–100). New York, NY: Oxford University Press.

Bruera, E., Sala, R., Spruyt, O., Palmer, L., Zhang, T., & Willey, J. (2005). Nebulized versus subcutaneous morphine for patients with cancer dyspnea: A preliminary study. *Journal of Pain Symptom Management, 25*(6), 613–618.

Cole, L., & Hanning, C. (1990). Review of the rectal use of opioids. *Journal of Pain Symptom Management, 52*, 118–126.

Coyle, N., Adelhardt, J., Foley, K., & Portenoy, R. (1990). Character of terminal illness in the advanced cancer patient: Pain and other symptoms during the last four weeks of life. *Journal of Pain & Symptom Management, 5*(2), 83–93.

Coyne, P., Hansen, L., & Watson, A. (2006). Compounded drugs: Are customized prescription drugs a salvation, snake oil, or both? *Journal of Hospice & Palliative Nursing, 8*(4), 222–226.

Davies, A., Sitte, T., Elsner, F., Reale, C., Espinosa, J., Brooks, D., & Fallon, M. (2011). Consistency of efficacy, patient acceptability and nasal tolerability of fentanyl pectin nasal spray compared with immediate-release morphine sulfate in breakthrough cancer pain. *Journal of Pain and Symptom Management, 41*(2), 358–366.

Davis, M., Walsh, D., LeGrand, S., & Naughton, M. (2002). Symptom control in cancer patients: The clinical pharmacology and therapeutic role of suppositories and rectal suspensions. *Supportive Care in Cancer, 10*(2), 117–138.

DiSalvo, W., Joyce, M., Tyson, L., Culkin, A., & Mackay, K. (2007). Putting evidence into practice: Evidence-based interventions for cancer-related dyspnea. *Clinical Journal of Oncology Nursing, 12*(2), 341–352.

Doyle, D. (2005). Palliative medicine in the home: An overview. In D. Doyle, G. Hanks, N. Cherny, & K. Calman (Eds.), *Oxford textbook of palliative medicine* (3rd ed., pp. 1097–1114). New York, NY: Oxford University Press.

Fohr, S. (1998). The double effect of pain medication:Separating myth from reality. *Journal of Palliative Medicine, 1*(4), 315–328.

Furst, C., & Doyle, D. (2005). The terminal phase. In D. Doyle, G. Hanks, N. Cherny, & K. Calman (Eds.), *Oxford textbook of palliative medicine* (3rd ed., pp. 1119–1133). New York, NY: Oxford University Press.

Hagen, N., Elwood, T., & Ernst, S. (1997). Cancer pain emergencies: A protocol for management. *Journal of Pain and Symptom Management, 14*(1), 45–50.

Hanks, G., De Conno, F., Cherny, N., Hanna, M., Kalso, E., McQuay, H., . . . Ventafridda, V. (2001). Morphine and alternative opioids in cancer pain: the EAPC recommendations. *British Journal of Cancer, 84*, 587–593.

Heidrich, D., & English, N. (2010). Delirium, confusion, agitation, and restlessness. In B. Ferrell & N. Coyle (Eds.), *Oxford textbook of palliative nursing* (3rd ed., pp. 449–467). New York, NY: Oxford University Press.

Higginson, I., & Murtagh, F. (2010). Cancer pain epidemiology. In E. Bruera & R. Portenoy (Eds.), *Cancer pain: Assessment and management* (2nd ed., pp. 37–52). New York, NY: Cambridge University Press.

Jacobsen, J. (2009, May). *Topical opioids for pain.* Retrieved from http://www.eperc.mcw.edu/EPERC/FastFactsIndex/ff_185.htm

Jansen, J. (2010). Disambiguating clinical intentions: The ethics of palliative sedation. *Journal of Medicine & Philosophy, 35*(1), 19–31.

Kadian Package Insert. (2010, February). Retrieved from http://www.kadian.com/NR/rdonlyres/805E2900-ADBA-4FE4-A69E-173E4B9C151B/577/KADIAN_Prescribing_Information.pdf

Kirklin, D. (2005). The role of the humanities in palliative medicine. In D. Doyle, G. Hanks, N. Cherny, & K. Calman (Eds.), *Oxford textbook of palliative medicine* (3rd ed., pp. 1182–1189). New York, NY: Oxford University Press.

Knight, P., & Espinosa, L. (2010). Sedation for refractory symptoms and terminal weaning. In B. Ferrell & N. Coyle (Eds.), *Oxford textbook of palliative nursing* (3rd ed., pp. 525–543). New York, NY: Oxford University Press.

Koh, M., & Portenoy, R. (2010). Cancer pain syndromes. In E. Bruera & R. Portenoy (Eds.), *Cancer pain: Assessment and management* (2nd ed., pp. 53–85). New York, NY: Cambridge University Press.

Lazanda Package Insert. (2011). Retrieved from http://www.lazanda.com/common/pdfs/Lazanda_Prescribing_Information.pdf

Manfredi, P., Morrison, R., & Meier, D. (1998). The rule of double effect. [Ltr to Editor]. *New England Journal of Medicine, 338*(19), 1389–1390.

McQuay, H. (1990). The logic of alternative routes. *Journal of Pain and Symptom Management, 5*(2), 75–77.

Meier, D., Back, A. L., & Morrison, R. (2001). The inner life of physicians and care of the seriously ill. *Journal of the American Medical Association, 286*(23), 3007–3014.

Mercadante, S. (2007). Opioid titration in cancer pain: A critical review. *European Journal of Pain, 11*(8), 823–830.

Miaskowski, C., Bair, M., Chou, R., D'Arcy, Y., Hartwick, C., Huffman, L., . . . Manwarren, R. (2008). *Principles of analgesic use in the treatment of acute pain and cancer pain* (6th ed.). Glenview, IL: American Pain Society.

Moryl, N., Coyle, N., & Foley, K. (2008). Managing an acute pain crisis in a patient with advanced cancer. "This is as much of a crisis as a code." *Journal of the American Medical Assoction, 299*(12), 1457–1467.

Muller-Busch, H., Andres, I., & Jehser, T. (2003). Sedation in palliative care – A critical analysis of 7 years experience. *BMC Palliative Care, 2*(2), 1–9.

Nee, D. (2006). *Rectal administration of medications at end of life.* Retrieved from http://www.hpna.org/PicView.aspx?ID=461

Old, J., & Swagerty, D. (2007). *A practical guide to palliative care.* Philadelphia, PA: Wolters Kluwer.

O'Leary, N., Stone, C., & Lawlor, P. (2010). Multidimensional assessment: Pain and palliative care. In E. Bruera & R. Portenoy (Eds.), *Cancer pain: Assessment and management* (2nd ed., pp. 105–129). New York, NY: Cambridge University Press.

Paice, J. (2010). Pain at the end of life. In B. Ferrell & N. Coyle (Eds.), *Oxford textbook of palliative nursing* (3rd ed., pp. 161–185). New York, NY: Oxford University Press.

Pasero, C., & McCaffery, M. (2011). *Pain assessment and pharmacologic management.* St. Louis, MO: Mosby Elsevier.

Patterson, J., & Hodges, M. (1998). The rule of double effect. *New England Journal of Medicine, 338*(19), 1389.

Quill, T. E., Holloway, R. G., Shah, M. S., Caprio, T. V., Olden, A. M., & Storey, J. C. (2010). *Primer of palliative care* (5th ed.). Glenview, IL: American Academy of Hospice and Palliative Medicine.

Quill, T., Dresser, R., & Brock, D. (1997). The rule of double effect-a critique of its role in end-of-life decision making. *New England Journal of Medicine, 337*(24), 1768–1771.

Radbruch, L., Trottenberg, P., Elsner, F., Kaasa, S., & Caraceni, A. (2011). Systematic review of the role of alternative application routes for opioid treatment for moderate to severe cancer pain: An EPCRC opioid guidelines project. *Palliative Medicine, 25*(5), 578–596.

Roth, A., & Massie, M. (2009). Anxiety in palliative care. In H. Chochinov & W. Breitbart (Eds.), *Handbook of psychiatry in palliative medicine* (2nd ed., pp. 69–80). New York, NY: Oxford University Press.

Salacz, M., & Weissman, D. (2009, April). *Controlled sedation for refractory suffering - Part II.* Retrieved from http://www.eperc.mcw.edu/fastFact/ff_107.htm

Steinhauser, K., Christakis, N., Clipp, E., McNeilly, M., McIntyre, L., & Tulsky, J. (2000). Factors considered important at the end of life by patients, family, physicians, and other care providers. *Journal of the American Medical Association, 284,* 2476–2482.

Vachon, M., & Huggard, J. (2010). The experience of the nurse in end-of-life care in the 21st century: Mentoring the next generation. In B. Ferrell & N. Coyle (Eds.), *Oxford textbook of palliative nursing* (3rd ed., pp. 1131–1151). New York, NY: Oxford University Press.

Vascello, L., & McQuillan, R. (2006). Opioid analgesics and routes of administration. In O. de Leon-Casasola (Ed.), *Cancer pain: Pharmacological, interventional and palliative care approaches* (pp. 171–193). Philadelphia, PA: Saunders.

von Gunten, C. (2009, April). *Teaching the family what to expect when the patient is dying.* Retrieved from http://www.eperc.mcw.edu/EPERC/FastFactsIndex/ff_149.htm

Walsh, D., & Tropiano, P. (2002). Long-term rectal administration of high-dose sustained-release morphine tablets. *Supportive Care in Cancer, 10*(8), 653–655.

Wilson, K., Lander, M., & Chochinov, H. (2009). Diagnosis and management of depression in palliative care. In H. Chochinov & W. Breitbart (Eds.), *Handbook of psychiatry in palliative medicine* (2nd ed., pp. 39–68). New York, NY: Oxford University Press.

20

Psychosocial Aspects of Cancer Pain

Yvonne D'Arcy

OVERVIEW

The diagnosis of cancer is a life-altering event that affects not only the body but the mind and spirit as well. This interconnection can help to promote positive effects such as healing, or stress that can lead to increased pain. Patients must face the impact of the diagnosis both on themselves and others in their lives. They are made aware of their mortality and how this new diagnosis affects their future. How patients cope with the diagnosis of cancer is not only a reflection of their emotional resources but also of the support they receive from family and friends. Since there is a multifactorial effect with cancer pain, it is best treated with a biopsychosocial model that includes not only medication but the following:

- Pain coping and adjustment to the pain
- The relationship of psychologic distress to pain
- The social context of pain
- Psychosocial pain management protocols (Porter & Keefe, 2011)

One of the biggest fears that newly diagnosed cancer patient is the fear of having unrelieved pain (American Pain Society [APS], 2005; Gorin et al., 2012). The estimated prevalence of pain in patients with cancer is 53% (Gorin et al., 2012). The pain can be caused by the following:

- Tumor involvement, metastases to bones or organs
- Treatment toxicity such as chemotherapy-induced mucositis
- Diagnostic procedures such as bone marrow biopsies and lumbar punctures

In approximately one-third of patients, the pain intensities are reported to be moderate to severe. Undertreated cancer pain due to inadequate prescriptions is reported to range from 8% to 82% with a mean of 43% (Chen, Tang, & Chen, 2011). The pain can interfere with sleep, the activities of daily living, enjoyment of life, ability to work, and social interactions (Gorin et al., 2012).

As a graduate nursing student, I spoke with a family member caring for her husband at home who was dying from cancer. I was interested in knowing how the impact of the disease had affected the patient and family and the changes in their quality of life. Her first comments to me were that the first thing to disappear was their social contacts: "If you can't go bowling on Fridays with your team, the group tends to continue without you. We slowly lost touch with those of our friends who could still do the activity." She spoke to me about how her world slowly changed from someone who spent a great deal of time out of her home or at work to someone who was basically homebound: "It's not that I would change things to be out of the house; I want to be here for my husband, but at night it gets so very lonely and it feels like your world has gotten so much smaller." The burden of caregiving can have profound effects on the patient, family relationships, and the caregiver themselves. In some cases, there is even a higher incidence of physical and mental morbidity in the caregivers (Williams & McCorkle, 2011).

As treatments improve, the number of patients who survive cancer treatment has grown dramatically. In 1971, there were 3 million cancer survivors in the United States, while today there are over 12 million (Valdivieso, Kujawa, Jones, & Baker, 2012). Demographically, the majority of cancer survivors are adults, with two-thirds over the age of 65 and two-thirds alive after 5 years (Valdivieso et al., 2012). Cancer survivors are those who survive after their diagnosis and treatment, becoming former patients who are no longer under treatment (Haylock, 2010). A broader definition includes the concept of diagnosis as the beginning of survivorship "from the time of its discovery and for the balance of life, an individual diagnosed with cancer is a survivor" (Haylock, 2010).

How the patient with cancer pain copes with the stress and anxiety of the pain, the effect it can have on the caregiver, and the residual pain that some survivors are left with after treatment, are all important issues to discuss. This chapter will examine the important aspects about caregivers, spirituality, culture, and coping with the stress of cancer pain.

| *Clinical Pearl* | The way the patient with cancer pain responds to the pain is more than just a physical response, it is a combination of mind, body, and spirit that affects the way the patient experiences, processes, and copes with the pain. |

ROLE OF STRESS AND ANXIETY IN ACTIVATING THE PAIN RESPONSE

Recent research has been developing around the concept of a symptom cluster including pain, depression, and fatigue. Although the literature is incomplete at this point, there is sufficient evidence to suggest that stress hormones are a common co-occurrence of pain, depression, and fatigue (Porter & Keefe, 2011). In a study with advanced stage breast cancer patients, findings indicated elevated levels of hypothalamic–pituitary–adrenal hormones, and the sympathetic nervous system hormones had high correlations with pain, depression, and fatigue (Thornton, Anderson, & Blakely, 2010).

Patient expectations and fears also can affect the way pain is perceived. In a study with patients who were preparing for surgery for breast cancer, the researchers assessed the patients for anxiety and tension and asked how much pain the patient expected to have after surgery. There was a high positive correlation between higher levels of pain postoperatively, in patients who reported higher levels of tension and anxiety preoperatively, and who expected to have more pain postoperatively (Montgomery, Schnur, Erblich, Diefenbach, & Bovbjerg, 2010).

One way for clinicians to deal with this effect on pain is to increase the self-efficacy of the patient. If patients feel they have more control over their pain, they can minimize the hormonal and other stress effects and help to decrease the symptom cluster of pain, fatigue, and depression. One of the strongest findings for self-efficacy is that patients who have high levels of self-efficacy for pain control report much lower levels of pain (Porter & Keefe, 2011). Techniques for increasing self-efficacy for controlling pain by enhancing communication include the following:

- Modeling of skills, such as showing a video of a similar patient describing his or her pain to the health care provider
- Role-playing with feedback on the patient's performance provided by the health care provider
- Applying learned skills with pain descriptors when calling to report pain flares (Porter & Keefe, 2011)

The important aspect here is the use of effective communication to reduce stress and anxiety about the pain by communicating to the health care provider information that the provider can use to provide effective pain control strategies.

Another emerging technique for decreasing stress and anxiety about pain is acceptance of pain. This is for patients where pain persists despite all efforts and interventions to control it. Researchers found that acceptance of pain resulted in positive adaptation to pain (Gauthier et al., 2009). In a study with 129 outpatients in a pain clinic, patients with advanced cancer were screened using a variety of measures including the McGill Pain Questionnaire-SF, BPI, SF-36, Karnofsky Performance Scale, and other tools. Findings indicate that for 63% of the patients, their worst pain was moderate to severe, and 60% had moderate to severe interference with daily activities. Those patients who scored high on the pain willingness scale (willingness to tolerate higher levels of pain) had less pain catastrophizing and higher scores on activity engagement and had fewer depressive symptoms (Gauthier et al., 2009). Overall, the findings indicated that acceptance of pain resulted in better psychologic well-being (Gauthier et al., 2009). Pain acceptance was not associated with pain quality, duration, or severity. For cancer survivors with chronic pain, enhancing the acceptance of pain may provide a key to increasing coping and quality of life while decreasing stress, anxiety, and pain.

Caregiver Issues With Cancer Pain Management

Caregiving can be informal, provided by family and friends, or formal, where care is provided by hospice, skilled nursing facilities, or at home with health care providers (Hassett, 2011). In either situation, many families are very focused on controlling any pain that they perceive the patient is experiencing or the pain that the patient reports. Misunderstandings about the use of opioid medications can hamper the treatment of cancer pain and, when medications for pain are prescribed, the patient and family will need adequate education so that medications are given appropriately (Meeker, Finnell, & Othman, 2011).

The constant vigilance of caregivers can be extremely fatiguing and many caregivers experience periods of physical and emotional burnout where respite care (if available) can provide a brief period of time where the patient's care is given over to health care professionals. The fatigue that caregivers can experience can affect their relationship to the patient and how effectively the patient's complaints of pain are treated (Meeker et al., 2011).

In a review of the literature on caregiving and cancer pain management, Meeker and colleagues found that the majority (70%) of caregivers for patients with cancer pain were female, with the majority of these being spouses or adult children (2011). The average age of the caregiver was 55.8 years. Further studies revealed that pain management was seen as a primary function of caregivers, with 67% in the United States, and 95% in Australia, with 70% reporting their involvement as moderate to extensive.

Unfortunately, the Meeker review found that caregivers' attitudes were often classified as barriers to effective pain management. Ratings of caregivers' knowledge about pain management ranged from 55% to 60% in the studies included in the review. Fears and concerns about pain management were also found to be a source of inadequate pain relief for patients. These fears identified by the Barriers Questionnaire included the following:

- Fear about side effects
- Addiction
- Tolerance
- Discomfort of injections
- Belief in the inevitability of pain with a cancer diagnosis
- Belief that it is wrong to complain about pain
- Fear that raising the issue of pain will distract the health care provider from the primary task of disease treatment
- Fear that an increase in pain signals disease progression (Meeker et al., 2011)

Caregivers who were questioned using this questionnaire reported that there was some correlation; most of the questions were considered valid to some extent, with the least correlation with the injection question.

Because there is such a burden both physically and emotionally on caregivers for patients with cancer pain, a tool has been developed to ascertain the quality of life for caregivers, the Caregiver Oncology Quality of Life Questionnaire (CarGOQoL). To validate this questionnaire, 837 caregivers of cancer patients completed the 75-item tool. Findings indicated that women overall had a more negative impact on their quality of life than men and had a heavier caregiver burden (Minaya et al., 2011). Adult children also reported heavy caregiver burden, while duration of caregiving and caregiver age were not correlated to a decreased quality of life in all the respondents (Minaya et al., 2011). This reinforced findings that caregivers will adapt over time to the caregiving when the duration of time is extended, but the caregiving does take a toll on the caregivers themselves.

In a survey study of caregivers to determine if caregivers had higher levels of depression, poor health, or social isolation, reports from the 4,041 respondents indicated that caregiving alone did not produce greater depression, poor health, or social isolation (Robison, Fortinsky, Kleppinger, Shugrue, & Porter, 2009). The indicators that caused more negative impact on the caregiver's lives were living with the care receiver, inadequate income, and unmet needs for community-based, long-term care services (Robison et al., 2009).

In order to ensure that patients with cancer pain receive the best pain control while in a caregiving situation, the caregiver should receive education about medications and side effects, and that medication effects can have a positive impact (e.g., using morphine to ease respiratory distress). Providing caregivers with community resources and support from respite agencies and physical and mental health professionals will lessen the burden of caregiving and help promote a better quality of life for both caregiver and patient.

SPIRITUALITY IN CANCER PAIN

Not all patients with cancer pain can be classified as religious or having a religious affiliation but most have some type of spiritual connection that makes life worth living, a form of spirituality (Son et al., 2012). There are some identifiable relationships among religion, spirituality, and psychological well-being (Schreiber & Brockopp, 2011). In a systematic review with breast cancer survivors, three variables were identified, as follows:
1. Religious practice, religious coping, and perception of God
2. Spiritual distress, spiritual reframing, spiritual well-being, and spiritual integration
3. Combined measures of both the religion and spirituality constructs (Schreiber & Brokopp, 2011)

The findings of this review indicate that health care providers should conduct a brief, clinically focused assessment of the patient's belief system and the importance the patient places on this aspect of his or her life (Schreiber & Brokopp, 2011).

Implications of the Schreiber and Brokop review are that survivors of breast cancer indicate that a positive impact on psychologic well-being may be experienced by those who have a belief system, while a negative impact may be experienced by those without a significant prior relationship with God or who question a belief system early in the survivorship period. Overall, a patient with a relationship with a religious belief and self-forgiving nature will experience a better sense of well-being.

In a review of patients with hematologic malignancies, psychosocial well-being was positively influenced by a sense of coherence, self-esteem, health locus of control, coping strategies, and social support (Allart, Soubeyran, & Cousson-Gelie, 2012). The relationship to a global sense of well-being considering these factors had only weak evidentiary support.

The spiritual connection to pain is best considered as the physical pain aspect and the emotional suffering of the patient, e.g., "why me?" (Wein, 2011). Having a spiritual view of cancer pain can allow patients to reconcile their negative feelings and focus on those aspects that provide positive support. For patients who make a "contract with God" for a certain type of outcome, failure of the desired outcome can lead to a serious spiritual crisis that can have an adverse effect on the patient or family.

IMPACT OF CULTURE ON CANCER PAIN

The culture of the patient or the patient family dyad can impact the reporting and treatment for cancer pain dramatically. It can have both a positive or negative effect on how the pain is treated and resolved. Myths and fears about opioid use can create a situation where, despite the health care providers providing the patients and family with correct information, cancer pain remains inadequately treated. For some ethnic groups, pain is seen as a way to atone for past sins or indiscretions and needed as a means to attain forgiveness. For others, pain is seen as negative and something that should be eliminated as quickly as possible. Culture provides meaning for every person and it can help the person cope with or resolve the meaning of pain and suffering (Wein, 2011).

Some aspects of culture can be difficult for the health care provider to deal with during the active treatment phase of the cancer. Beliefs in folk remedies or herbs, or special waters or other culturally significant compounds can lead to distraction from the standard-of-care treatments that current society recognizes as essential for the treatment to be successful. This can be very difficult to address with the patients and family as pain persists despite the use of what the patient sees as valuable contributions to treating the pain and disease.

In an example of how culture can affect cancer pain, Chen and colleagues conducted a meta-analysis of 22 studies on the differences between Asian and Western cultures related to barriers to cancer pain treatment (2011). There were reports of more undertreated pain in the Asian patient group. The authors of the meta-analysis hypothesized that, since Asian patients saw other patients suffering from cancer pain, they themselves became less interested in cancer pain treatment. The authors felt these findings merited more investigation.

They also found that Asian patients had higher barrier scores on the Barrier Questionnaire than Western patients. A basic finding in this study was that in contrast to the Western culture, Asian cultures do not support the disclosure of the patients' cancer diagnosis to the patient. This results in a hypervigilance to pain and a more difficult-to-treat pain syndrome as pain is left undertreated for longer periods of time (Chen et al., 2011). Overall findings from this analysis indicated that as opposed to Western culture, Asian patients with cancer pain were more fatalistic and perceived cancer pain as a universal, natural, and inevitable reaction of the body to cancer (Chen et al., 2011).

Although there are many other cultural differences among patients with cancer pain, this analysis sends the right message that cultural differences should be examined and addressed when treatment options are being considered. Working with the patient's cultural beliefs for treating pain can provide a better, more positive outcome than ignoring the presence of these differences.

SUMMARY

Patients who have cancer pain have a great number of concerns and issues to consider. They are not just people with specific types of cancer where treatments are driven by standards of care. They are people who are individuals, have family members, and come from a variety of cultures and beliefs. Instead of treating these differences as impediments, using these differences to strengthen the communication with and acceptance of these differences can put a positive light on patient interactions. Cancer pain truly does have a mind–body–spirit effect that can be used to reduce barriers and improve overall patient outcomes in cancer pain treatment.

Case Study

Jeremy is a 56-year-old patient with end-stage lung cancer. His wife Judy is his primary caregiver and they have four adult children who live locally. Before his illness, Jeremy was an electrician and had many local ties to the community he lives in. After his last hospitalization, he decided that enrolling in hospice was the best option for his care. His wife remains at home and she is managing to treat the pain that Jeremy reports with morphine. The hospice nurse helps his wife decide when he needs to have more pain medication and if he is getting all the pain relief possible. Because of his respiratory status, his wife feels that, at times, the pain medication makes Jeremy's breathing too slow. She is afraid to give him medications that affect his breathing. Occasionally, one of the adult children comes into the house to relieve Judy and to allow her to go grocery shopping or do errands. The worst times are at night when Judy feels alone and powerless to help Jeremy. She often asks, "Why is this happening to us?" She shares these feelings with the hospice nurse who tries to come later in the day to provide support. Judy knows that family and friends would stay with her at night but she does not want to continue to ask for help.

Questions to Consider

1. What could the hospice nurse tell Judy that would make it easier for her to administer pain medications?
2. How could family, friends, and community organizations help Judy with her need for support?
3. Is there a cultural or spiritual effect in this case?

REFERENCES

Allart, P., Soubeyran, P., & Cousson-Gelie, F. (2012). Are psychosocial factors associated with quality of life in patients with haematological cancer? A critical review of the literature. *Psycho-Oncology*. Retrieved from www.wileyonlinelibrary.com

American Pain Society (APS). (2005). *Guidelines for the management of cancer pain in adults and children*. Glenview, IL: Author.

Chen, C. H., Tang, S. T., & Chen, C. H. (2011). Meta-analysis of cultural differences in Western and Asian patient-perceived barriers to managing cancer pain. *Palliative Medicine*, 1–16. Retrieved from http://pmj.sagepub.com/content/early/2011/04/07/0269216311402711

Gauthier, L., Rodin, G., Zimmerman, C., Warr, D., Moore, M., Shepherd, F., & Gagliese, L. (2009). Acceptance of pain: A study of patients with advanced cancer. *Pain*, *143*, 147–154.

Gorin, S., Krebs, P., Badr, H., Janke, E. A., Jim, H., Spring, B., . . . Jacobsen, P. (2012) Meta-analysis of psychosocial interventions to reduce pain in patients with cancer. *Journal of Clinical Oncology*, *30*, 1–14.

Hassett, M. (2010). The full burden of cancer. *The Oncologist*, *15*(8), 793–795.

Haylock, P. (2010) Advanced cancer: A mind-body-spirit approach to life and living. *Seminars in Oncology Nursing*, *26*(3), 183–194.

Meeker, M. A., Finnell, D., & Othman, A. K. (2011). Family caregivers and cancer pain management: A review. *Journal of Family Nursing, 17*(1), 29–60.

Minaya, P., Baumstarck, K., Berbis, J., Goncalves, A., Barlesi, F., Michel, G., . . . Auquier, P. (2011). The Caregiver Oncology Quality of Life Questionnaire (CarGOQoL) development and validation of an instrument to measure the quality of life of caregivers of patients with cancer. *European Journal of Cancer.* Retrieved from www.sciencedirect.com

Montgomery, G., Schnur, J., Erblich, J., Diefenbach, M., & Bovbjerg, D. (2010). Presurgery psychological factors predict pain, nausea, and fatigue one week after breast cancer surgery. *Journal of Pain and Symptom Management, 39*(6), 1043–1052.

Porter, L., & Keefe, F. (2011). Psychosocial issues in cancer pain. *Current Pain and Headache Report, 15*, 263–270.

Robison, J., Fortinsky, R., Kleppinger, A., Shugrue, N., & Porter, M. (2009). Broader view of family caregiving: Effects of caregiving and caregiver conditions on depressive symptoms, health, work, and social isolation. *Journal of Gerontology Social Sciences, 64B*(6), 788–798.

Schreiber, J., & Brockopp, D. (2011). Twenty-five years later-what do we know about religion/spirituality and psychological well-being among breast cancer survivors? A systematic review. *Journal of Cancer Survivors.* Retrieved from www.springerpub.com

Son, K., Lee, C., Park, S., Lee, C., Oh, S., Oh, B., ...Lee, S. H. (2012) The factors associated with the quality of life of the spouse caregivers of patients with cancer: A cross-sectional study. *Journal of Palliative Medicine, 15*(2), 1–9.

Thornton, L., Anderson, B., & Blakely, W. (2010). The pain, depression, and fatigue symptom cluster in advanced breast cancer: Covariation with hypothalamic-pituitary-adrenal axis and the sympathetic nervous system. *Health Psychology, 29*(3), 333–337.

Valdivieso, M., Kujawa, A., Jones, T., & Baker, L. (2012). Cancer survivors in the United States: A review of the literature and a call to action. *International Journal of Medical Sciences, 9*(2), 163–173.

Wein, S. (2011). Impact on culture on the expression of pain and suffering. *Journal of Pediatric Hematology Oncology, 33*(2), S105–S107.

Williams, A. L., & McCorkle, R. (2011). Cancer family caregivers during the palliative, hospice, and bereavement phases: A review of the descriptive psychosocial literature. *Palliative and Supportive Care, 9*(3), 315–325.

ADDITIONAL RESOURCES

Bahti, T. (2010). Coping issues among people living with advanced cancer. *Seminars in Oncology Nursing, 26*(3), 175–182.

Cora, A., Partinico, M., Munafa, M., & Polombo, D. (2012). Health risk factors in caregivers of terminal cancer patients. *Cancer Nursing, 35*(1), 38–47.

Northfield, S., & Nebauer, M. (2010). The caregivers journey for family members of relatives with cancer: How do they cope? *Clinical Journal of Oncology Nursing, 14*(5), 567–577.

Pearce, M., Coan, A., Herndon, J., Koenig, H., & Abernathy, A. (2011). Unmet spiritual care needs impact emotional and spiritual well-being in advanced cancer patients. *Supportive Care in Cancer.* Retrieved from www.springerpub.com

A

Selected Websites for Additional Information

www.ampainsoc.org	The American Pain Society publishes Clinical Practice Guidelines, and has information on acute pain, chronic pain, cancer pain, and pain management in primary care.
www.theacpa.org	The American Chronic Pain Association has information on support groups for patients with chronic pain and general information on chronic pain.
www.aspmn.org	The American Society for Pain Management Nursing provides certification in pain management nursing, hosts annual and regional conferences, advocates for persons in pain, and generates position statements on topics related to pain management.
www.ons.org	The Oncology Nursing Society (ONS) is a large organization with multiple publications, and many resources for cancer pain management.
www.americangeriatrics.org	The American Geriatrics Society has guidelines and position statements on pain management in older patients.
www.nccn.org	The National Comprehensive Cancer network has guidelines for cancer pain management.
www.aahpm.org	The American Academy of Hospice and Palliative Care Medicine has information on hospice and palliative care.

www.hpna.org

The Hospice and Palliative Care Nurses Association has information on end-of-life care and cancer pain management, and offers certification in the field.

http://www.s4om .moonfruit.org/

The Society for Oncology Massage has information on using massage to help relieve cancer pain.

Equianalgesic Conversion Table

Equianalgesic Table for Opioid Conversion

Analgesics	Generic	Brand Name	Oral Dose	Parenteral	
Immediate release	Morphine	Roxanol, MSIR	30 milligrams	10 milligrams	Parenteral to oral relative potency: 1:6 with acute dosing and 1:3 with chronic dosing
	Oxycodone	Roxicodone, Oxy IR	20 milligrams	NA	
	Hydromorphone	Dilaudid	7.5 milligrams	1.5 milligrams	
	Oxymorphone	Opana, Numorphan	10 milligrams	1 milligram	Oxymorphone short-acting oral form has an extended half-life of 4-6 hours
	Hydrocodone	Vicodin, Lortab	30 milligrams	NA	
	Fentanyl	Sublimaze	NA	100 micrograms	
	Methadone	Dolophine	5–10 milligrams	10 milligrams	Use methadone with caution: Half-life of 12-150 hours accumulates with repeated dosing. Non-linear pharmacokinetics, seek expert consultation when converting from morphine oral equivalent doses of 100 mg per day or higher.
	Meperidine	Demerol	NR	NR	Meperidine is not recommended. Use with caution. Toxic metabolite normeperidine can cause seizures.
Controlled Release Not recommended for opioid-naïve patients	Morphine	MSContin, Avinza, Kadian	30 milligrams		
	Oxycodone	Oxycontin	20 milligrams		
	Fentanyl transdermal	Duragesic	NA	12 micrograms transdermal	

Basic intravenous conversion: Morphine 1 milligram = Dilaudid 0.2 milligrams = Fentanyl 10 micrograms.

Basic oral and transdermal conversion: morphine 30 mg = oxycodone 20 mg = hydrocodone 30 mg = hydromorphone 7.5 mg = fentanyl transdermal 12 mcg/hr.

NR = not recommended.

When switching from one opioid to another, reduce the dose by 25% to 50% with adequate breakthrough medication.

When switching to methadone, reduce the equianalgesic dose by 75% to 90%.

Breakthrough medication should be available when controlled-release medications are being used.

All opioid medications should be carefully dosed and titrated with consideration for the individual patient and the medical condition of the patient. Use caution in older adults, those with renal or hepatic impairment, respiratory conditions (asthma, sleep apnea, impaired ventilation) and opioid-naive patients.

Sources: Miaskowski, C., Bair, M., Chou, R., D'Arcy, Y., Hartwick, C., Huffman, L., et al. (2008). *Principles of analgesic use in the treatment of acute pain and cancer pain*; Fine, P., & Portenoy, R. (2007). *Opioid analgesia*; Inturrisi, C., & Lipman, A. (2010). *Bonica's management of pain*, pp. 1174–1175; McPherson, M. L. (2010). *Demystifying opioid conversion calculations: A guide for effective dosing*. Bethesda, MD: American Society of Health-System Pharmacists. Smith, H., & McCleane, G. (2009). *Current therapy in pain*. Adapted with permission from D'Arcy, Y. (2011). *Compact clinical guide to chronic pain management*. New York: Springer Publishing Company.

Index

367